BODY CT

SECRETS

BODY CT

SECRETS

John G. Strang, MD
Associate Professor
Department of Radiology
University of Rochester School of Medicine
Director
PET/CT University Imaging at
    Science Park
Rochester, New York

Vikram Dogra, MD
Professor of Radiology
Associate Chair of Education
    and Research
University of Rochester
    School of Medicine
Rochester, New York

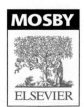

MOSBY

ELSEVIER

1600 John F. Kennedy Boulevard
Suite 1800 Philadelphia, PA 19103-2899

Body CT Secrets

ISBN-13: 978-0-323-03404-3
ISBN-10: 0-323-03404-7

NOTICE

Knowledge and best practice in this field are constantly changing. As new research and experience broaden our knowledge, changes in practice, treatment and drug therapy may become necessary or appropriate. Readers are advised to check the most current information provided (i) on procedures featured or (ii) by the manufacturer of each product to be administered, to verify the recommended dose or formula, the method and duration of administration, and contraindications. It is the responsibility of the practitioner, relying on his or her own experience and knowledge of the patient, to make diagnoses, to determine dosages and the best treatment for each individual patient, and to take all appropriate safety precautions. To the fullest extent of the law, neither the Publisher nor the Editor assumes any liability for any injury and/or damage to persons or property arising out or related to any use of the material contained in this book.

Library of Congress Cataloging-in-Publication Data
Body CT secrets / [edited by] John G. Strang, Vikram Dogra.
     p. cm. – (Secrets series)
   ISBN 0-323-03404-7
     1. Diagnostic imaging–Miscellanea. 2. Diagnostic imaging–Examinations, questions, etc. I. Strang, John G. II. Dogra, Vikram. III. Series.

RC78.7.D53B64 2006
616.07'54–dc22

                                                                        2006041879

Vice President, Medical Education: Linda Belfus
Developmental Editor: Stan Ward
Project Manager: Mary Stermel
Marketing Manager: Kate Rubin

Printed in China.

Working together to grow
libraries in developing countries

www.elsevier.com | www.bookaid.org | www.sabre.org

ELSEVIER   BOOK AID International   Sabre Foundation

Last digit is the print number: 9 8 7 6 5 4 3 2 1

CONTENTS

CONTRIBUTORS

Osbert Adjei, MD
Department of Radiology, University of Rochester Medical Center, Rochester, New York

Elizabeth J. Anoia, MD
Department of Urology, Case Western Reserve University School of Medicine, Cleveland, Ohio

Nami Azar, MD
Assistant Professor, Department of Radiology, Case Western Reserve University School of Medicine, Cleveland, Ohio

Arun Basu, MD
Department of Radiology, University of Rochester Medical Center, Rochester, New York

Shweta Bhatt, MD
Department of Imaging Services, University of Rochester Medical Center, Rochester, New York

Matthew Cham, MD
Department of Radiology, University of Rochester Medical Center, Rochester, New York

Kedar Chintapalli, MD
Professor of Radiology, University of Texas Health Sciences Center at San Antonio, San Antonio, Texas

Joseph Crawford, MD
Assistant Professor, Department of Radiology, Case Western Reserve University School of Medicine; University Hospitals of Cleveland, Cleveland, Ohio

Baz Debaz, MD
Assistant Professor, Department of Radiology, Case Western Reserve University School of Medicine; University Hospitals of Cleveland, Cleveland, Ohio

Vikram Dogra, MD
Professor of Radiology, Associate Chair of Education and Research, University of Rochester School of Medicine, Rochester, New York

Mahadevappa Mahesh, MS, PhD
Chief Physicist, Department of Radiology, The Johns Hopkins Hospital, Baltimore, Maryland

Suleman Merchant, MD
Department of Imaging Services, University of Rochester Medical Center, Rochester, New York

Igor Mikityansky, MD
Department of Radiology, University of Rochester Medical Center, Rochester, New York

Kevin Garrett Miller, MD
Department of Radiology, Case Western Reserve University School of Medicine, Cleveland, Ohio

Hugh T. Morgan, PhD
Senior Staff Scientist, Philips Medical Systems, Cleveland, Ohio

Dean Nakamoto, MD
Assistant Professor, Department of Radiology, Case Western Reserve University School of Medicine; Section Chief, Body Imaging, University Hospitals of Cleveland, Cleveland, Ohio

Sherif G. Nour, MD
Assistant Professor of Radiology and Biomedical Engineering, Case Western Reserve University School of Medicine; Director, Interventional MRI Therapy Program, Department of Radiology, University Hospitals of Cleveland, Cleveland, Ohio

Paul Okunieff, MD
Professor, Department of Radiation Oncology, University of Rochester Medical Center, Rochester, New York

Margaret Ormanoski, DO
Assistant Professor, Department of Radiology, University of Rochester Medical Center, Rochester, New York

Jeffrey S. Palmer, MD
Director of Minimally Invasive Pediatric Urology, Rainbow Babies and Children's Hospital; Assistant Professor of Urology and Pediatrics, Case Western Reserve University School of Medicine, Cleveland, Ohio

Raj Mohan Paspulati, MD
Assistant Professor, Department of Radiology, Case Western Reserve University School of Medicine; University Hospitals of Cleveland, Cleveland, Ohio

Kalpesh Patel, MD
Department of Radiology, University of Rochester Medical Center, Rochester, New York

Srinivasa R. Prasad, MD
Associate Professor of Radiology, University of Texas Health Sciences Center at San Antonio, San Antonio, Texas

David John Prologo, MD
Department of Radiology, Case Western Reserve University School of Medicine, Cleveland, Ohio

P. Sridhar Rao, PhD
Assistant Professor, Department of Radiology, Case Western Reserve University School of Medicine; University Hospitals of Cleveland, Cleveland, Ohio

Deborah Rubens, MD
Professor, Department of Radiology, University of Rochester Medical Center, Rochester, New York

Nael E. A. Saad, MBBCh
Department of Radiology, University of Rochester Medical Center, Rochester, New York

Wael E. A. Saad, MBBCh
Assistant Professor, Department of Radiology, University of Rochester Medical Center, Rochester, New York

Waqar Shah, MD
Department of Radiology, University of Rochester Medical Center, Rochester, New York

Kristina Siddall, MD
Department of Radiology, University of Rochester Medical Center, Rochester, New York

John G. Strang, MD
Associate Professor, Department of Radiology, University of Rochester School of Medicine; Director, PET/CT University Imaging at Science Park, Rochester, New York

Susan Voci, MD
Associate Professor, Department of Radiology, University of Rochester Medical Center, Rochester, New York

Rajashree Vyas, DMRD
Radiology Fellow, Department of Imaging Sciences, University of Rochester Medical Center; Strong
Memorial Hospital, Rochester, New York

Andrea Zynda-Weiss, MD
Department of Radiology, University of Rochester Medical Center, Rochester, New York

PREFACE

The first book in The Secrets Series, *Surgical Secrets,* came out when I (JS) was a medical student about to start clinical rotations. Everyone (it seemed) in my class read it. Its Socratic format made it manageable, readable, and memorable. It was portable and to the point. It was so practical. It was not the compendium of all surgical knowledge—there are other masterful works for that—but *Surgical Secrets* was a place to start. It was—at least in a small way—revolutionary.

It is, therefore, an honor to edit *Body CT Secrets.* Computed tomography (CT) is the second revolution in medical imaging. The first—plain projectional x-ray—is so powerful that it has been fundamental to medical diagnosis for more than a century. Few technologies of 1895 can make that claim. But it has a major flaw—the superimposition of structures. CT introduced cross-sectional imaging. CT let us handle that third dimension, making imaging more understandable and much more powerful. Imaging now lies at the crux of so many more diagnostic pathways because of CT and the cross-sectional way of thinking.

We would like to give thanks and acknowledgment to the people who made this book happen. First, to the authors and co-authors as listed in the table of contents; they should all be proud. However, we especially want to thank those who cannot be seen in the table of contents: our production team, Margaret Kowaluk and Holly Stiner at the University of Rochester, whose skill, professionalism, and good cheer are unmatched; Dr. Deborah Rubens, who shared the secrets she learned in editing *Ultrasound Secrets*; our editors, Linda Belfus and Stan Ward, at Hanley and Belfus (now Elsevier), for their patience and support; and our chairmen, Dr. David Waldman and Dr. John Haaga, for balancing clinical and academic demands in a truly difficult and often thankless job.

I (JS) would particularly like to thank my family—my wife, Susie, for her loving partnership since the first day of medical school; my children, Kathryn, Alex, Scott, and Jack, for letting me see anew through their eyes; my brothers, David and Robert, my lifelong friends; and my parents, Gil and Jill, for more than there are words to say.

I (VD) would also like to thank all of the authors, who deserve my sincere appreciation for their hard work. I would also like to acknowledge assistance of Dr. Shweta Bhatt in the preparation of this book.

We also thank our patients—that we may all learn to make better diagnoses for their benefit. They are who *Body CT Secrets* is for.

John G. Strang, MD
Vikram Dogra, MD

TOP 100 SECRETS

These secrets are 100 of the top board alerts. They summarize the concepts, principles, and most salient details of CT body scans.

1. Computed tomography (CT) differs from conventional radiography by forming a cross-sectional image, eliminating the superimposition of structures that occurs in plain film imaging because of compression of three-dimensional body structures onto the two-dimensional recording system.

2. The sensitivity of CT to subtle differences in x-ray attenuation is at least a factor of 10 higher than normally achieved by film screen recording systems because of the virtual elimination of scatter.

3. Radiation doses in CT range from 15–50 mGy, depending on exam type. In general, these doses are at least 10 times higher than in radiographic exams.

4. Always seek to optimize scan parameters to minimize patient dose consistent with diagnostic image quality: Minimize mAs, minimize kVp, maximize pitch, maximize slice thickness, and maximize collimator setting.

5. When scanning children, be sure to use pediatric protocols, not adult protocols. In pediatric protocols the CT scan parameters should be reduced so that radiation doses are optimized according to patient size.

6. Pregnant women should be scanned only if there is adequate justification to avoid unnecessary fetal irradiation.

7. Many of the side effects of contrast media are entirely or mainly due to high osmolality. The other causes of side effects due to contrast media are chemotoxicity (allergic-like symptoms), ion toxicity (interference with cellular function), and those caused by a high dose.

8. The major risk factor for contrast-induced nephropathy is underlying renal dysfunction. Other risk factors include diabetes mellitus, dehydration, poor renal perfusion, nephrotoxic medications, and the volume of contrast injected.

9. Four main categories of drugs can be used to treat adverse contrast reactions: antihistamines, corticosteroids, anticholinergics, and adrenergic agonists.

10. Radiation therapy stops tumor from growing, but it may not totally disappear on CT. Growth after radiation therapy is presumed to be recurrence.

11. Radiation therapy is most demanding for precise localization of tumor because it is effectively percutaneous surgery.

12. Gross tumor volume (GTV) for radiation oncology is the tumor that you see and know is present. Clinical target volume (CTV) includes subclinical or microscopic tumor and thus is larger than GTV. Planning target volume (PTV) is CTV plus a margin for technical variation of XRT delivery. The entire PTV should receive the planned treatment dose.

13. Irradiated tissue first goes through a flare phase of edema over days to weeks, then fibrosis over weeks or months.

14. PET/CT is more powerful than PET alone because of improved tumor characterization and localization. Hypometabolic tumors are a PET blind spot filled in by PET/CT.

15. PET/CT is more powerful than CT because of small lesion detection, high lesion conspicuity, and early lesion response to therapy. Bone and soft tissue lesions are CT blind spots filled in by PET/CT.

16. Look for traumatic pseudoaneurysms below the aortic arch, anterior to the descending thoracic aorta.

17. Do a chest CT to look for aortic injury if you see infarcts on an abdominal CT or a periaortic hematoma at the diaphragm.

18. Some large pneumothoraces may not visible on supine, portable, trauma chest x-rays.

19. Multidetector CT is a major advance for the detection of pulmonary emboli compared to single-slice CT. MDCT provides thinner images with more coverage faster, minimizing respiratory motion and bolus mistiming. It has become the de facto gold standard for the diagnosis of pulmonary emboli.

20. With care, the mimics of pulmonary emboli (mucus plugs, poor opacification of veins, partial volume averaging of air and lymph nodes) can be distinguished from pulmonary emboli. Make sure your suspected embolus is in a pulmonary artery.

21. CT has a number of different roles to play in chest infection, including determining site, cause, likely infectious organisms, and complications. Empyema and lung abscess must be distinguished.

22. The major forms of tuberculous infection are primary, reactivation, miliary, endobronchial, and extrapulomonic.

23. Fungal infections often mimic cancer in their appearance (nodular masses with lymphadenopathy) and behavior when untreated (subacute indolent progression).

24. AIDS patients can get a number of pulmonary infections and conditions (e.g., Kaposi's sarcoma). They often have mixed disease and scarring from prior disease, making specific diagnosis difficult.

25. High-resolution chest CT has specific findings that correlate to underlying anatomic structures. Multidetector CT potentially makes every chest CT a "high–resolution" CT.

26. Pneumoconioses are occupationally acquired diseases due to particulate inhalation. The fact that they are occupationally acquired leads to a high political and legal profile.

27. Coal worker's pneumoconiosis, silicosis, and asbestos-related diseases are the most important pneumoconioses.

28. Asbestos causes a range of pulmonary diseases including calcified pleural plaques (asbestos exposure), rounded atelectasis, asbestosis, malignant mesothelioma and is a major risk factor for lung cancer.

29. Sarcoidosis causes changes which include adenopathy and pulmonary nodules and interstitial lung disease. The appearance can be characteristic but also can mimic and needs to be differentiated from lung cancer.

30. Scleroderma causes esophageal dysmotility and characteristic basal and posterior fibrosis of lung secondary to aspiration.

31. Wegener's granulomatosis causes pulmonary nodules, some cavitated. It must be differentiated from lung metastases.

32. Lung cancer is incredibly common, and the radiologist is often the first to know. Always suspect it. Most symptomatic patients at time of diagnosis will die of their disease.

33. Carefully distinguish between "work-up" and "follow-up." Work up more suspicious nodes (i.e., determine the need for resection *now*, through biopsy, PET, etc.). Follow up smaller, less suspicious nodes(i.e., rescan for growth in several months). The size threshold is approximately 1 cm. Don't say follow-up when you mean work-up.

34. Significant growth in small tumors can be difficult to measure with present tools because of the volumetric nature of growth.

35. Lung cancer screening trials are in progress. The ELCAP study showed that CT screening can down-stage lung cancer. Randomized trials are evaluating whether long-term morbidity and mortality are also changed.

36. Computer-assisted detection has promising results for the detection of pulmonary nodules and virtual colonoscopy. It improves sensitivity for nodule detection. The number of false-positive nodules detected, however, remains high.

37. Coronary artery calcification measurement is a third application for CAD. CAD is already widely used with mammography. These are the leading causes of neoplastic and nonneoplastic death.

38. CAD is a partial answer to growing image overload. It should let us take advantage of the high-quality thin-slice data sets produced by MDCT.

39. The four Ts of the anterior mediastinum: thyroid tumor, thymoma, teratoma, and terrible lymphoma.

40. The thymus varies in appearance with age but should appear "soft" and arrowhead-shaped.

41. Anterior mediastinal masses of thyroid origin connect to the thyroid.

42. Middle mediastinal masses are most commonly of lymph node origin. Their distribution and appearance (egg-shell calcification, low-density) can be a clue to their etiology. The differential diagnosis of middle mediastinal masses also includes vascular masses/aneurysms and bronchogenic or pericardial cysts.

43. Neurogenic tumors often present as smoothly marginated posterior mediastinal masses.

44. Esophageal carcinoma has high morbidity and mortality rates. CT is usually done for staging rather than for diagnosis and for detection of local spread, metastases, and lymphadenopathy. PET/CT is an alternative staging modality.

45. Check for coronary artery anomalies on MDCT. Think of vascular variants before you biopsy mediastinal masses.

46. Incomplete mixing of opacified blood from the side of the injection with unopacified blood from the contralateral side and/or the azygous vein mimics SVC thrombosis.

47. Venous collaterals usually indicate obstruction, but retrograde filling of peripheral veins can occur with high injection rates, poor cardiac function, and dependently due to gravity.

48. Stanford type A dissection require surgical repair due to risk of rupture, cardiac tamponade, and myocardial infarction.

49. Stanford type B dissections are medically managed (control of hypertension) but occasionally need operative repair too. They should be followed to watch for potential aneurysm development, as surgical indication.

50. For first-pass imaging, the degree of contrast opacification depends on how fast you inject iodinated contrast, not how much you inject.

51. Intramural hematomas are separate entities but share some of the pathogenesis and treatment of true aortic dissections.

52. Pay attention to aortic streak and motion artifacts in patients who are not at risk for dissections, so you can differentiate them when you have a patient who is suspected to have dissection.

53. Helical unenhanced CT is the best imaging modality for the diagnosis of urinary tract calculi.

54. Signs of urinary obstruction include presence of a calculus, ureteral dilatation, perinephric stranding, and unilateral absence of white pyramids.

55. It is important to identify ACKD because of an increased risk of renal cell carcinoma (12–18 times higher than in the general population).

56. Striated nephrogram is characteristic of pyelonephritis. It is also seen in ARPKD, renal vein thrombosis, contusion, and tubular obstruction.

57. Pyonephrosis is a true urologic emergency requiring urgent intervention and is identified on CT by increased pelvic wall thickness, perinephric inflammatory changes, and layering of contrast and pus in the dilated pelvis on CECT, along with clinical signs of infection.

58. Renal cell carcinoma is the most common primary malignant renal neoplasm.

59. Nephrographic phase is the best phase for diagnosing RCC and is identified by less enhancement than surrounding normal parenchyma. Venous extension of RCC is best diagnosed on the corticomedullary phase.

60. CECT-triple phase is the best modality for evaluating patients with blunt or penetrating abdominal trauma.

61. CT urography is preferred over excretory urography and has following advantages:
    - Both renal parenchyma and urothelium can be evaluated in single exam.

- It has a shorter duration.
- Renal masses can be characterized in the same exam.

62. Neuroblastoma demonstrates calcification in approximately 90% of cases on CT scans whereas Wilms tumor calcifies in 5% of cases. Neuroblastoma tends to encase rather than displace major vessels, while the opposite occurs with Wilms tumor.

63. Fifty percent of adrenal carcinomas present as functioning tumors, usually secreting cortisol and associated with Cushing's syndrome.

64. Primary hyperaldosteronism is associated with decreased plasma rennin level, whereas secondary hyperaldosteronism is associated with elevated plasma rennin level.

65. Lung carcinoma is the most common source for adrenal metastatic disease.

66. Gastrointestinal stromal tumor (GIST) is the most common nonepithelial neoplasm of the stomach and small bowel. It is rare in the colon and rectum.

67. Conventional CT scanning is not sensitive in early gastric cancer (reported sensitivity of about 50%).

68. Small bowel malignant tumors are uncommon and account for less than 3% of GI malignancies. The most common is adenocarcinoma, followed by malignant carcinoid, lymphoma, and sarcomas.

69. GI malignancies in AIDS include Kaposi's sarcoma (most common) and non-Hodgkin lymphoma.

70. In children intussusception is the most common cause of intestinal obstruction, while in adults it is responsible for less than 5% of bowel obstructions. Unlike childhood intussusception, which is usually idiopathic, the adult form is associated with a cause, such as a mass or polyp.

71. If the appendix is not obvious, locate the tip of the cecum and search around it.

72. When you consider bowel ischemia, look at the supplying vessels for occlusion.

73. Perforated colon carcinoma can mimic diverticulitis with thickened bowel and pericolonic stranding. Look for the offending diverticulum itself. Do a follow-up colonoscopy when the patient has recovered if it is not clearly diverticulitis.

74. In bowel obstruction, the distal bowel is seldom totally evacuated.

75. The total iodine load determines peak hepatic enhancement.

76. Late arterial phase is the optimal phase for detection of hypervascular liver tumors.

77. Multiphase CT is crucial to optimal hepatic imaging and permits characterization of liver lesions.

78. CT is not the primary imaging modality of gallbladder.

79. Mirizzi's syndrome should be considered when acute cholecystitis is associated with biliary obstruction.

80. Porcelain gallbladder is associated with high incidence of carcinoma.

81. Delayed enhancement is characteristic of cholangiocarcinoma.

82. The extent of pancreatic necrosis detected by CT has good correlation with morbidity and mortality of acute pancreatitis.

83. Groove pancreatitis is a segmental form of chronic pancreatitis in the groove between the duodenum and head of pancreas.

84. Focal chronic pancreatitis and carcinoma of pancreas cannot be distinguished by imaging. IPMT and chronic pancreatitis have similar CT appearances.

85. Functioning islet cell tumors enhance in the arterial phase of the CT scan.

86. Malignant splenic lesions are more common than benign lesions, and the most common malignant tumor of the spleen is lymphoma. Up to one-third of all patients with lymphoma (Hodgkin and non-Hodgkin) have splenic involvement.

87. Splenomegaly in a patient with lymphoma does not always indicate splenic lymphoma. Up to 30% of enlarged spleens in lymphoma patients are benign in origin.

88. The most common solid or mixed solid and cystic mass in an asymptomatic patient is hemangioma. However, up to 25% of splenic hemangiomas may rupture or cause symptoms of hypersplenism.

89. An incidentally noted, large subcapsular cystic lesion with septations and small mural nodules in the spleen of a child raises the possibility of lymphangioma.

90. CT is the gold standard for the imaging of the retroperitoneum.

91. The most common cause of retroperitoneal fibrosis is idiopathic. Only retroperitoneal fibrosis causes medial deviation of the ureters. Other masses cause lateral deviation of ureters.

92. CT cannot differentiate benign from malignant retroperitoneal lymphadenopathy.

93. Aortic aneurysm more than 5 cm in diameter should be surgically repaired.

94. CT scan in ovarian cancer is more effective at detecting retroperitoneal lymph node disease rather than intra-abdominal disease.

95. A thickened bladder wall on CT scan may be simply due to nondistention.

96. Mucus in the urine should raise the suspicion of a patent urachus with possibility of urachal carcinoma.

97. Since urethral carcinoma is more common in females, those with irritative symptoms should not be dismissed as having overactive bladder.

98. The main indications for CT of the male pelvis are evaluation of the prostate gland, seminal vesicles, urinary bladder, and rectosigmoid region.

99. In most cases of prostatic cancer, diagnostic accuracy with CT is poor. Only stage T3b (invasion of the seminal vesicles) and stage T4 prostate cancer can be distinguished from BPH.

100. The most common type of prostate trauma is grade 3. Fluid (urine) is seen below the urogenital diaphragm on CT. This is inferior and lateral to the levator ani muscles cradling the prostate. In grade 2 injuries, fluid is seen above the urogenital diaphragm in the extraperitoneal space.

I. BASIC CONCEPTS

CT PHYSICS

Mahadevappa Mahesh, MS, PhD

1. **What is CT?**
   CT is a method for acquiring and reconstructing an image of a thin cross section of an object. It is based on measurements of x-ray attenuation through the section using many different projections. This is achieved by rotating both x-ray tube and detectors around the patient.

2. **How is CT different from conventional radiographs?**
   CT differs from conventional radiography in two significant ways:
   - CT forms a cross-sectional image, eliminating the superimposition of structures that occurs in plain film imaging because of compression of three-dimensional (3D) body structures onto the two-dimensional recording system.
   - The sensitivity of CT to subtle differences in x-ray attenuation is at least a factor of 10 higher than normally achieved by film screen recording systems because of the virtual elimination of scatter.

3. **What are the basic principles of CT?**
   Fundamentally a CT scanner makes many measurements of attenuation through the plane of a finite thickness cross section of the body. The system uses these data to reconstruct a digital image of the cross section in which each pixel in the image represents a measurement of the mean attenuation of a box-like element (voxel) extending through the thickness of the section. An attenuation measurement quantifies the fraction of radiation removed in passing through a given amount of a specific material of thickness Δx, as shown in Fig. 1-1. Attenuation is expressed as:

   $$I_t = I_0 e^{-\mu \Delta x}$$

   where, I_t and I_0 are the x-ray intensities measured with and without the material in the x-ray beam path, respectively, and μ is the linear attenuation coefficient of the specific material (*see* Fig. 1-1). The image reconstruction process, such as the filtered back-projection method and many other methods, are applied to derive the average attenuation coefficient (μ) values for each voxel in the cross section, using many rays from many different rotational angles around the cross section.

4. **How is CT signal produced?**
   A CT signal results from tissue discrimination based on the variations in attenuation between "voxels," which depends on differences in voxel density and atomic number of elements present and is influenced by the detected mean photon energy.

5. **What is a CT image?**
   A CT image as shown later is composed of *pixels* (picture elements). Each pixel on the image represents the average x-ray attenuation in a small volume (*voxel*) that extends through the tissue section. In Fig. 1-2, the pixel size is exaggerated. In addition, in a real CT image, all tissues within a single pixel would be the same shade of gray.

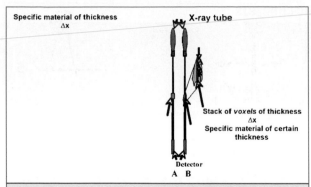

Figure 1-1. An attenuation measurement quantifies the fraction of radiation removed in passing through a given amount of a specific material of thickness Δx.

6. What is pitch?

The concept of "pitch" was introduction with the arrival of helical or spiral CT scanners. Pitch is defined as the ratio of table travel per gantry rotation to the x-ray beam width.

$$Pitch = l/W$$

where l is table feed per gantry rotation (mm/rotation) and W is x-ray beam width (mm). Accordingly,

- **Pitch = 1:** Implies contiguous slice similar to conventional step-and-shoot scan, for example: 10-mm slice thickness with 10-mm slice interval
- **Pitch > 1:** Implies extended imaging and reduced patient dose with lower axial spatial resolution
- **Pitch < 1:** Implies overlapping and higher patient dose with higher axial spatial resolution

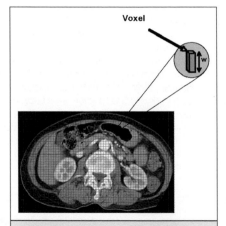

Figure 1-2. A CT image is composed of pixels. Each pixel on the image represents the x-ray attenuation in a small volume (voxel) that extends through the tissue section. w = section width.

With single-row detector CT (SDCT) scanners, the concept of *pitch* is straightforward. With multiple-row detector CT (MDCT), the concept of pitch was muddled with the introduction of two different definitions for pitch with following variations:

- **Beam pitch or collimator pitch similar to the previously defined pitch:** Typical values are 0.75, 1, 1.25, ...
- **Detector pitch:** Ratio of table feed per gantry rotation to width of single DAS channel width. Typical values are 4, 6, 12, 18, ...

However, with recent international agreement, pitch is again defined as simply ratio of table travel to total x-ray beam width. Adopting the usage of common definition of *pitch* would be applicable equally to both SDCT and MDCT and eliminates confusion existing between the relationship of radiation dose and various definitions of pitch (Fig. 1-3).

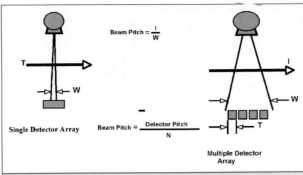

Figure 1-3. With recent international agreement, pitch is again defined as simply ratio of table travel to total x-ray beam width. I = table travel (mm)/rotation, W = beam width (mm), T = single data acquisition channel width (mm), N = number of active data acquisition channels.

7. **What is "field of view" (FOV) in CT?**

The FOV in CT is the area of scan region that is included in the image reconstruction. There are two types of FOV: scan FOV (SFOV) and display FOV (DFOV). SFOV is the region within the gantry opening, the anatomy that is included in the reconstruction. SFOV is less than the physical opening of the CT gantry, which is the reason why part of the anatomy is cut off in scanning larger patients. On the other hand, DFOV is area of reconstructed image that can be displayed. Smaller DFOV results in larger image size. The SFOV influences the physical dimensions of image pixel. A 10-cm FOV in a 512×512 matrix results in pixel dimensions of approximately 0.2 mm, and a 35-cm FOV produces pixel widths of about 0.7 mm (Fig. 1-4).

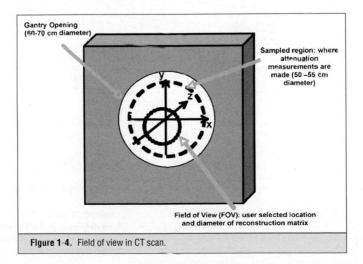

Figure 1-4. Field of view in CT scan.

8. What does gantry rotation speed mean?

It is the speed at which the CT gantry rotates once around the patient. It is often called "scan time." Scan time is consistently decreasing with increasing demand for higher temporal resolution. Scan time of 1 second was normal in SDCT, and with MDCT the gantry rotation speed has become less than 400 milliseconds to provide the very high temporal resolution required for stopping physiologic motion. This is especially critical in cardiac CT imaging. However, to maintain similar image noise with faster gantry rotation speed, the tube current (mA) has to be operated at a very high level.

For certain scan protocols (cardiac), partial gantry rotation (less than complete rotation) is utilized to achieve higher temporal resolution (250 milliseconds).

9. Explain CT generations.

From the time of first CT scanners, a variety of CT geometries have been developed to acquire x-ray transmission data for image reconstruction. These geometries are commonly called *generations* and are useful in differentiating scanner design, especially among the conventional CT scanners that do not have helical/spiral scanning capability (Fig. 1-5). With helical/spiral CT scanners, CT generations can be further grouped as single-row detector helical CT scanners (SDCT, sixth generation) and multiple-row detector helical CT scanners (MDCT, seventh generation). Also, despite fundamental scanning differences, the electron beam CT (EBCT) is often classified as fifth generation.

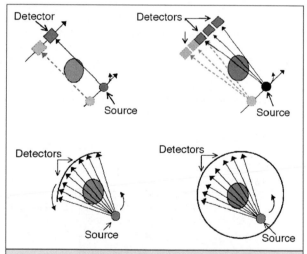

Figure 1-5. Four generations of CT scanners. **Upper left,** First generation with parallel x-ray beam and translate-rotate motion. **Upper right,** Second generation with translate-rotate motion. **Bottom left,** Third generation with rotate-rotate motion. Data are acquired by rotating both the x-ray source with a wide fan beam geometry and the detectors around the patient. **Bottom right,** Fourth generation with rotate-stationary motion. Data are acquired by rotating the x-ray source with a wide fan beam only; the detectors are stationary.

10. What is a helical or spiral CT scan?

Helical or spiral CT scan is the method of acquiring data continuously through several complete gantry rotation while the CT table is translated in and out of the gantry. Three technological advances were critical in the development of helical CT scans: development of slip-ring technology, high-power x-ray tubes, and interpolation algorithms.

11. **What is slip-ring gantry?**

Slip rings are electromechanical devices consisting of circular electrical conductive rings and brushes that transmit electrical energy across a moving interface. All power and control signals from the stationary parts of the scanner system are communicated to the rotating frame through the slip ring. The slip-ring design consists of sets of parallel conductive rings concentric to the gantry axis that connects to the tube, detectors, and control circuits by sliding contractors. These "sliding contractors" allow the scan frame to rotate continuously with no need to stop between rotations to rewind system cables.

12. **What are interpolation algorithms?**

Interpolation algorithms are special algorithms developed to generate projections in a single plane so that conventional back projections can be used for image reconstruction. With helical CT scans, all data did not lie in a single plane; therefore, conventional reconstruction methods could not be applied in image reconstruction.

The helical data set is first interpolated into a series of planar image data sets prior to applying conventional reconstruction methods. There were several important benefits to this development. First, the reconstruction planes could be placed in any arbitrary position along the scanned volume encompassed by the table traverse during multiple rotations. This meant that sections could be overlapping along the scan axis thus greatly improving data sampling and making 3D reconstructions practical. Second, because images can be acquired in a single breath-hold, the 3D reconstructions are free of the misregistration artifacts caused by involuntary motion that bedevil conventional CT. True 3D volumes could be acquired that can be viewed in any perspective, making the promise of true 3D radiography a practical reality. A final benefit was that because overlapping slices were generated by mathematical methods rather than overlapping x-ray beams, the improved z-axis sampling was obtained without a radiation dose penalty to the patient.

13. **What is MDCT?**

MDCT is a commonly used acronym that stands for multiple-row detector computed tomography. The other commonly used term is MSCT, or multiple slice computed tomography.

14. **What is the difference between SDCT and MDCT?**

The principal differences between single and multiple-row detector helical scanners are illustrated in Fig. 1-6. In both cases, both the x-ray tube and the detectors rotate around the patient to collect multiple projection data (similar to third-generation conventional CT scanners) while the patient table is translated through the CT gantry. The differences are in the number of detector rows in the z-direction of the patient and the number of multiple slices obtained at the isocenter. By late 1998, all major CT manufacturers launched MDCT scanners capable of providing at least four slices per section per rotation with minimum gantry rotation times of 0.5 second.

As shown in the figure, the difference between SDCT and MDCT is the number of detector arrays available in the z-direction. In SDCT, there was only single row of detectors arrays in the z direction, and therefore, it yielded only single axial slice per each CT gantry rotation. On the other hand, in MDCT, there are multiple rows of detector arrays yielding multiple axial slices per each CT gantry rotation.

15. **What are the different detector arrays designs available in four-section MDCT scanners?**

Figure 1-7 shows the detector design of all major MDCT scanners that were capable of providing a maximum of four slices per gantry rotation. Even though the detector design consists of multiple row of detectors, the maximum number of slices obtained per gantry rotation was limited by the number of data acquisition channels (DAS). In this case, the maximum number of slices was four due to the availability of 4 DAS channels.

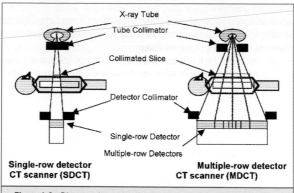

Figure 1-6. Diagram shows the difference between single-row detector and multiple-row detector CT designs. The multiple-row detector array has elements of unequal dimension and represents the design of one particular manufacturer.

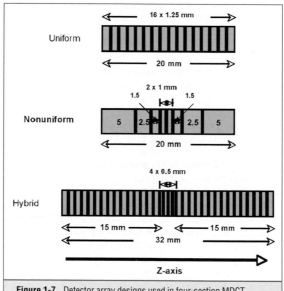

Figure 1-7. Detector array designs used in four-section MDCT scanners.

16. **What are the advantages of MDCT?**

The clinical advantages of multiple-row detector technology can be broadly divided into three categories:

- The ability to obtain large number of thin slices resulting in higher spatial resolution in both axial and longitudinal direction. This is important in terms of obtaining isotropic spatial resolution, that is, cubic voxels, so that the images are equally sharp in any plane traversing the scanned volume. This capability is reasonably obtained with multiple sections of sub-millimeter thickness. Ideally the true 3D radiograph would have cubic voxels of less than 1 mm in size, over large volumes, acquired with very short times (at least within a reasonable breath-hold). Cardiac imaging, which was possible with the SDCT scanners, became practical with multiple-row detector scanners.

- The speed can be utilized for fast imaging of large volume of tissue with variable slice thickness. This is particularly useful in studies in which patient motion is a limiting factor. With a four-slice system and a 0.5-section rotation, the volume data can be acquired eight times faster than with the single slice, 1-second scanner. Because 16- and 64-slice MDCT systems have rotation times less than 0.4 sec, the volume data are acquired at even higher rates than with first-generation MDCT scanners.

- The other main advantage of MDCT systems is their ability to cover large volumes in short scan times. The volume coverage and speed performance in MDCT scanners are better than their counterparts in SDCT without compromises in image quality. The fast rotation times and large volume coverage provide improved multiplanar reconstruction and 3D images with reduced image artifacts.

17. **What are the various detector array designs in four-slice MDCT scanners?**

- **Uniform element arrays:** In this type of detector array designs, several solid-state small detectors of same dimension are arranged in rows of identical thickness (e.g., 16 rows of 1.25 mm). The image acquired depends on the x-ray beam width, selection of detector rows, and how the two are coupled. It is possible to acquire four simultaneous slices of 1.25 mm each, or to increase the slice thickness by coupling rows of detectors, for example, coupling two, three, and four detector rows together, to obtain four slices of 2.5-, 3.75-, and 5-mm thick, respectively.

- **Nonuniform element arrays:** In this type of detector arrays, the detector width gradually increases in thickness as they move away from the center of axis of rotation. The two detector rows in the center of the array are 1 mm each, whereas the detectors adjacent to the central row are of increasing thickness with the outermost detector row of 5 mm thick.

- **Hybrid element arrays:** The third type of design incorporated features of uniform and nonuniform design. This detector arrays is composed of 4 thin detectors of 0.5 mm at center and 15 detectors of 1 mm width on either side of the central detectors for the total z-axis coverage of 32 mm per x-ray tube rotation around the gantry (see Fig. 1-7).

18. **What is sequential or axial scan mode?**

This is similar to conventional "step-and-shoot" scanning, in which, after each tube rotation, the patient is translated to the next position for subsequent scans. Compared with SDCT scanners, the volume of data acquired with each rotation is enhanced nearly four to eight times with 0.5-second rotation time scanners. Also, thicker slices can be reconstructed retrospectively using data from multiple data channels. Reconstructing thicker slices has inherent advantage in situations required to avoid streak artifacts due to partial volume averaging or to improve low contrast detection with improved image noise. With x-ray tube rotation at 0.5 second and anatomical coverage of 10 mm per rotation, MDCT scans are significantly faster than SDCT scanners with enhanced capability to perform a wide variety of clinical scans.

19. **What is spiral or helical scan mode?**

It is analogous to the SDCT helical scanning mode, with multiple data channels simultaneously obtaining data as the patient is translated into the gantry. The data from all four channels contribute to each of the four reconstructed slices. The interpolation algorithms can be adjusted to trade off longitudinal resolution against noise and artifacts. One can reconstruct to different slice thickness by adjusting the slice profiles retrospectively according to the desired image quality. For example, scanning at 4×2.5 mm mode, one can retrospectively reconstruct slices of thickness equal to or greater than 2.5 mm.

20. **What are the detector array designs in 16-slice MDCT scanners?**

One common feature of the detector array designs of 16-slice MDCT compared with 4-slice MDCT is that all major manufacturers have migrated toward the "hybrid" detector design with thin detectors (16) in the center and thick detectors (4) at either sides. The scan acquisition modes are obtained as either 16 thin slices or 16 thick slices per gantry rotation (Fig. 1-8).

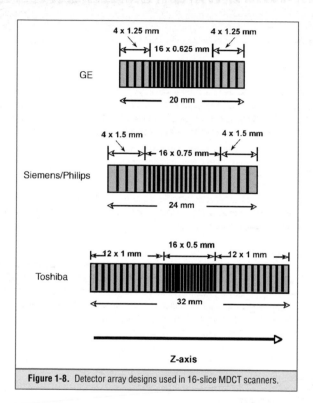

Figure 1-8. Detector array designs used in 16-slice MDCT scanners.

BIBLIOGRAPHY

1. Bushberg JT, Siebert JA, Leidholdt EM, et al: The Essential Physics of Medical Imaging. Baltimore, Lippincott Williams & Wilkins, 2002.

2. McNitt-Gray MF: AAPM/RSNA physics tutorial for residents: Topics in CT. Radiation dose in CT. Radiographics 22:1541–1553, 2002.

3. Mahesh M: Search for isotropic resolution in CT from conventional through multiple-row detector. Radiographics 22:949–962, 2002.

4. Pannu HK, Flohr TG, Corl FM, Fishman EK: Current concepts in multi-detector row CT evaluation of the coronary arteries: Principles, techniques, and anatomy. Radiographics 23:S111–S125, 2003.

5. Prokop M: General principles of MDCT. Eur J Radiol 45:S4–S10, 2003.

CHAPTER 2

RADIATION DOSE IN CT

P. Sridhar Rao, PhD, and Hugh T. Morgan, PhD

1. **What is radiation dose?**
   In the context of CT, dose can be loosely described as the energy absorbed from the x-rays used in the imaging procedure. More precisely, dose is the energy absorbed by an object, like a block of tissue, divided by the mass of that object. The modern unit of absorbed dose is the gray (abbreviated as Gy). It is equal to 1 joule (J) per kg. Often the subunit milligray (mGy) is used, where 1000 mGy equal 1 Gy. An older unit of absorbed dose is the rad, where 100 rads are equal to 1 Gy.

2. **Can radiation exposure to two different parts of the body be added to obtain the total radiation dose to a patient?**
   Not directly. In a CT scan series, for example, if the dose to the abdomen is 10 mGy and the dose to the pelvis is 10 mGy, one *cannot* add them to get a total of 20 mGy. They must be considered as separate doses to separate parts of the body.

3. **What is effective dose?**
   The effective dose is a hypothetical dose from a uniform whole body irradiation that would cause the same biologic harm as an actual nonuniform partial body irradiation, as in a CT scan series. It is a weighted average of the doses to all the various parts of the body. It is obtained by multiplying each organ dose by a "weighting factor" and adding the products. The numerical values of the factors are roughly proportional to the biologic sensitivities of the corresponding organs. The effective dose has a separate unit, the sievert (Sv).

4. **How does CT dose compare with dose from ordinary radiographic views?**
   CT doses are higher by a factor of 10 or more. The distribution of the dose is also more uniform in CT than in radiographs. The advantage gained from the higher dose is improved contrast resolution and the tomographic view.

5. **Are the biologic effects from CT the same as those from other x-ray procedures?**
   The effects are the same, because both are x-rays and are ionizing radiation. However, the degree of the effect will be greater for CT, because it delivers higher doses.

6. **How are image noise and dose related?**
   Qualitatively, as dose increases, image noise decreases. Quantitatively, if everything else is the same, this is expressed as:

$$\sigma \, \alpha \, (1 / \sqrt{dose})$$

where σ is the standard deviation of the CT numbers in a homogenous portion of the image and is a measure of noise. Good judgment should be used to choose an optimal set of scan parameters that will minimize dose at an acceptable level of noise.

7. **What differences in dose are there between axial scans and helical scans?**
   Helical scans with a pitch factor of 1 are like axial scans that are contiguous. The dose is almost the same. The difference is at the ends of the scan length, where an extra half or one full rotation is performed by helical scanners but not imaged.

8. **What differences in dose are there between single-slice and multislice helical scans?**
   Everything else being equal, the dose will be slightly higher (~10%) for multislice technology due to the multislice "over-beaming" phenomenon. This follows from the finite size of the focal spot in the x-ray tube. The x-ray beam therefore has penumbras at the edges of the beam where the x-rays are not as intense as in the main beam. The transmission data in the penumbra are not generally used for image reconstruction. The penumbra irradiates the patient, but to no purpose.
   Because penumbra width is constant, its proportion to collimator width increases as the collimation decreases. Patient dose also increases.

9. **Is the dose higher with increasing scan length?**
   This question must be answered carefully. Increasing the scan length means more of the body is exposed to x-rays. Therefore, more organs will absorb x-ray energy and receive doses that will be the same (to a first approximation). However, because more organs have been affected, the *effective* dose will be higher. Doubling the scan length will approximately double the effective dose. The actual increase will depend on the organs affected and their relative radiosensitivities.

10. **If an organ is not in any of the views, does it still get a dose?**
    In general, yes. Organs that are in the direct x-ray beam and that are imaged will get the highest dose. Nearby organs will experience scattered radiation and will therefore get a smaller dose. The actual dose will depend on how far it is from the tissues affected by the primary x-ray beam.

11. **What scan parameters affect CT dose?**
    The kVp, mAs, pitch factor, slice thickness, collimation, scan angle, and filtration all affect the dose in CT.

12. **How does kVp affect CT dose?**
    The kVp (kilovoltage-peak) of the x-ray beam determines how well the beam penetrates the patient. The higher the kVp, the more penetrating is the x-ray beam and the more uniformly the dose is distributed in the patient. If all other parameters remain the same, higher kVp causes higher dose. Changing from 120 to 140 kVp will increase the dose by about 40%.

13. **How does mAs affect dose?**
    The mAs is the tube current in milliamperes (mA) times the duration of one rotation in seconds. Either the current or the rotation time can be varied. The mAs is proportional to the number of photons directed at the patient. Therefore, dose is directly proportional to the mAs. More mAs will give a better (less noisy image) but at higher dose.

14. **How does pitch factor affect dose?**
    The dose is inversely proportional to pitch, provided you do not adjust the mAs. Pitch is the ratio of table travel per tube rotation to collimation (for a single-slice scanner). Going from a pitch of 1 to a pitch of 2 by doubling the table speed means that the x-ray is on for half as long, and so the dose is halved. Note that as pitch increases, image noise increases. However, in some scanners the x-ray tube current (the mA) may increase proportionally with pitch so that the noise remains the same. Then the dose is unchanged.

15. How does slice thickness affect dose?

Slice thickness does not necessarily affect the dose directly. However, for the same scan parameters, thin slices are reconstructed from less data than thick slices and therefore have more noise. A higher mAs is usually required for thin slices to keep the image noise reasonable. Therefore, in practice thin slices are associated with higher dose.

16. How does collimation affect dose?

Collimation determines the x-ray beam width. Narrower beams increase dose because of the overlap or overbeaming effect. A 4×1.5 mm collimation will result in higher dose than for a 16×1.5 mm collimation, everything else being equal (*see* question 8).

17. How does scan angle affect dose?

For axial scans, a single slice may be reconstructed from data acquired in a full 360-degree rotation (normal scan), or more (overscan), or less (underscan). Dose varies accordingly.

18. How does filtration affect dose?

Filters placed near the x-ray tube reduce dose in two ways. A beam-shaping filter (e.g., wedge filter, bow tie filter) shapes the beam intensity to reduce the dose gradually toward the edges of the radiation field. Additional flat filters remove soft or low-energy x-rays and thereby reduce skin dose, as in other types of x-ray machines.

19. Which parameters can be easily adjusted to minimize dose?

The easiest to adjust are the mA (or mAs) and the pitch. They should be chosen to optimize the balance between the quality of the image and the dose to the patient. Modern multislice scanners have dose reduction schemes that cause the mA to vary during the scan based on the varying attenuation of the patient (thorax vs. abdomen, or lateral vs. anterior-posterior). These dose reduction schemes can reduce dose by 30% or more and produce the same image quality as fixed mA scans.

20. What is automatic exposure control as it relates to CT?

The goal of automatic exposure control (AEC) is to automatically vary the scan parameters to maintain a preselected image signal-to-noise ratio for a given exam type regardless of patient size. The dose reduction scheme described in question 19 is one example of AEC.

21. How is the patient dose in CT determined?

Because the dose is difficult to measure in an actual patient, it is sometimes measured in anthropomorphic "phantoms" or models that mimic human anatomy. Usually measurements are made in two cylinders of well-defined dimensions, and from the data the dose to patients is inferred. The cylinders are made of polymethyl methacrylate (PMMA, also called acrylic). One is 32 cm in diameter and is called a CTDI body phantom; the other is 16 cm in diameter and is called a CTDI head phantom. Both are 15 cm long.

22. What is meant by "dose profile"?

In the context of CT scanners, a dose profile is the distribution of the dose along a line parallel to the scan length. It is measured inside the plastic phantoms described previously. Five grooves are cut into the cylinders, one along the axis and four symmetrically placed at the periphery (actually 1 cm in from the periphery). Measurement devices such as special x-ray film or thermoluminescent dosimeters are placed inside them. The final results are displayed graphically with dose on the y-axis and distance on the x-axis (Fig. 2-1).

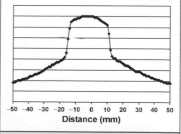

Distance (mm)

Figure 2-1. Dose profile for a Philips Brilliance scanner operated in the 16×1.5 mm collimation mode.

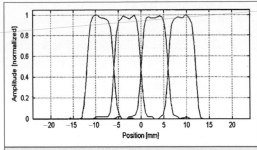

Figure 2-2. Slice sensitivity profiles for the four slices from a Philips Brilliance scanner operated in the 4 × 6 mm collimation mode. Each SSP has a FWHM of approximately 6 mm.

23. What is a slice sensitivity profile?

The slice sensitivity profile (SSP) is a plot of the relative system response in the direction of the scan length (Fig. 2-2). The slice thickness (T) is defined as the full width at half maximum (FWHM) of the SSP.

24. What does CTDI mean?

The computed tomography dose index (CTDI) is a measure of a CT scanner's dose performance and is derived from a CTDI phantom dose profile for a single axial scan. There are several variants of CTDI , each with a slightly different meaning.

25. What is CTDI (FDA)?

The CTDI (FDA) was defined by the U.S. Food and Drug Administration in 1984. It is directly related to the total area under a dose profile between two symmetric points at −7 and +7 slice thicknesses from the center (Fig. 2-3). It is defined mathematically as:

$$\text{CTDI(FDA)} = \frac{1}{nT} \int_{-7T}^{+7T} D(Z)dz$$

where $D(z)$ is the dose profile, T is the slice thickness, and n is the number of tomographic slices produced in a single axial scan.

Figure 2-3. Illustration of CTDI (FDA). The curve is a body dose profile for a scanner operated in a 4 × 6 mm collimation mode. Because the slice thickness is 6 mm, the area under the curve and between the vertical lines x = −42 mm and x = +42 mm must be evaluated.

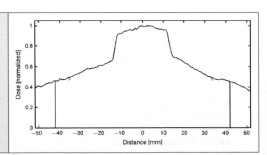

26. What is CTDI (100)?

The CTDI (100) was defined later to simplify measurements. It is also the area under the dose profile, but measured between two symmetric points that are always at −50 mm and +50 mm from the center (Fig. 2-4). The definition is as follows:

$$\text{CTDI (100)} = \frac{1}{nT} \int_{-50mm}^{+50mm} D(Z)\, dz$$

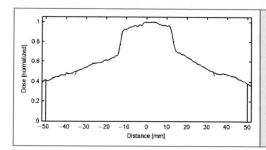

Figure 2-4. Illustration of CTDI (100). The curve is the same as in Fig. 2-3. The area under the curve and between the vertical lines x = –50 mm and x = +50 mm is evaluated.

27. What is CTDI$_w$?
CTDI$_w$ is defined as:

$$\text{CTDI}_W = (1/3)\, \text{CTDI}(100)_{center} + (2/3)\, \text{CTDI}\,(100)_{peripheral}$$

It is regarded as the average dose within a scan plane.

28. What is CTDI$_{vol}$?
CTDI$_{vol}$ is an approximation of the patient dose averaged over the entire scan volume. It is likely to be displayed on the operator's console.
- For helical scans,

$$\text{CTDI}_{vol} = \text{CTDI}_w /\text{pitch factor}$$

- For axial scans,

$$\text{CTDI}_{vol} = \text{CTDI}_w\,(N\,T\,/\,\Delta d)$$

where N is the number of slices produced in a single axial scan, T is the thickness of each slice, and Δd is the distance traveled by the patient support or table between consecutive scans. CTDI$_{vol}$ extends CTDI$_w$ to noncontiguous scans.

29. What is DLP?
Dose-length product (DLP) is defined as:

$$\text{DLP} = \text{CTDI}_{vol} \times \text{scan length}$$

Its value is related to the effective dose and therefore to the probable biologic harm of a procedure. It also may be displayed on the operator's console.

30. Where is information on CTDI and DLP available?
Manufacturers' literature will always list numerical values for CTDI (FDA) and CTDI (100), measured in both the body phantom and the head phantom. The CTDI (100) measured in air at the axis of the gantry may also be listed. This last value is often the starting point for calculating patient doses. Modern scanners also display CTDI$_{vol}$ and DLP for every scan protocol on their user consoles.

31. How close is CTDI to patient dose?
If there is no other information, the CTDI$_w$ or CTDI$_{vol}$ can be assumed to be the dose to the patient's organs that are in the direct beam. This can at best be only an approximation, because it is really the dose to the CTDI plastic phantoms.

Several authors have written software that use CTDI (100) measured in air. By entering this number and various scan parameters into their computer programs, one can calculate doses to different organs and the resulting effective dose. These calculations are also limited by the models on which the calculations are based.

32. **What are typical numerical values for CT doses?**

The doses in Table 2-1 have been excerpted from data published by a European study group of radiologists and physicists who gathered data from several countries. Exact values of patient dose for any particular procedure will vary considerably depending on CT manufacturer, model, scan parameters, and actual patient size. Note that the standard deviations are large, so that the actual values for $CTDI_w$ and DLP vary over a wide range. Nevertheless, the mean values serve as good indicators of typical patient doses.

TABLE 2-1. TYPICAL NUMERICAL VALUES FOR CT DOSES		CTDIw (mGy)		DLP (mGy cm)	
Examination Type	Sample Size	Mean	SD	Mean	SD
Head	102	50.0	14.6	882	332
Face and sinuses	20	31.7	15.9	259	118
Vertebral trauma	20	44.1	21.5	392	214
Chest	88	20.3	7.6	517	243
HRCT of lung	20	31.7	14.9	200	71
Abdomen	91	25.6	8.4	597	281
Liver and spleen	15	26.1	11.3	658	293
Pelvis	82	26.4	9.6	443	233
Osseous pelvis	16	24.7	17.8	514	426

CTDI = computed tomography dose index, DLP = dose-length product, HRCT = high-resolution CT.

33. **Why is CT dose higher for children than for adults?**

The dose will be higher for children only if the same scan parameters (kVp, mAs, pitch) are used for children as for adults. Because the smaller bodies of children attenuate less of the x-ray beam, the dose at the center of their bodies is almost the same as at their skin, whereas for adults it is two to three times less. Therefore, although the skin dose for children will be slightly smaller because the skin is slightly farther away from the x-ray source, the average dose will be much higher. This is why CT scanners should have dose-reduced pediatric protocols for scanning children.

34. **Can pregnant women undergo CT scans?**

In general, women who are pregnant should not undergo x-ray procedures of the abdomen or pelvis unless there are compelling reasons for doing so. This is especially true of CT because doses are far higher than in conventional radiography. Thoracic scans are also undesirable because radiation can be scattered by tissues in the primary beam toward the fetus. Head CT is much safer because there will be far less scatter. If a CT scan must be carried out on a pregnant patient, informed consent should be obtained.

35. **What is the range of doses a fetus may get in a CT scan?**

If the fetus is in the direct x-ray beam, its dose will be in the range of 10–30 mGy, depending on the size of the patient and the parameters chosen for the CT scan. Thoracic scans will deliver a lower dose because only secondary radiation will reach the fetus. Head scans will deliver a still lower dose.

If it is known that a fetus will not be in the CT images, then wrapping a lead apron around the pelvis will be of some help. However, one should bear in mind that it will only protect against leakage radiation from the gantry and not against scatter from within the patient's body.

36. **What are the consequences of radiation exposure from CT to a fetus?**

Within 14 days of conception, radiation exposure has an all-or-nothing effect; either the conceptus is aborted, or it will suffer no effect and will develop normally.

Beyond the first 14 days, exposures in the first trimester carry the risk of malformations and mental retardation. For fetal doses up to about 250 mGy, the risk is about 0.1% per mGy, or lower.

After the first trimester, radiation exposure may result in an elevated risk of childhood cancer. The risk is estimated to be between 0.07% and 0.88%, depending on the actual dose and the stage of pregnancy.

37. **What are the ways in which a patient's dose can be reduced?**

The most obvious ways are to eliminate unnecessary scans and to scan only the organs of interest. For scans that are performed, optimal scan parameters (kVp, mAs, pitch) should be chosen.

- Decreasing the kVp will decrease the dose, if everything else remains the same. However, noise will also increase.
- The pitch should be as large as possible, bearing in mind that too large a pitch will make for a noisy image.
- The mAs should be as small as possible, consistent with a good usable image with adequate contrast and noise.
- Another factor that can be altered is gantry angulation. Tilting the gantry during a head scan will avoid directly irradiating the eyes and thereby reduce the dose to the eyes.

38. **How can an optimal mAs be chosen before performing a CT scan?**

One way of doing this is to adopt a scheme in which a reference mAs is first determined as the optimal value for a standard-sized patient. When scanning a real patient, the actual mAs is increased or reduced from the reference value according to a chart tabulating the increase or decrease according to that patient's true size. The use of automatic exposure control can substitute for use of such a chart (*see* question 20).

39. **Does the use of electron beam computed tomography (EBCT) have an effect on a patient's dose?**

No. EBCT differs from conventional CT only in how it generates the x-ray beam and directs it at a patient. For the same scan parameters, the dose is approximately the same in both modalities.

40. **Will operators and other personnel near a CT scanner also receive a dose from the radiation?**

If the CT room is properly shielded from radiation, the personnel outside the room will receive a negligible dose. However, inside the room there will be considerable scattered radiation from the patient. The exact amount will depend on the scan parameters (e.g., kVp, mAs, slice thickness). There will also be a very small contribution from leakage of x-radiation through the housing of the x-ray tube and the gantry.

KEY POINTS: RADIATION DOSE IN CT

1. Radiation doses in computed tomography (CT) range from 15–50 mGy, depending on exam type. In general these doses are at least 10 times higher than in radiographic exams.

2. Always seek to optimize scan parameters to minimize patient dose consistent with diagnostic image quality: Minimize mAs, minimize kVp, maximize pitch, maximize slice thickness, maximize collimator setting.

3. When scanning children, be sure to use pediatric protocols, not adult protocols. In pediatric protocols the CT scan parameters should be reduced so that radiation doses are optimized according to patient size.

4. To avoid unnecessary fetal irradiation, pregnant women should be scanned only if there is adequate justification.

41. What is a stray radiation dose map?

It is a map of the maximum scatter radiation around a CT scanner, obtained by scanning the CTDI body phantom under near worst case conditions—maximum kVp and widest collimator setting (Fig. 2-5). Notice that the dose is much lower directly to the side of the gantry.

The map should be symmetric about the axis of rotation of the gantry. Actual measured values may show small discrepancies, as in the figure. In that case, the asymmetric values can be averaged to yield a usable number.

42. How is the map used?

One use is to estimate radiation doses to individuals who may be in the immediate vicinity of the scanner, such as personnel participating in a biopsy procedure or members of a patient's family. Another use is for calculating the amount of radiation shielding that should be built into the walls when the room is being designed.

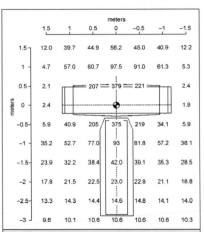

Figure 2-5. IEC stray radiation dose map for the Philips Brilliance 16/10/6 family of CT scanners. The numbers in the map are radiation levels in μGy/1000 mAs when the scanner is operated at 140 kVp and 24 mm collimation. The CTDI body phantom (cylindrical PMMA phantom of 32 cm diameter and 15 cm length) is positioned centrally in the beam and serves as the scatter medium.

43. The map only shows doses in one plane. What about other directions and planes?

Because the map is symmetric about the axis of rotation of the gantry, it can be rotated through any angle about this axis to estimate doses in any other plane or direction.

44. This map only shows doses up to a limited distance. What about locations farther away?

For greater distances, the inverse square law of radiation fall-off can be used to estimate the dose from the data in the map. For example:

Dose at 5 meters = $(3/5)^2 \times$ dose at 3 meters

BIBLIOGRAPHY

1. Boone JM, Geraghty EM, Seibert JA, Wootton-Gorges SL: Dose reduction in pediatric CT: A rational approach. Radiology 228:352–360, 2003.

2. European Commission Study Group: European Guidelines on Quality Criteria for Computed Tomography. EUR 16262 EN. Office for Official Publications of European Communities: 2000. Available at www.drs.dk/guidelines/ct/quality/index.htm

3. Imaging Performance Assessment of CT: ImPACT CT Patient Dosimetry Calculator. ImPACT, London, 2004. www.impactscan.org/ctdosimetry.htm

4. International Electrotechnical Commission: Medical Electrical Equipment–Part 2-44: Particular Requirements for the Safety of x-ray Equipment for Computed Tomography. International Electrotechnical Commission (IEC) 60601-2-44: 2002.

5. Kalender WA, Schmidt B, Zankl M, Schmidt M: A PC program for estimating organ dose and effective dose values in computed tomography. Eur Radiol 9:555–562, 1999.

6. McCullough CH, Hoffman A, Kofler J, et al: Dose Optimization in CT: Creation, Implementation and Clinical Acceptance of Size-Based Technique Charts. In RSNA 2002. Available at archive.rsna.org/index.cfm?ACTION=EVENT &id=66601&p_navID=272&em_id=3104016

7. Morgan HT: Dose reduction for CT pediatric imaging. Pediatr Radiol 32:724–738, 2002.

8. U.S. FDA Code of Federal Regulations: Diagnostic X-ray Systems and Their Major Components. Washington, DC, Government Printing Office, 1984, 21 CFR 1020.33.

9. Wagner LK, Lester RG, Saldana LR: Exposure of the Pregnant Patient to Diagnostic Radiations, 2nd ed. Madison, WI, Medical Physics Publishing, 1997, pp 88–93.

CHAPTER 3

ADVERSE CONTRAST REACTIONS

Vikram Dogra, MD, and Shweta Bhatt, MD

1. **How are iodinated contrast media classified?**
   Classification of iodinated contrast media can be done from many different perspectives, that is, ionic versus nonionic, low osmolality versus high osmolality, monomers versus dimers, and grams of iodine. However, the most practical way is classification according to osmolality (Table 3-1).

TABLE 3-1. CLASSIFICATION OF CONTRAST MEDIA BY OSMOLALITY	
High osmolality	
Ionic (monomers)	Iothalamate (Conray)
	Diatrizoate (Renovist, Hypaque, all others)
Low osmolality	
Ionic (dimers)	Ioxaglate (Hexabrix)
Nonionic (monomers)	Iohexol (Omnipaque)
	Iopamidol (Isovue)
	Ioversol (Optiray)
	Iopromide (Ultravist)
	Ioxilan (Oxilan)
Nonionic (dimer)	Iodixanol (Visipaque)

2. **What is meant by high-osmolar contrast media?**
   High-osmolar contrast media are ionic salts with an osmolality significantly higher than serum. Ionic media dissociate into a cation and anion in solution. "Ionic" and "nonionic" are often used synonymously with "high osmolar" and "low osmolar," but in fact they are not quite synonymous.

3. **What are the units of iodine concentration?**
   Milligrams of iodine (mgI) per milliliter of solution (mL). A typical CT dose is 100 mL of "300" concentration (300 mgI/mL of solution). Therefore, you are injecting 30 gm of iodine—about an ounce!

4. **Why do contrast media result in side effects?**
   Many of the side effects of contrast media are entirely or mainly due to high osmolality. The high-osmolar contrast media (diatrizoate and iothalamate) have a relatively high osmolality (1500–2100 mosm/kg water) compared to serum (300 mosm/kg water). The other causes of side effects due to contrast media are chemotoxicity (allergic-like symptoms), ion toxicity (interference with cellular function), and those caused by a high dose.

5. **What patients are at risk for an adverse contrast reaction?**
   The following patients are at a higher risk for an adverse contrast reaction:
   - Previous history of idiosyncratic reaction (5 times relative risk)
   - Patients with history of asthma (2–5 times)

- Multiple food or drug allergies (2 times)
- Patients with azotemia and cardiac disease
- Patients on beta blockers (2.7 times)

6. **Can radiographic contrast be administered to patients taking metformin?**
   Metformin is an oral antihyperglycemic agent with renal excretion. Contrast-induced nephropathy in a diabetic patient continuing to take metformin can lead to metformin build-up, hypoglycemia, coma, and death. Metformin use should be stopped when an iodinated contrast agent is administered, and the patient should wait 48 hours before resuming use of metformin while being monitored for acute renal failure.

7. **Define contrast-induced nephropathy.**
   An increase in serum creatinine (SCr) of 0.5 mg/dL or 25% above baseline at 48 hours after contrast dosing is defined as contrast-induced nephropathy.

8. **What are the risk factors for contrast-induced nephropathy?**
   The major factor is underlying renal dysfunction. Diabetes mellitus is an additional contributory factor in the presence of renal dysfunction. Other factors include dehydration, poor renal perfusion, nephrotoxic medications, and the volume of contrast injected.

9. **How do you prevent contrast-induced nephropathy?**
   - Good hydration should be maintained before and after contrast administration.
   - N-Acetylcysteine, 600 mg orally twice daily for 2 days, before contrast administration has been shown to reduce contrast-induced nephropathy in outpatients with renal insufficiency.

10. **What are the relative contraindications for contrast administration?**
    The following is a list of relative contraindications for the administration of contrast medium:
    - Pheochromocytoma (hypertensive crisis with ionic contrast; nonionic contrast can be used)
    - Multiple myeloma (renal failure)
    - Sickle cell disease (sickle cell crisis)
    - Hyperthyroidism (thyroid storm)
    - Insulin-dependent diabetes mellitus (contrast-induced renal failure)
    - Myasthenia gravis (acute exacerbation)
    - Paroxysmal nocturnal hemoglobinuria
    - Patients on interleukin–2

KEY POINTS: ADVERSE REACTIONS TO CONTRAST MATERIALS

1. Many of the side effects of contrast media are entirely or mainly due to high osmolality.

2. The other causes of side effects due to contrast media are chemotoxicity (allergic-like symptoms), ion toxicity (interference with cellular function), and those caused by a high dose.

3. An increase in serum creatinine (SCr) of 0.5 mg/dL or 25% above baseline at 48 hours after contrast dosing is defined as contrast-induced nephropathy.

4. The major risk factor for contrast-induced nephropathy is underlying renal dysfunction. Other risk factors include diabetes mellitus, dehydration, poor renal perfusion, nephrotoxic medications, and the volume of contrast injected.

11. **What are adverse contrast reactions to intravenous (IV) iodinated contrast media?**
    The adverse effects of IV iodinated contrast media can be divided into two categories:
    1. **Adverse physiologic effects:** Most commonly nausea, a metallic taste (iodine is a metal), and sensation of warmth. An intra-arterial injection of contrast media can also cause a passing sensation of pain and intense heat due to peripheral vasodilatation. These reactions are much more common with high-osmolar contrast. Some uncommon physiologic reactions include the following:
        - Neurotoxicity (seizure)
        - Contrast nephropathy
        - Cardiac depression
        - Arrhythmias
        - Inhibition of clotting mechanisms
        - Increased airway resistance
    2. **Anaphylactoid reactions:** Idiosyncratic and unpredictable adverse reactions caused by a number of possible mechanisms including histamine release, central nervous system (CNS) toxicity, and cardiac toxicity. These reactions are not dose- or concentration-dependent, unlike physiologic reactions.

12. **What is meant by the term *anaphylactoid reaction*?**
    Anaphylactoid reactions are the non–IgE-mediated reactions, unlike anaphylaxis, which follows antigen-IgE mediated release of mediators from mast cells and basophils and may result in the release of identical mediators with similar end-organ responses. The clinical features and the induced biochemical alterations are indistinguishable from true anaphylaxis.

13. **What is the most common anaphylactoid reaction to contrast media?**
    The most common anaphylactoid reaction to contrast is limited to the skin and subcutaneous soft tissue. Pruritus is the most prominent complaint. Local vasodilatation causes erythema, and leaky capillaries are responsible for the raised wheals (hives).

14. **What is the etiology of adverse idiosyncratic (anaphylactoid) reactions?**
    The exact etiology of idiosyncratic reactions is not fully understood. There are three possible etiologies:
    - Histamine release from basophils and mast cells
    - Complement activation, which results in the release of histamine and more powerful agents such as kallikreins and leukokinins via the complement activation system
    - Allergic reaction may or may not require a sensitizing exposure

15. **What are the findings in an anaphylactoid syndrome?**
    The various findings in an anaphylactoid syndrome are as follows:
    - **Skin:** Pruritus, urticaria, angioedema, erythema
    - **Eyes:** Pruritus, conjunctival congestion
    - **Nose:** Sneezing, congestion, rhinorrhea
    - **Mouth:** Pruritus, edema
    - **Upper airway:** Hoarseness, stridor, laryngeal edema
    - **Lower airway:** Dyspnea, tachypnea, wheezing, rales, bronchospasm, pulmonary edema
    - **Cardiovascular:** Hypotension, tachycardia, arrhythmia
    - **Gastrointestinal:** Abdominal pain, cramping, diarrhea, nausea, vomiting

16. **What are the possible methods to prevent a contrast reaction?**
    Adequate patient screening for the presence of risk factors for adverse contrast reactions, such as renal insufficiency, previous life-threatening reaction, active bronchospasm, asthma, hypotension, or shock from an underlying illness, may help prevent contrast reactions in these patients.

Premedication with steroids prior to contrast administration will also decrease the incidence of moderate and severe anaphylactoid reactions.

17. **What are the pretreatment protocols to prevent contrast reactions in at-risk patients?**
    There are two recommended protocols available for the pretreatment of patients who are at risk and who require contrast media. These regimens have been shown to lower the incidence of subsequent contrast reactions compared to nontreated individuals:
    - **Lasser approach:** 32 mg of Medrol orally 12 hours and 2 hours prior to IV administration of contrast medium
    - **Greenberger regimen:** Prednisone, 50 mg orally 13 hours, 7 hours, and 1 hour prior to the exam; Benadryl, 50 mg orally 1 hour prior to the exam; ephedrine, 25 mg orally 1 hour prior to the exam (contraindicated in the presence of heart disease)

18. **What should be the initial response in the treatment of acute adverse contrast reaction?**
    Initial response in a case of adverse contrast reaction includes six basic steps:
    1. Release abdominal compression.
    2. Check pulse.
    3. Ensure an adequate airway.
    4. Start oxygen supplementation at a relatively high rate of 6–10 L/min.
    5. Elevate the patient's legs.
    6. Secure IV line.

19. **What is the cause of hypotension in a case of adverse contrast reaction? What is the treatment?**
    Hypotension is caused by the lowering of systemic vascular resistance due to diffuse vasodilatation. Leaky capillary beds allow plasma to pour into the extravascular space, lowering blood pressure, and causing reflex tachycardia.
    Immediate treatment of hypotension includes leg elevation to augment venous return, oxygen supplementation, and rapid administration of isotonic IV fluid.

20. **What is the technique for administering oxygen in a case of adverse contrast reaction?**
    Oxygen is very important in the initial treatment of all reactions to intravascular contrast media. Oxygen should be administered at a high rate of about 10–12 L/min via face mask. A "rebreather" mask is optimal for delivering good oxygenation, whereas nasal prongs are much less effective. High concentrations of oxygen should be administered to any patient in respiratory distress regardless of his or her preexisting condition.

21. **What is the role of intravascular fluid replacement in a case of adverse contrast reaction?**
    Intravascular fluid replacement is very important and is the single most effective treatment for hypotension. Therefore, early intervention with IV fluids before starting drug therapy should be reemphasized as the highest priority in treating hypotension. Normal saline or lactated Ringer's solution is preferred for acute, initial intravascular fluid expansion. Within the first 20 minutes 500–700 mL can be instilled. As much as 2–3 L of fluid may be needed over several hours. Iso-oncotic colloid solutions such as 5% human albumin are selected if the hypotension is unresponsive to initial fluid therapy.

22. **Why raise the patient's legs in a case of hypotension?**
    Because this provides an **immediate** bolus of fluid. Legs should be raised high, flexed at the patient's hips, and held by an assistant. Placing the ankles on a pillow is not sufficient. The point

is to speed venous return in a patient with acute vasodilation and hypotension not to provide comfort.

23. **What are the drugs that can be used in an adverse contrast reaction?**
Four main categories of drugs can be used:
- Antihistamines
- Corticosteroids
- Anticholinergics
- Adrenergic agonists

24. **What is the role of antihistamines in an adverse contrast reaction?**
Antihistamines are the histamine-1 (H1) receptor antagonists and are the most frequently used drugs by radiologists for treatment of reactions to contrast media; however, they have limited therapeutic roles. They are used primarily to reduce symptoms from skin reactions such as pruritus and as second-line drugs for respiratory reactions after use of epinephrine. They are not first-line drugs in patients having a respiratory or a hypotensive reaction.

25. **What is the role of corticosteroids in the treatment of an acute adverse contrast reaction?**
High-dose IV corticosteroids do not play a significant role in the treatment of an acute reaction because of the slow onset of action. However, they may be effective in reducing recurrent delayed symptoms that can be observed for as long as 48 hours after an initial reaction.

26. **What is the dose for the administration of steroids?**
IV doses of 100–1000 mg of hydrocortisone have been recommended. The initial dose can be followed by a continuous infusion of 300–500 mg in a 250 mL solution of saline or D5W at a rate of 60 mL/h.

27. **What is the role of epinephrine in the treatment of an adverse reaction to radiographic contrast media?**
Epinephrine is the most important single medication in the treatment of anaphylactoid reactions. Epinephrine is a powerful sympathomimetic agent. It activates both alpha- and beta-adrenergic receptors. The alpha-agonist effects of epinephrine increase blood pressure and reverse peripheral vasodilation. These vasoconstrictive effects also decrease angioedema and urticaria. The beta-agonist actions of epinephrine reverse bronchoconstriction, produce positive inotropic and chronotropic cardiac effects, and may increase intracellular cyclic adenosine monophosphate (AMP), which inhibits mediator release from inflammatory cells.

28. **What are the various modes of administration of epinephrine and its indications?**
Epinephrine is mainly administered subcutaneously, intramuscularly, or intravenously. It may also be administered as an aerosolized mist endotracheally or even transtracheally. Subcutaneous or intramuscular injections of epinephrine can be used effectively in an acutely reacting patient provided that the patient is not hypotensive. If the patient is hypotensive, the tissue perfusion will be poor and the pharmacologic effects delayed and diminished. IV epinephrine should be utilized whenever there is rapid progression of symptoms or when the patient is significantly hypotensive (systolic blood pressure < 90 mmHg).

29. **What epinephrine preparations are available? What doses should be administered?**
Epinephrine is manufactured in two dilutions.
- 1:1000 dilution = 1 mg of epinephrine in 1 mL of fluid. This is intended for subcutaneous and intramuscular administration. Subcutaneous epinephrine is generally administered at a dose

of 0.1–0.3 mg. The dose can be repeated every 10–15 minutes until a total dose of 1 mg is administered; however, repeat injections can be provided at shorter intervals if a responding patient's symptoms begin to recur before the 10 or 15 minutes have elapsed.

- 1:10,000 dilution = 1 mg of epinephrine in 10 mL of fluid. Intended for IV use. It is administered at the same dose of 0.1–0.3 mg; however, owing to its greater dilution, this requires injection of 1 to 3 mL per dose. IV epinephrine should be administered slowly whenever possible. An infusion of 10–20 μgm/min is preferred unless a respiratory or cardiac arrest appears imminent.

30. **What is the dose of epinephrine in a case of cardiac arrest?**
The 1:10,000 epinephrine comes in a prepared total dose of 1 mg for use in a cardiac arrest situation. The total dose is injected intravenously if the patient is in cardiac arrest.

31. **What is the dose of epinephrine in infants and children?**
A subcutaneous dose of 1:1000 epinephrine is 0.01 mg/kg of body weight up to a maximum of 0.3 mL (0.3 mg); for IV administration, a lower dose of 1:10,000 dilution is used, for example, 1–5 μgm/kg. You should have weight-based tables ready for reference; do not attempt to calculate this in a emergent chaotic situation.

32. **What are the possible complications arising due to epinephrine administration?**
Epinephrine is powerful and even young healthy patients can develop potentially life-threatening complications as a result of its use, including hypertensive crises, myocardial ischemia, and infarction. These occur most commonly when large doses are administered (0.5–1 mg).

In individuals with a fragile intracerebral or coronary circulation, the alpha agonist effects of a large dose of epinephrine may invoke a hypertensive crisis that could produce a stroke or myocardial ischemia. Hypertensive crisis is more likely to develop in a patient receiving beta blockers for any reason because such individuals exhibit primarily an alpha adrenergic vasoconstrictive response. Additionally, the sympathomimetic effects of epinephrine have been observed to be exacerbated in patients receiving tricyclic antidepressants.

33. **Can epinephrine be safely used in pregnant patients?**
There is disagreement about the use of epinephrine in pregnant women who have anaphylactic or anaphylactoid reactions. Epinephrine should be avoided when possible when treating pregnant patients with a severe contrast reaction and hypotension. As uterine vessels are extremely sensitive to alpha-adrenergic stimulation, administration of epinephrine to a pregnant patient can severely compromise fetal blood flow, thus leading to poor fetal outcome. Ephedrine (25–50 mg IV push) is suggested as an alternative medication.

34. **What are the specific treatment plans for the following more frequently occurring adverse reactions after radiographic contrast administration?**
1. **Nausea and vomiting:** 20% of fatal contrast reactions begin with nausea and vomiting. Therefore, patients should be observed closely for systemic symptoms while IV access is maintained.
   - Position the patient to avoid aspiration.
   - Observe closely.
2. **Urticaria**
   - **Mild:** Observe until resolution.
   - **Moderate:** H1 receptor blocker (diphenhydramine); H2 receptor blocker (cimetidine) may be added. Observe until resolution.
   - **Severe urticaria, angioedema, or diffuse erythema:** Administer (1) alpha-adrenergic agonist (low-dose epinephrine, 0.1 mg, 1.0 mL 1:10,000, slowly over 2–5 minutes; repeat as necessary), (2) IV fluids (normal saline or lactated Ringer's solution), (3) H1

receptor blocker plus H2 receptor blocker, (4) corticosteroids (e.g., hydrocortisone, 200 mg; prednisone, 100 mg; methylprednisolone, 80 mg).

3. **Bronchospasm:** Tends to occur in patients who already have a history of bronchospasm. Treatment includes the following:
   - Administer oxygen by mask 6–10 L/min.
   - Use beta$_2$ agonist inhaler, for example, albuterol–metered dose inhaler or nebulized.
   - Administer IV epinephrine 1 mL of 1:10,000 or 0.1 to 0.3 mL of a 1:1000 dilution subcutaneously if unrelieved by inhaled bronchodilators.

4. **Laryngeal edema:** Presents with hoarseness or coughing.
   - **Mild:** Provide oxygen by mask, 6–10 L/min; epinephrine 1:1000 dilution 0.1–0.3 mL subcutaneous.
   - **Severe:** Administer IV epinephrine 1 mL of 1:10,000 dilution slowly over one to several minutes.

5. **Isolated hypotension:** Elevate legs (immediately returns about 700 mL of fluid to the central circulation); provide oxygen by mask, 6–10 L/min; administer IV fluids (normal saline or lactated Ringer's solution).

6. **Secondary hypotension:** Epinephrine, 1:10,000, 1 mL (0.1 mg), given slowly over 2–5 minutes or IV drip infusion of 1-4 µgm/min; if response to initial therapy is poor, call a code.

7. **Vasovagal reaction:** Characterized by sinus bradycardia and hypotension. Treatment includes the following:
   - Elevate legs.
   - Administer IV fluids.
   - Provide oxygen by mask.
   - For atropine, larger doses are indicated. 1.0 mg initially by slow push, additional doses of 0.6–1.0 mg given every 3–5 minutes to a total dose of 3 mg in adults. Atropine should never be used in doses less than 0.6 mg because it may worsen the existing bradycardia.

8. **Pulmonary edema:** Patients are short of breath with crackles or rales at the lung bases. Treat as follows:
   - Elevate patient's head.
   - Administer high-dose oxygen by mask, 6–10 L/min.
   - Monitor electrocardiogram.
   - Administer furosemide, 40 mg IV slowly.
   - Administer morphine, 1–3 mg IV, repeated every 5–10 minutes.

9. **Hypertensive crisis:** Treatment includes the following: (1) oxygen by mask, (2) nitroglycerine (0.4 mg tablet sublingually or topical application of a 1- to 2-inch strip of 2% ointment), (3) call for assistance.
   - **For hypertension related to autonomic dysreflexia:** Administer nifedipine, 10-mg capsule; puncture or bite and swallow contents.
   - **For hypertension caused by pheochromocytoma:** Administer phentolamine, 5 mg IV, or labetalol, 20 mg IV push followed by 20–80 mg IV every 10 minutes up to a total of 300 mg.

10. **Seizures/convulsions:** Often due to a severe hypotensive reaction but may also be due to contrast irritating an underlying abnormal focus. Treatment includes the following:
    - Avoid aspiration.
    - Provide oxygen by mask, 6–10 L/min.
    - Treat hypotension or vagal reaction if present.
    - Administer IV diazepam, 5 mg.

35. **What is the management of a pulseless patient due to an adverse reaction following contrast administration?**
    This patient requires the same treatment as a presumed cardiac arrest patient:
    1. Establish unresponsiveness.
    2. Airway

- Open airway.
- Suction if needed.
3. Breathing
   - Provide supplemental oxygen.
   - Provide ventilation support.
4. Circulation
   - Elevate legs.
   - Administer isotonic fluids.
5. Provide cardiopulmonary resuscitation (CPR).
6. Perform electrocardiographic evaluation as soon as possible.
7. Defibrillation if appropriate. Defibrillation should precede CPR if a defibrillator can be obtained immediately. If ventricular fibrillation or pulseless ventricular tachycardia is recognized, shock the patient at 200 J. If no change, shocks should be repeated at 300 J and then at 360 J.

36. **What is the cause of contrast media extravasations?**
    Contrast media extravasations result either from the creation of two holes in a vein (double-wall puncture or multiple consecutive punctures) or from actual placement of the needle or catheter tip outside of a vein.

37. **What are the risk factors for extravasation and extravasation injuries?**
    1. Abnormal circulation in limb to be injected
       - Atherosclerotic peripheral vascular disease
       - Connective tissue disease
       - Diabetic vascular disease
       - Previous radiation
       - Tourniquets
       - Venous thrombosis
    2. Noncommunicative patient (unable to complain about pain at the injection site)
       - Demented
       - Elderly
       - Infants and children
       - Unconscious
       - Foreign language speakers
    3. Problems at the site to be injected
       - Injections through needles rather than catheters

- Injections on dorsum of hand, foot, or ankle
- Multiple punctures of the same vein
4. Use of indwelling IV lines (particularly when in place for more than 20 hours)

38. **What is the mechanism of injury due to extravasation of contrast media?**
Hyperosmolality of contrast media is primarily responsible for its extravascular toxicity. When large volumes are extravasated, simple mechanical compression may also be a factor. In addition, once skin ulceration and necrosis occurs, the extravasation site may become superinfected.

39. **How does one diagnose the occurrence of extravasation of contrast?**
Patients often complain of stinging or burning pain, and the affected site may become erythematous, swollen, and tender.

40. **How do you treat extravasation injuries?**
1. Immediate treatment
   - Elevation of affected extremity (above heart)
   - Ice packs (15–60 minute application)
   - Call referring physician (if more than 5 mL of extravasation)
   - Observation for 2–4 hours
   - Local hyaluronidase injections (seldom done)
2. Indications for plastic surgery consultation
   - Extravasated volume exceeds 30 mL ionic or 100 mL nonionic contrast
   - Patient develops any of the following: skin blistering or ulceration; altered tissue perfusion, sensation, or temperature; increasing or persistent pain
3. Daily phone calls by nurse or radiologist until manifestations resolve
4. Documentation

41. **What are the best ways to avoid extravasation injuries?**
   - Close monitoring of the patient and injection site during test injections and during the injection of the bolus before the CT scan begins
   - Use of hypo-osmolar contrast

BIBLIOGRAPHY

1. Almen T: The etiology of contrast medium reactions. Invest Radiol 29(Suppl 1):S37–S45, 1994.
2. Bettmann MA: Frequently asked questions: Iodinated contrast agents. Radiographics 24:S3–S10, 2004.
3. Bielory L, Kaliner MA: Anaphylactoid reactions to radiocontrast materials. Anesth Clin 23(3):97–118, 1985.
4. Bush WH, McClennan BL: Epinephrine administration for severe adverse reactions to contrast agents [letter]. Radiology 196:879, 1995.
5. Bush WH, Swanson DP: Acute reactions to intravascular contrast media: Types, risk factors, recognition, and specific treatment. AJR Am J Roentgenol 157:1153–1161, 1991.
6. Curry N, Schabel S, Reiheld C, et al: Fatal reactions to intravenous non-ionic contrast material. Radiology 178:361–362, 1991.
7. Katayama H, Yamaguchi K, Kozuka T, et al: Adverse reactions to ionic and non ionic contrast media. Radiology 175:621–628, 1990.
8. Katzberg RW (ed): The Contrast Media Manual. Baltimore, Lippincott, Williams & Wilkins, 1992.
9. McClennan BL: Adverse reactions to iodinated contrast media. Recognition and response. Invest Radiol 29(S1):S46–S50, 1994.

CHAPTER 4

CT RADIATION TREATMENT PLANNING

Rajashree Vyas, DMRD, John G. Strang, MD, and Paul Okunieff, MD

1. **Why is there a chapter on radiation treatment planning in *Body CT Secrets*?**
   Think of radiation therapy (XRT) as percutaneous surgery. Ionizing radiation is the knife that destroys malignant cells. To plan XRT, it is essential first to accurately identify tumor and then to anatomically localize that tumor relative to the external body surface. No one needs to know more precisely where the tumor is (and where the tumor is not) than the radiation oncologist!

   XRT techniques—like imaging—have moved from two-dimensional to 3D treatment techniques for many applications. Three-dimensional treatment techniques need 3D planning techniques such as CT (Fig. 4-1). Interpreters of CT must know the terminology of XRT and the concerns of the radiation oncology team.

2. **How does XRT work?**
   XRT is a clinical treatment modality. XRT causes cellular reproductive inactivation. Tumor cells ultimately die by necrosis or apoptosis or during aberrant mitosis. The irradiated tumors often do not disappear because the inflammation and supporting stroma of the tumor do not resorb. Thus, reproductive sterilization of the tumor (stopping its ability to divide immortally) leads to permanent tumor control even if the tumor does *not* totally disappear on follow-up CT scans.

3. **What tumors are commonly treated with XRT?**
   Cervical, lung, breast, prostate, head, neck, and central nervous system tumors, sarcomas, and metastases from various primary malignancies are commonly treated with

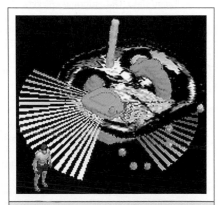

Figure 4-1. Arcs of 3D XRT conformal to hepatic adenocarcinoma metastasis within the right lobe of the liver.

XRT. Nonmalignant indications for XRT use include treatment of intracranial arterial-venous malformations, prevention of coronary artery restenosis, and prevention of heterotopic bone formation.

4. **What are common dose-limiting organs?**
   Depending on the body region undergoing XRT, common dose-limiting organs include spinal cord (in cervical, thoracic, and upper abdominal XRT), kidney, liver, orbits (lens and optic nerves in brain XRT), and lung (in lung and mediastinal XRT). Less sensitive but still important organs that limit radiation dose include brain stem, heart, small bowel, and skin.

5. **What terms should be in my XRT vocabulary?**
   - **Brachytherapy:** *Brachy* = short (referring to distance). The source of radiation is very close to treated tissue or may even be embedded within it (e.g., prostatic seed implants, intracavitary XRT for rectal or gynecologic tumors).

- **Teletherapy:** Source of radiation is at some distance from the patient, such as an x-ray beam. The usual distance is 100 cm for linear accelerators.
- **Adjuvant therapy:** A treatment used in conjunction with primary treatment for patients with localized disease. Typically the local disease has been surgically resected and is thus no longer detectable. Adjuvant treatments may include chemotherapy, hormone therapy, biologic therapy, or XRT.
- **Neoadjuvant therapy:** This is adjuvant therapy given prior to anticipated curative surgery.
- **Stereotactic radiosurgery (SRS):** Nonsurgical procedure in which a single high-dose of precisely localized radiation is used. "Stereotactic" refers to image guidance using a 3D reference system attached to the patient. The radiation is typically delivered using arcing fields or through a large number of fixed fields focused on the target.
- **Stereotactic radiotherapy (SRT):** When SRS is administered in fractionated doses over a period of days/weeks, it is termed SRT.
- **Gross tumor volume (GTV):** Gross palpable or CT-visible tumor tissue. This is what you see and know is tumor.
- **Clinical target volume (CTV):** GTV + subclinical/microscopic tumor tissue that is presumed to be extend from the gross tumor volume. This volume also includes potential lymph-node drainage patterns.
- **Planning target volume (PTV):** This is CTV + surrounding margin to compensate for minor variations in daily treatment set-up or other anatomic movements such as breathing.
- **Conformal XRT:** Conformal XRT refers to fractionated radiation wherein the radiation is delivered via multiple fields. The shape of each field conforms to the silhouette of the tumor from the projection of the radiation field.
- **Intensity-modulated radiation therapy (IMRT):** A newer form of conformal 3D XRT. IMRT is sometimes called "dose painting." In IMRT the dose is calculated using inverse dose algorithms. It can be thought of as an inverse CT scan in which the algorithm calculates the microbeam doses that must be delivered to create a dose image. IMRT differs from conformal XRT in that different doses are delivered in each microbeam that makes up each of the conformal fields.
- **Gamma knife:** Form of SRS using multiple beams of highly focused gamma rays to kill tumor cells. Gamma rays are produced by 201 cobalt-60 sources aimed at a point. The patient's tumor is positioned at this focus point using a rigid frame fixed to their skull.
- **Isodose curve:** Curve passing through points of equal dose, related to the planned treatment dose. For example, there are isodose curves for 70%, 80%, 90%, 100%, and so forth, of treatment dose.
- **Treatment simulation:** Essentially a "dress rehearsal" for the actual XRT procedure. The planned field arrangement is verified using a simulator that mimics the geometry of the XRT machine to produce diagnostic quality images. Simulators use plain film, fluoroscopy, or CT imaging.
- **Dose-limiting tissue:** Normal tissue surrounding or in close proximity to tumor tissue. It limits the radiation dose due to lower radiation tolerance. The dose limits for different tissues are based on their individual radiosensitivities and on the volume of the organ that must be included in the radiation field.
- **Fractionation:** This is the division of the total dose into multiple treatment sessions.
- **Localization:** This is a procedure in which target volume and dose-limiting normal tissues in the region to be treated are delineated with respect to the patient's external surface.

6. **Who is on the radiation oncology team?**
   - **Radiation oncologists:** MD or DO responsible for management of the XRT for cancer patients. They evaluate patient disease, prescribe and develop treatment plans, ensure accurate XRT delivery, identify and treat XRT side effects, monitor patient progress, and adjust treatment as necessary.
   - **Radiation physicists:** Usually a PhD, the radiation physicist works directly with the doctor in treatment planning and delivery, oversees the work of dosimetrists, is responsible for developing

and directing quality control programs for equipment and procedures, measures radiation beam characteristics, and performs safety tests. Radiation physicists are board-certified by the American Association of Physicists in Medicine and are licensed by the Department of Health in many states.

- **Dosimetrists:** Usually have a BS degree in the physics. They perform complex computations to deliver a prescribed radiation dose to a defined tumor volume, supervise and/or assist in preparation of beam-modifying devices and immobilization devices, work with radiation therapists in treatment plan implementation, and assist medical physicists in quality assurance and radiation safety programs. Dosimetrists are licensed in most states.

- **Radiation therapists:** Administer daily XRT per prescription and are specifically trained in the operation of the linear accelerators, simulators, and other equipment. They work under the physician's supervision, maintain daily records, and check treatment machines regularly to ensure that the table, gantry, and lasers are operating properly. They are licensed in most states.

- **Radiation oncology nurses:** They care for patients during the course of treatment and educate patient about potential side effects of XRT and their management.

7. **What are the types of external radiation beam machines?**
   - Orthovoltage units (OVU) (seldom used now)
   - Linear accelerators
   - Machines that expose isotopes such as cobalt-60 (also rarely used aside from the gamma knife)

   A few institutions have cyclotrons for delivery of proton beams, neutron beams, or heavy particles. Unlike other external beam radiation machines, the cobalt-60 source emits radiation constantly. Hence, the source must be shielded when the machine is in the "off" position to protect personnel.

8. **What is an OVU?**
   Used primarily in the past, OVUs are a third type of external beam machine that features kilovoltage photons. They typically operate in the range of 50–250 kVp. Lower energy beams are absorbed to a greater degree by the skin than high-energy beams. Thus, they are useful only for fairly superficial tumors. For deep tumors they cause severe complications. They have largely been abandoned in favor of electrons for superficial cancers. Some sites still use OVUs for treatment of dermal basal and squamous cell tumors or for some low superficial rectal tumors, which can be exposed by rigid proctosigmoidoscopy.

9. **What is a linear accelerator?**
   Medical linear accelerators are widely used external beam radiation machines (x-ray machines). They use high-frequency electromagnetic waves to accelerate electrons to high energies. Accelerated electrons may either be used directly to radiate superficial tumors or may be fired at a target to produce high-energy x-rays to treat deep-seated tumors (Fig. 4-2).

10. **What is IMRT?**
    IMRT is an advanced form of 3D conformal XRT. Computer-controlled x-ray accelerators deliver precise radiation doses of

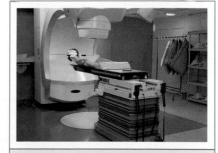

Figure 4-2. Linear accelerator. The beam is above the head of the bed. The beam is on a C-arm that can rotate around the patient. The patient and patient's bed can rotate the C-arm and table about the same point, and that central point is marked by orthogonal lasers mounted on the walls.

varying intensity to the tumor from multiple angles. The shape and the dose of radiation may be varied within a single beam. Thus, the net effect is that precise radiation dose distribution can be tightly wrapped around the tumor volume while avoiding sensitive structures such as the spinal cord.

IMRT is planned using 3D CT images in conjunction with computerized dose calculations to determine the dose intensity pattern that best conforms to the contour of the tumor. Typically, a combination of several intensity-modulated fields from different beam directions tailors maximum radiation dose to the tumor while minimizing dose to adjacent normal tissues. By irradiating from many directions, the dose is high at the intersection of the rays and falls off rapidly away from the treatment volume (Fig. 4-3).

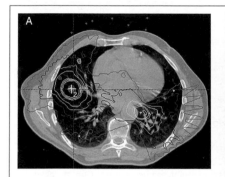
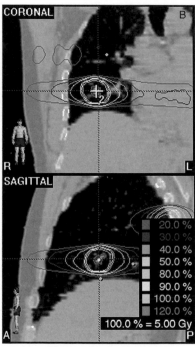

Figure 4-3. Isodose distributions with the maximum dose concentrated to right lower lobe pulmonary adenocarcinoma in axial images *(A)* and coronal and sagittal *(B)* reconstructions.

11. **What are the advantages of IMRT and 3D conformal XRT over conventional XRT?**
    IMRT and 3D conformal XRT differ from conventional radiotherapy in that the radiation dose is designed to conform to the 3D shape of the tumor by using movable multileaf collimators (Fig. 4-4). In IMRT, the intensity of the radiation field is divided into beamlets, which can each be adjusted to focus higher radiation dose to the tumor while minimizing radiation exposure to the surrounding normal tissues. Conformal 3D XRT also treats a 3D volume, but IMRT differs from it by modulating the beamlets within the field. IMRT is also sometimes called "dose painting."

12. **What is a potential disadvantage of IMRT compared to conventional XRT?**
    A tighter dose distribution centered on the tumor makes accurate targeting critical because portions of the tumor volume may be missed if either the localization is inadequate or the definition

of the volume at risk is imperfect. The benefits of IMRT can only be achieved with accurate image evaluation.

13. **What does CT radiation treatment planning involve?**
CT radiation treatment planning finds the GTV, CTV, and PTV, does dose calculation and fractionation, decides the field of arrangement to be used, designs beam-modifying devices, and produces appropriate isodose distribution. Volumetric dose information is calculated for the tumor and normal tissues. This allows the radiation oncologist to both maximize tumor control and to estimate risk to organs such as the lung and kidney.

14. **What is the expected course of events in XRT?**
Decision to implement XRT → positioning and immobilization → treatment simulation in the simulator → data acquisition by CT/magnetic resonance imaging (MRI) → planning (GTV,CTV, and PTV) technique and dose calculations → treatment verification on the treatment machine (dry run) → treatment delivery → follow-up.

15. **What XRT planning equipment is commonly used?**
An acquisition device (CT/MR scanner), a treatment simulator (fluoroscopic or CT device), and a 3D radiation treatment planning computer and software. Positron emission tomography (PET) scans are becoming standard.

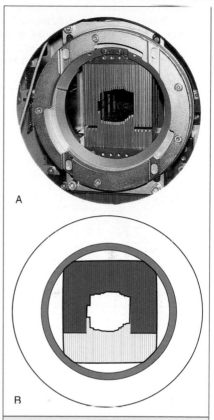

A

B

Figure 4-4. *A* and *B,* Multileaf collimator mounted on the linear accelerator for 3D conformal therapy. There are multiple pairs of leaves that can be adjusted by computer to shape the treatment field.

16. **How is accurate localization of target volume reproduced at each session of XRT?**
Beam alignment laser systems mounted within the CT scanner and immobilization devices achieve consistent patient positioning (Fig. 4-5). Permanent tattoos are placed on the patient's skin to serve as landmarks to which the lasers are aligned for the daily treatments. Radiodense markers can be placed on the tattoos for CT imaging (Fig. 4-6).

17. **What 3D imaging modalities are used in radiation treatment planning?**
Three-dimensional modalities localize the 3D target volume of tissue better than conventional x-ray methods. Understanding the 3D anatomy of the target volume allows for directing a conformal field at the target from arbitrary angles. Understanding the anatomy of the nontarget normal tissues in three dimensions likewise allows for avoidance of these structures.
- For identification of tumor and normal tissues in the brain, **MR images** are critical. Special sequences to distinguish necrosis from tumor and high versus low perfusion, as well as those that accentuate edema, vascular voids, and cranial nerves are fused together to obtain treatment plans.

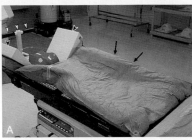

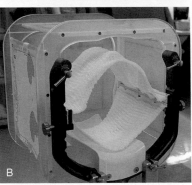

Figure 4-5. *A,* Body immobilization devices: vacuum bag, headrest, side wings, and handholds *(above head).* The vacuum bag contains polymer beads and is initially filled with air. The patient lies on the bag, and the beads mold to the shape of the patient. The air is withdrawn from the bag, causing the beads to stick together and harden, thus creating a patient-specific form. The bag is reusable after reinflation. Vacuum bags of individual patients can be seen hanging at the side in Fig. 4-2. *B,* Brain and head immobilization device. The mesh softens when warmed in water and is molded to the patient's face and skull. The mask is used during CT planning and during radiation treatment. With use of the mask, the reproducibility of patient repositioning can be better than 2 mm.

- **CT images** have become critical for detecting and targeting tumors in the lung and chest. CT also out performs MR for most cases in the abdomen and pelvis. The respiratory variation and geometric distortions in MR limit its use stereotactic targeting. This is true even for cranial radiosurgery. Thus MR becomes useful in separating malignant from nonmalignant structures when the separation is not clearly delineated by CT. Modern CT can easily be done in a single breath-hold, even with thin slices, and has greatly impacted the radiation of even small tumors. To be most useful the CT scans must be performed with the patient immobilized in the same

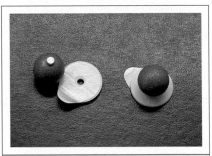

Figure 4-6. Close-up view of surface markers. The hole in the pad of the surface marker is placed over the tattoo. The ball with the metal button is then inserted into the pad. The button shows on radiography, the ball shows on CT and on MR.

devise and with the same laser points as will be used for treatment. This can be achieved with either a dedicated CT simulator or with a specially modified diagnostic radiology CT suite.

- **Nuclear medicine bone scans** are sensitive to detect tumor tissue. However, it can be difficult to localize tumor extent with respect to external body surface. Ordinary planar images in conjunction with the nuclear images are usually sufficient to target the tumor. Although in some cases MR might be more sensitive than other imaging techniques, they are still insufficiently specific to allow for targeting in the absence of bone scans and x-rays.

- **PET scans** have good tumor detection and can be very specific, but geometric and anatomic localization is suboptimal. As with MR, respiration and other needed immobilization is difficult with PET compared to CT. PET-CT will likely have a major role in XRT planning. The coregistration of the images allows the radiation oncologist to take advantage of the strengths of the individual imaging modalities.

18. **Are CT images obtained for treatment planning different from diagnostic CT images?**
Yes. XRT planning images must be performed with the patient in a reproducible position in addition to being diagnostically accurate. They are obtained with the patient in the *treatment position* on a flat table insert. They also use external reference marks visible on CT images, such as plastic markers. In addition to the orthogonal orientation, the rotation (rock, roll, yaw) of the patient on the table is corrected using lasers in combination with the tattoos and plastic markers.

Because of the positioning requirements of the imaging, diagnostic images (with oral and intravenous contrast) are sometimes also obtained and fused to the treatment planing CT to help with the plan.

19. **How was XRT planning performed before there was CT?**
Localization procedures used a diagnostic-type x-ray machine to acquire anterior and lateral radiographs with a device on the patient's skin surface or graticule built into the fluoroscope. A radiopaque marker (lead wire) indicated ink marks on the patient's skin. Recognizable internal structures were demagnified from the orthogonal films and outlined with respect to the skin marks indicated on the contour of the patient. Bone landmarks were used along with soft tissue shadows on the planar x-rays to target the treatment fields.

Technical limitations included difficulty in accurately determining distances to patient and cassette and unreliability of using the patient's external contour/skin mark as a reference point. Of course, it was also harder to locate the tumor and treatment volume. Because of the potential for error in targeting by this approach, radiation field orientations were largely limited to lateral fields and AP-PA fields.

20. **Should I, the radiologist, circle gross tumor volume (GTV), clinical target volume (CTV), or planning target volume (PTV) on XRT planning images?**
Talk to the radiation oncologist so that you have the same plan and expectations. Usually we trace GTV. Ultimately the radiation oncologist is responsible for the volume delineation, but best patient care results when we work together.

21. **Are involved lymph nodes included in the GTV?**
Yes. GTV includes primary tumor, metastatic lymphadenopathy, or other metastases. It does not include lymph-node regions that are at risk but not diagnostically involved with tumor by imaging criteria.

22. **What is the role of CT after treatment planning?**
It is used for detecting recurrence of tumor and complications of XRT.

23. **What happens after XRT?**
In general, irradiated tissue first goes through a phase of edema and inflammation (like a sunburn), then in some patients a fibrosis phase of scarring (hopefully not like any sunburn you may have had!). This has different appearances in different tissues. The tumor may become obscured initially by the surrounding acute and subacute reaction, before re-emerging in the fibrosis phase.

24. **What is the spectrum of radiographic changes expected within lung tumors after XRT?**
Within lung tumors in the immediate and early post-XRT period, a faint fluffy/cotton-wool opacity surrounding the primary tumor is common (Fig. 4-7). After XRT, lung tumors may either regress, leaving behind fibrotic tissue, or remain stable in size. Some tumors may show central

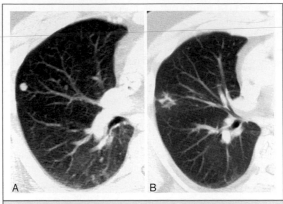

Figure 4-7. Typical fluffy "cotton-wool" appearance of irradiated metastatic nodule at 4 months. These can wax and wane in time and are easily confused with tumor recurrence. They are usually negative on PET scan.

necrosis suggested by central hypodensity with lack of enhancement on postcontrast images. Some tumors disappear without a trace. The inflammation (cotton-wool change) can wax and wane with time and can be confused with tumor recurrence. Radiation inflammatory reactions are more intense along pleural surfaces, and a flare extending along these surfaces suggests an inflammatory state rather than recurrence (Fig. 4-8).

25. **What are some patterns of radiation fibrosis in the lung?**
It depends on the radiation port arrangement and dose. Classical paramediastinal and tangential breast ports are common and easy to recognize (Fig. 4-9). Conformal ports can produce more complex shapes (Fig. 4-10).

26. **What is the spectrum of radiographic changes expected within liver tumors after XRT?**
In the immediate/early post-XRT period, liver tumors may show a surrounding zone of hypodensity consistent with hepatocellular edema. This usually is maximum about 6 weeks after treatment and normally subsides by 6 months. The tumor will usually become very hypoattenuating and well demarcated during this period, surrounded by the less hypodense and less demarcated edema.

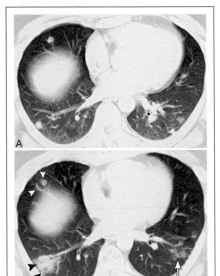

Figure 4-8. Metastatic colorectal carcinoma. **A,** Three metastatic nodules are shown on the pre-XRT scan. **B,** Typically there are no immediate changes, although tumor regression is common. Changes that occur 2–6 months after irradiation are called early reactions and can include fluffy/cotton-woolly opacity surrounding the tumor *(white arrow)*, surrounding zone of consolidation *(black arrowheads)*, and stable size of the tumor with surrounding rim of fibrosis conforming to the arc of radiation *(white arrowheads)*. These changes can persist indefinitely and progress to fibrosis.

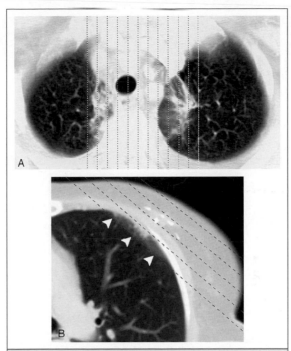

Figure 4-9. Radiation fibrosis. *A,* Paramediastinal fibrosis delineates the irradiated field. *B,* Linear fibrosis *(arrowheads)* in tangential treatment field in an irradiated breast tumor. These changes usually occur 6 months or more after irradiation.

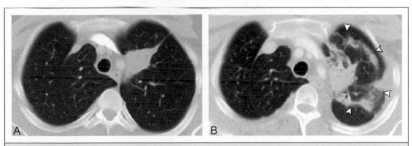

Figure 4-10. Radiation fibrosis after conformal therapy. *A,* Baseline scan showing left upper lobe bronchioloalveolar carcinoma. *B,* Seven-month follow-up scan showing surrounding fibrosis conforming to the arcs of 3D conformal XRT *(arrowheads).*

Nonirradiated portions of the liver might hypertrophy during this period. It can be very difficult to differentiate damaged liver from tumor. Like tumor, the regenerating liver surrounding the hypointense damaged liver will often enhance. Over time (over 9 months), the tumor may either remain stable or regress in size. The combination of liver damage and regeneration results in a change in liver shape (Fig. 4-11).

27.   **Define XRT failure, XRT success, and XRT recurrence.**
      An important point to remember is that the desirable end point of XRT is either "reproductive inactivation" of tumor cells or cellular death. Reproductive inactivation will not necessarily cause

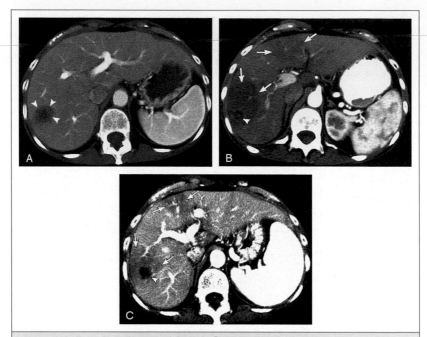

Figure 4-11. Expected changes within the liver after XRT in a patient with metastatic colorectal carcinoma who underwent XRT for six metastatic hepatic lesions. *A,* Baseline scan shows one of the lesions within the right posterior hepatic lobe *(arrowheads).* Another lesion within the medial segment of the left hepatic lobe is not visualized on the same image. *B,* At 3 months after XRT, blooming/flare of the surrounding zone *(arrows)* secondary to radiation damage within the right and left hepatic lobes. There is some shrinkage of the lesion itself *(arrowhead).* **C,** Four-month follow-up shows interval decrease in surrounding zone of radiation injury *(arrows)* with stable size of metastatic lesion *(arrowhead).* The six treated lesions were stable at 4-month follow-up with interval development of a new left hepatic lobe metastasis.

disappearance of tumor tissue. Because this is a microscopic process, a realistic expectation of XRT success would be a lesion that stops growing.

Thus, after XRT we would like to see a stable/regressing lesion. Any growth of tumor tissue after XRT is considered treatment failure (Fig. 4-12). If the lesion initially remains stable/regresses after XRT but begins to grow at a later point in time, it is considered as tumor recurrence.

New metastases that occur outside the radiation target volumes are not XRT failure because they were never irradiated and are presumed to exist microscopically before XRT (Fig. 4-13).

28. **How can tumor recurrence be differentiated from post-XRT fibrosis?**
On CT images, differentiation of tumor recurrence from post-XRT fibrosis can be difficult—again, growth indicates recurrence. On PET/PET-CT, hypermetabolic activity beyond 3 months is suspicious for recurrence. Interpreting scans during the inflammatory phase after irradiation or before tumor cell death has occurred is difficult. When in doubt, it can be very important to perform biopsies and careful correlation with anatomic imaging techniques, such as CT. Serial PET scans are also very helpful because increasing glucose metabolism over time strongly indicates tumor recurrence.

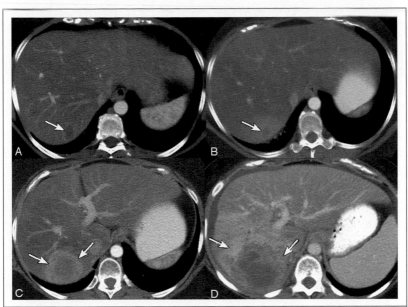

Figure 4-12. Continued growth of metastases over 6 months from a primary ampullary adenocarcinoma. *A,* Baseline scan showing right posterior lobe metastasis *(arrows)*. Images after 3D conformal XRT (*B, C,* and *D*) show increasing size of the lesion *(arrows)*. Growth in tumor size after XRT is considered treatment failure, but during the first 3–6 months after irradiation it can be difficult to differentiate transient hepatic damage from increased tumor size using just anatomic imaging. The role of PET for clarifying difficult cases is promising but not yet proven.

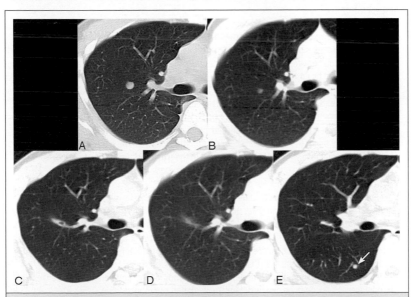

Figure 4-13. Scans of the lung done before and after radiotherapy for metastatic adenocystic carcinoma of the minor salivary gland. *A,* Pre-XRT scan showing right upper lobe metastatic nodule. Scans after 3D conformal XRT show interval regression of nodule with faint residual tumor at 3 months *(B),* 6 months *(C),* and 2 years *(D).* At 2 years and 2 months *(E)* there was development of a new pulmonary metastasis *(arrow).* This lung nodule was also treated with success.

KEY POINTS: CT RADIATION TREATMENT PLANNING

1. Radiation therapy stops tumor from growing, but it may not totally disappear on CT. Growth after radiation therapy is presumed to be recurrence.

2. Radiation therapy is most demanding for precise localization of tumor because it is effectively percutaneous surgery.

3. Gross tumor volume (GTV) for radiation oncology is the tumor that you see and know is present.

4. Clinical target volume (CTV) includes subclinical or microscopic tumor and thus is larger than GTV.

5. Planning target volume (PTV) is CTV plus a margin for technical variation of XRT delivery. The entire PTV should receive the planned treatment dose.

6. Irradiated tissue first goes through a flare phase of edema over days to weeks, then fibrosis over weeks or months.

29. **What are the acute side effects of XRT?**
    Side effects of XRT are directly proportional to the volume of irradiated tissues, XRT dose, and the time over which it was delivered. Reactions may be more severe if accompanied by chemotherapy, especially Adriamycin. Common generalized complications include loss of appetite, malaise, and hair loss. Depending on the body region undergoing XRT, localized side effects include superficial skin erythema, soreness and increased dermal sensitivity, esophagitis, dysphagia, cough, shortness of breath, nausea, vomiting, diarrhea, and enterocolitis. With pelvic XRT in females, vaginal itching/burning/dryness may occur, whereas in males, reduction in sperm number and function may occur. Also, bladder irritation may cause frequent urination or discomfort.

30. **What are the delayed complications of XRT?**
    Delayed complications of XRT are more common with older forms of XRT than newer targeted XRT and protocols. As with the early complications, they increase with dose and field size. They are also worsened by comorbidities such as diabetes, collagen vascular disease, cardiovascular disease, and obstructive pulmonary disease. There is an increased risk of ischemic heart disease that begins about 8 years after mediastinal irradiation, particularly in survivors of childhood Hodgkin's disease treated several decades ago. Bowel strictures can occur, particularly when the radiation dose exceeds 50 Gy. After pulmonary XRT, radiation fibrosis may occur. Early menopause may occur in women with pelvic irradiation. XRT can be carcinogenic, causing secondary malignancies within tissues included in the treatment field (Fig. 4-14).

31. **What does the future hold for XRT?**
    Development of chemotherapeutic agents that serve as *sensitizers* of tumor tissue, such as 5-fluorouracil (5-FU) and Adriamycin, have already had beneficial impacts on patient outcome. Biologic modifiers of DNA repair and growth factor inhibitors will likely have important interactions with radiation. Radiation protectors of normal tissues remarkably can also be radiosensitizers of tumor. Progress is expected in this area of clinical research. Examples of agents in this class include cyclo-oxygenase-2 (COX-2) inhibitors and curcumin.
    Metabolic imaging modalities that better detect tumor will greatly benefit XRT, because XRT can only target a lesion if we can find it for the radiation oncologist.

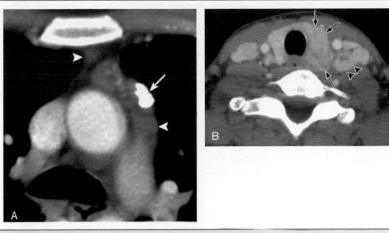

Figure 4-14. A 28-year-old woman who had neck and mediastinal irradiation for Hodgkin's lymphoma at age 13 now presents with a neck mass. ***A,*** Note calcified lymph nodes consistent with successfully treated Hodgkin's lymphoma *(arrow)*, but also note noncalcified anterior lymphadenopathy *(arrowheads)*. ***B,*** CT through neck shows a large heterogeneously enhancing left thyroid mass *(black arrows)* that was papillary carcinoma of the thyroid. There is also metastatic lymphadenopathy *(black arrowheads)*.

BIBLIOGRAPHY

1. Bentel GC: Radiation Therapy Planning, 2nd ed. New York, McGraw-Hill, 1995, pp 16 31, 98–267.
2. www.radiologyinfo.org/content/therapy/imrt.htm
3. www.radiologyinfo.org/content/therapy/gamma_knife.htm

CHAPTER 5

FUSION PET/CT IN ONCOLOGY

Arun Basu, MD, and John G. Strang, MD

1. **What is positron emission tomography (PET)? How does it work?**
   PET, a nuclear medicine modality, generates three-dimensional (3D) tomographic images showing the distribution of radiotracer within the human body. It uses positron-emitting isotopes, such as radioactive fluorine (F-18) bound to tracers. A PET tracer is injected (or inhaled), distributed, and then imaged. The unique biodistribution of the PET tracer is what makes it interesting.

2. **What is fluoro-2-deoxy-D-glucose (FDG)?**
   By far the most widely used PET radiotracer is fluoro-2-deoxy-D-glucose (FDG-F18). It is taken up by cells that take up glucose, but the "deoxy" group blocks phosphorylation. Imaging is done after a 1-hour period to allow uptake and distribution. There is markedly increased uptake of FDG in many malignancies.

3. **What is the half-life of FDG-F18?**
   Half-life is 110 minutes. This is shorter than the half-life of technicium-99 (Tc-99), allowing a higher percentage of the dose to be used for imaging. The 511-keV PET photons are also more energetic than Tc-99, so there is less absorption by overlying tissue.

4. **What are the major strengths of PET in oncology compared with CT?**
   In oncology, functional alteration can precede morphologic changes. Detection of altered function is often more sensitive than detection of changed morphology. PET has proven to be more sensitive for detection and staging for many cancers than CT. For example, a patient with nodal involvement of metastatic disease may present with normal-sized nodes, and the nodal involvement is thus not detectable without PET (Fig. 5-1).

   The other major strength of PET is the high contrast of pathology, leading to high conspicuity. Hypermetabolic tumors are very different from the surrounding tissue in many organs. This high contrast makes them stand out.

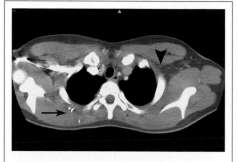

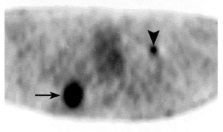

Figure 5-1. A patient with metastatic fibrosarcoma on CT and PET scan. In addition to a lytic right rib lesion *(arrow)*, the patient has metastasis to a normal-sized left subclavian lymph node *(arrowhead)*. (Courtesy of M. Cham, MD.)

Simple tools such as a maximum intensity projection (MIP) can be used to quickly get an overview of the distribution of hypermetabolic foci. In CT, tumors outside the lung lack that high conspicuity, and each axial image must be examined. The examination of individual images has become more difficult and time-consuming with multidetector CT and multiphase imaging.

5. What are the major weaknesses of PET compared with CT?
One major drawback regarding PET imaging is difficult anatomic localization. This may cause mislocalization of diseased tissue or misdiagnosis of sites of normal biodistribution and sites of disease. For example, skeletal muscle, brown (thermogenic) fat, and potentially abnormal lymph nodes lie intermingled in the neck. Determination of which structure has the increased PET uptake is key to interpretation but difficult to make on PET alone. Accurate localization permits biopsy when pathologic proof is needed (Fig. 5-2).

PET imaging also is extremely limited for characterizing increased uptake: A focus of malignant cells may appear similar to an abscess, and without an anatomic study, differentiation of these two pathologies may be difficult.

Not all tumors are hypermetabolic. PET imaging alone can be falsely reassuring in such cases (Fig. 5-3).

6. What is PET and CT fusion? How does it work?
PET/CT fusion imaging is the alignment of images from PET and CT. These modalities may be fused by the radiologist, software, or hardware techniques.

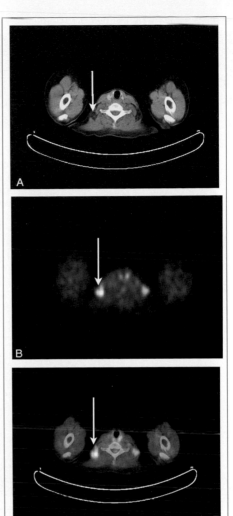

Figure 5-2. Brown fat. The symmetric hypermetabolic supraclavicular masses on the PET (B) correspond to supraclavicular fat on the CT (A). This is clearly delineated on the fustion PET/CT (C) image.

7. What is PET/CT fusion by the radiologist?
It is interpreting the two modalities together, without hardware or software. This is the first step to accurate diagnosis and can be quite effective, user-friendly (personality-dependent), portable, and robust. It avoids gross errors. However, its resolution is limited, it is dependent on acquiring all data sets, it can be quite tiring, and the work involved can scale exponentially.

8. **What is PET/CT software fusion?**

   Software fusion registers a PET image data set with a CT image data set when they are acquired separately on separate machines. Multiple software algorithms are available to accomplish software fusion. This technique is generally good for imaging intracranial abnormalities but has drawbacks for imaging parts of the body that do not come in their own rigid carrying case. Bowel movement, respiratory movement, bladder filling, and especially patient positioning cause inaccuracies in software fusion. Although techniques have been developed to minimize differences, such as 3D elastic transformations and nonlinear image warping, they are labor-intensive and are restricted to use in one body cavity.

   Tai YC, Lin KP, Hoh CK, et al: Utilization of 3D elastic transformation in the registration of chest x-ray CT and whole body PET. Trans Nucl Sci 44:1606–1612, 1997.

9. **What is PET/CT hardware fusion?**

   Hardware fusion acquires PET and CT together in one exam. This is what is meant by PET/CT. A PET/CT machine is one bed with two imaging systems: a PET system and a CT system. A scan is conducted in three basic steps. First, a topogram or scout image is acquired. From this image, the scan range for both modalities is determined. Second, the CT images are acquired. Finally, the patient is moved deeper into the gantry for PET data acquisition. The two sets of images are fused because they are acquired without the patient moving. The images may then be fused or viewed separately. Even with hardware fusion, there will be misregistration if there is motion of the organs between the CT and the PET (Fig. 5-4).

10. **What is the advantage of a PET/CT compared with a PET alone? (There better be some given the significant price difference!)**

    - PET/CT gives better fusions for soft tissues because the patient does not move between imaging. Hardware fusion does not eliminate internal organ motion (res-

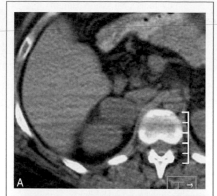
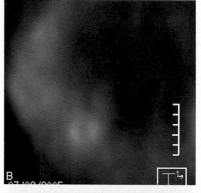
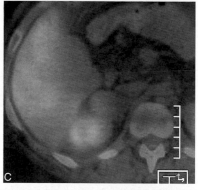

Figure 5-3. Metastatic melanoma with adrenal metastasis. The right adrenal mass was not hypermetabolic (PET image *B*). However, the mass was growing and was of similar appearance to a previously resected left adrenal metastasis (CT image *A*). The mass was resected and was also a melanoma metastasis. This mass would not have been apparent on PET alone. *C,* Fusion of the PET/CT image.

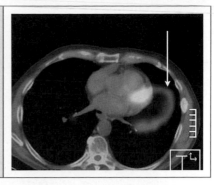

Figure 5-4. Cardiac creep on axial fusion image. There is misregistration of the heart on the CT and the left ventricular uptake *(arrow)* on the PET. Because the PET and the CT are not acquired simultaneously, organs can change positions—usually due to peristalsis or bladder filling. In this case, cardiac creep occurred—the heart shifted over time as the patient lay supine.

piratory/bowel motion), although differences can be further minimized through techniques such as respiratory gating. This is the true advantage because it allows more accurate diagnosis.

- PET/CT facilitates subsequent CT-guided biopsy by accurately determining precise site of disease on CT.
- PET/CT can further characterize some lesions that show increased metabolism, distinguishing some infections from malignancies.
- PET/CT can further characterize lesions that are not hypermetabolic. A common situation is a patient referred for evaluation of an ill-defined nodule found on earlier CT. If the PET is negative, is it because the nodule is gone (a resolved infiltrate) or not (it is benign or is a nonhypermetabolic malignancy)? CT can be compared with the earlier study and can answer this portion of the question.
- PET/CT is faster. Part of the PET process is the acquisition of a "transmission scan" to make an attenuation map. (The attenuation map is used to adjust the PET image for soft tissue attenuation.) In PET alone, the transmission is done with a slow external radiation source that takes minutes. In PET/CT, the CT gets the attenuation data in seconds.
- A PET/CT machine can be used as a CT machine when there are no PET patients.

11. **What are the major advantages of PET/CT over CT alone?**
    - CT determines residual disease by size and morphologic changes. However, it is possible to have complete resolution of disease without mass size or morphologic change. Metabolic response often precedes morphologic response.
    - It is useful for detecting disease in anatomically normal-sized tissue, such as nonenlarged lymph nodes.
    - Differentiating fibrosis or scar from active disease is often difficult. PET adds the dimension of function.
    - CT is a high-resolution but often low-conspicuity modality with hundreds of detailed images. PET is a high-conspicuity modality with relatively few images. FDG is a great contrast media for CT.
    - See Figure 5-5.

12. **Does staging accuracy increase when comparing PET with PET/CT?**
    Preliminary data in colorectal carcinoma staging demonstrate a 78% staging accuracy with PET alone, which increases to 89% with the fusion modality. These are fairly typical numbers reported for different tumors.

13. **How can PET/CT assist in patient diagnosis?**
    This fusion technology has proved to be helpful in characterizing lung nodules found incidentally on anatomic imaging by means of providing metabolic information. In the absence of symp-

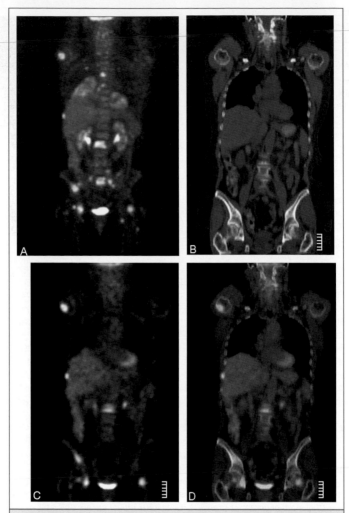

Figure 5-5. Widely metastatic right lower lobe lung cancer with bony metastases. The bony metastases are of high conspicuity on the PET maximum intensity projection *(A)*, allowing their easy detection on individual coronal sections with fusion to the CT for anatomic localization (*B, C,* and *D*).

toms, if imaging determines a hypermetabolic nodule, it is more likely a malignant etiology. However, the discovery of a nodule that demonstrates a normal metabolic profile does not exclude the presence of malignancy because some primary tumors demonstrate a relatively low metabolic requirement. PET/CT helps one choose the most suspicious nodule for biopsy (*see* Fig. 5-6).

14. **Describe patient preparation for a PET/CT fusion study.**
    The patient must fast for 6 hours prior to the examination but should drink plenty of water. Following injection of the calculated FDG dose, the patient must rest in a quiet room for

approximately 1 hour to minimize shunting of radiotracer to accessory musculature. Patients should also refrain from strenuous exercise 3 days prior to the exam. Diabetic patients require special preparation for the exam as well as a blood glucose check prior to examination because high insulin drives soft tissue uptake of FDG, potentially obscuring tumors.

Oral CT contrast is now given at many centers. Opacifying/distending the section bowel improves evaluation of the gastric mural component for metabolically active disease. This benefit is probably worth the potential effects of oral contrast on the attenuation correction.

15. What are common imaging pitfalls/technical considerations regarding PET/CT fusion?

The speed disparity between the fast CT acquisition (seconds) and the relatively slower PET acquisition (minutes) causes the attenuation correction map to be less accurate. When CT imaging is acquired during maximal inspiration,

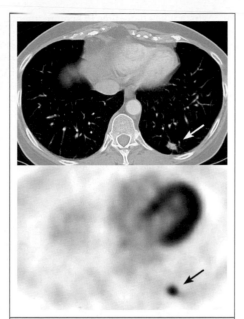

Figure 5-6. A solitary pulmonary nodule on CT with increased FDG uptake on PET scan *(arrow),* later determined to be metastatic colon carcinoma. (Courtesy of M. Cham, MD.)

there is potential misalignment of the PET and CT data sets secondary to diaphragmatic excursion/respiratory motion. Lesions in this area may be misregistered to the heart or lung base when in fact they are intra-abdominal or may not conform to a given anatomic structure. This problem can be minimized by acquiring CT images in expiration or shallow breathing.

16. Name three mechanisms by which oral and intravenous contrast cause attenuation correction artifacts.

- Oral contrast location can change between time of CT and time of PET.
- Intravenous contrast concentration can also change between time of CT and that of PET.
- Finally, the energy of photons used in CT (up to 120–140 kV) is less than that used in PET, so relative absorption is different.
- The trend, however, is toward using administered contrast for the CT advantages.

17. What is brown fat? Why does it take up FDG?

Brown fat is metabolically active fat that is found mostly in the axillary, supraclavicular, and pericoronary artery location. It is more commonly seen in women and is normal. It becomes metabolically active when the patient is cold, generating heat. It is found in a much greater proportion in bears, which are physically inactive during hibernating periods.

18. What is the imaging problem with brown fat?

Metabolically active brown fat in patients with PET alone would cause hypermetabolic areas in the supraclavicular regions. Of course, this is also a site where lymphadenopathy occurs. This finding creates a diagnostic dilemma and can make adjacent structures difficult to evaluate for metabolic activity. PET/CT fusion helps solve this problem. To eliminate this artifact, the patient must be warmed prior to and during the exam.

19. **Which takes more time to acquire images—PET or PET/CT?**
    PET/CT is a quicker acquisition because it saves time acquiring the attenuation correction maps. The attenuation maps for CT can be created in less than a minute compared with conventional PET, which can take 15–30 minutes using a radioisotope source. The PET emission acquisition time is comparable.

20. **What type of artifacts can hip prosthetics, dental fillings, and metallic foreign bodies cause?**
    On CT attenuated corrected images, they cause artifactually increased radiotracer uptake in attenuation-corrected images. The implants stop relatively more of the lower-energy CT photons (120–140 kV) than the high-energy positrons (511 keV). Misinterpretation can be minimized by correlation with the CT data and optimized acquisition protocols/data processing schemes.

    Oehr P, Biersack HJ, Coleman RE: PET and PET/CT in Oncology. Berlin, Springer, 2004.

KEY POINTS: FUSION PET/CT IN ONCOLOGY

1. PET/CT is a synergistic fusion of PET and CT.

2. PET/CT has greater diagnostic utility than PET alone because of improved tumor characterization and localization. Hypometabolic tumors are a PET blind spot filled in by PET/CT.

3. PET/CT has greater diagnostic utility than CT because of small lesion detection, high lesion conspicuity, and early lesion response to therapy. Bone and soft tissue lesions are CT blind spots filled in by PET/CT.

21. **How has PET/CT affected radiation therapy compared with treatment based on conventional CT alone?**
    There can be a decrease in the radiation treatment size field with improvement in the exact localization of the tumor.

    Koshy M, Paulino AC, Howell R, et al: The influence of F-18 FDG PET-CT fusion on radiotherapy treatment planning for head and neck cancer. ASCO Annual Meeting Proceedings (post-meeting edition). J Clin Oncol 22(14S):5534, 2004.

22. **What is the recommended interval for reimaging following chemotherapy in patients with lymphoma?**
    One month is the recommended time interval for reimaging to evaluate therapeutic efficacy. More rapid imaging is under investigation, because early metabolic nonresponders may benefit from a change in therapy.

23. **What is the recommended interval for reimaging following radiation therapy?**
    Wait at least 3 months after radiation therapy. During the 3 months after radiation therapy, FDG uptake can be due to the inflammation from the radiation therapy itself. After 3 months, if there is persistent uptake of radiotracer, residual or recurrent tumor should be suspected.

24. **What is respiratory gating in the setting of PET/CT fusion?**
    The scanner records the patient's normal respiratory cycle and only images during a relatively nonmobile portion of the cycle. This can be accomplished by use of an infrared camera to track a patient's normal breathing pattern coupled with fluoroscopic information regarding tumor motion.

25. What is the advantage of respiratory gating and is it essential for imaging?
Respiratory gating sharpens the appearance of lesions on PET images and thus increases ability to localize the lesion. Respiratory gating is presently not considered essential for PET/CT imaging and is not standard. This topic remains under investigation.

26. When is respiratory gating most advantageous?
Respiratory gating is most advantageous when used for radiation treatment.

27. What other radiotracers are there in addition to FDG-F18?
Many tracers are currently under investigation for PET applications. F-18 fluorocholine may be useful for prostate cancer. Fluorodeoxythymidine may be a useful tracer for the assessment of cellular proliferation in the setting of patients treated with antiproliferative chemotherapeutic agents. An amyloid agent is being tested for the detection of Alzheimer's disease. We are only at the beginning of more specifically targeted agents.

28. What are the clinical scenarios in which PET/CT fusion technology is used in the diagnosis and treatment of lymphoma?
Primary staging, restaging after treatment, and assessment of efficacy of treatment protocols for lymphoma patients. This modality is not commonly used in the setting of initial diagnosis.

29. What is a standardized uptake value (SUV)?
The SUV is a measure of the concentration of FDG in a region of interest standardized relative to the injected dose of FDG across the entire patient. An SUV of 1 would be average.

30. How do SUVs aid in patient diagnosis and treatment in lymphoma?
Transformation from a low-grade lymphoma to a higher grade often can manifest on imaging as a transition of once low-to-intermediate SUV to an intermediate-to-high value.

31. How does PET/CT contribute to management of primary brain tumors? What is the major shortcoming of intracranial FDG-PET imaging?
FDG-PET serves to complement anatomic imaging such as magnetic resonance imaging (MRI) and CT but is most useful for its diagnostic, prognostic, and therapeutic facets due to its high correlation between glucose metabolism and tumor grade. A major drawback of FDG-PET is the relatively high background activity of the gray matter and differentiation between normal tissue and low-grade tumors.

32. How useful is PET/CT in head and neck tumors?
PET/CT fusion is highly sensitive to most head and neck masses because the predominant histologic type of squamous cell carcinoma has high glucose metabolism.

Oehr P, Biersack HJ, Coleman RE: PET and PET/CT in Oncology. Berlin, Springer, 2004.

33. What are the clinical indications for PET/CT in thyroid carcinoma?
A common use in thyroid cancer patients is in those with known carcinoma suspected to have metastases (i.e., elevated thyroglobulin) but with a normal iodine-131 (I-131) scintiscan. In the case of suspected poorly differentiated tumor clone cells, PET/CT is also indicated.

Oehr P, Biersack HJ, Coleman RE: PET and PET/CT in Oncology. Berlin, Springer, 2004.

34. What is the sensitivity of PET/CT for evaluating a solitary pulmonary lung nodule for lung carcinoma? What histology types most commonly cause a false-negative result?
PET alone has a sensitivity of 96%. Factors that may effect or result in a false-negative result include (1) lesions smaller than 1 cm and (2) tumor types with low metabolic activity.

False-negative results can be minimized with use of CT images to evaluate morphology, location, and size of lesions. Carcinoid and bronchoalveolar cell carcinomas are two cell types that may result in a false-negative PET.

Oehr P, Biersack HJ, Coleman RE: PET and PET/CT in Oncology. Berlin, Springer, 2004.

35. **At what relative diameter size for breast cancer does PET become substantially less accurate?**
Masses of less than 1 cm are shown to have a marked decrease in sensitivity for detection by PET/CT. Small tumors have to accumulate a relatively higher proportion of FDG to be detectable.

36. **What clinical scenarios produce false-negative and false-positive PET/CT results when evaluating for pancreatic carcinoma?**
False-negative results may result from patients with neuroendocrine tumors, diabetes, or hyperglycemia. False-positive results may occur in inflammatory processes.

Oehr P, Biersack HJ, Coleman RE: PET and PET/CT in Oncology. Berlin, Springer, 2004.

37. **What is the detection rate of hepatocellular carcinoma with FDG-PET?**
The detection rate of hepatocellular carcinoma is only approximately 50%.

38. **In the setting of colorectal carcinoma, FDG-PET has proved highly effective for restaging purposes and response to treatment. What cell types of adenocarcinomas are less sensitive to detection?**
Mucinous adenocarcinomas and tumors less than 1 cm have been shown to have less sensitivity for detection by FDG-PET. Mucinous tumors contain large amounts of nonmetabolically active material. Small tumors, even if metabolically active, lose intensity due to partial volume effects.

Oehr P, Biersack HJ, Coleman RE: PET and PET/CT in Oncology. Berlin, Springer, 2004.

39. **What are some confounding factors in PET/CT results regarding malignancy of an ovarian mass?**
Early-stage tumors may demonstrate a low avidity for FDG, whereas many benign tumors may demonstrate a relatively high avidity for FDG.

40. **Regarding cancer of the urinary tract (kidney, ureter, bladder, prostate), what are the major drawbacks of PET/CT imaging?**
- There is relatively low glucose metabolism in these organs and some of their tumors.
- The urinary tract is the primary mode of excretion of FDG and thus may mask FDG avid disease.

41. **In what areas of management of musculoskeletal tumors has PET/CT proven most helpful?**
PET/CT has proved to be of great use in localization of a biopsy site with highest metabolic activity for initial diagnosis.

42. **How does F-18 sodium fluoride PET compare with routine Tc-99m bone scan?**
PET detects cellular activity of the tumor, whereas bone scan measures bone turnover. PET thus is often hypermetabolic in the aggressive, purely lytic tumors that can be falsely negative on bone scan. The overall sensitivity comparison for bone metastatic disease is thought to be increased compared with conventional bone scan for metastatic disease such as breast, lung, and prostate cancer. However, conclusive data are still pending.
PET/CT scan also offers increased spatial resolution, and of course fusion to the CT. The spatial resolution is approximately 5 mm, whereas it is 15 mm for conventional single-photon emission computed tomography (SPECT) imaging.

BIBLIOGRAPHY

1. Cohade C, Osman M, Pannu H, et al: Uptake in supraclavicular area fat ("USA-fat"): Description on 18FDG PET/CT. J Nucl Med 44:170–176, 2003.

2. Cook GJR, Wegner EA, Fogelman I: Pitfalls and artifacts in 18FDG PET and PET/CT oncologic imaging. Semin Nucl Med 2:122–133, 2004.

3. Dizendorf E, Hany T, Buck A, et al: Cause and magnitude of error induced by oral CT contrast agent in CT-based attenuation correction of PET emission studies. J Nucl Med 44:732–738, 2003.

4. Goerres G, Kamel E, Heidelberg TN, et al: PET-CT image co-registration in the thorax: Influence of respiration. J Nucl Med 29:351–360, 2002.

5. Goerres G, Kamel E, Seifert B, et al: Accuracy of image coregistration of pulmonary lesions in patients with non-small cell lung carcinoma using an integrated PET/CT system. Radiology 226:906–910, 2003.

6. Goerres G, Ziegler S, Burger C, et al: Artifacts at PET and PET/CT caused by metallic hip prosthetic material. Radiology 226:577–584, 2003.

7. Hany TF, Steinert HC, Goerres GW, et al: PET diagnostic accuracy: improvement with in-line PET-CT system—initial results. Radiology 225:575–581, 2002.

8. Heiko S, Erdi YE, Larson SM, Yeung HWD: PET/CT: A new imaging technology in nuclear medicine. J Nucl Med 30:1419–1437, 2003.

9. Heiko S, Larson SM, Yeung HWD: PET/CT in oncology: Integration into clinical management of lymphoma, melanoma and gastrointestinal malignancies. J Nucl Med 45:72S–81S, 2004.

10. Jerusalem G, Warland V, Najjar F, et al: Whole-body 18F-FDG PET for the evaluation of patients with Hodgkin's disease and non-Hodgkin's lymphoma. Nucl Med Commun 20(1):13–20, 1999.

11. Kamel E, Hany TF, Burger C, et al: CT versus 69Ge attenuation correction in a combined PET/CT system: Evaluating the effect of lowering the CT tube current. Eur J Nucl Med 29:346–350, 2002.

12. Kinahan PE, Townsend DW, Beyer T, Sashin D: Attenuation correction for combined 3D PET/CT scanner. Med Phys 25:2046–2053, 1998.

13. Koshy M, Paulino AC, Howell R, et al: The influence of F-18 FDG PET-CT fusion on radiotherapy treatment planning for head and neck cancer. ASCO Annual Meeting Proceedings (post-meeting edition). J Clin Oncol 22(14S):5534, 2004.

14. Maisey MM, Wahl RL, Barrington SF: Atlas of Clinical Positron Emission Tomography. London, Arnold Publishers, 1999.

15. Metser UR, Goor O, Lerman H, et al: PET–CT of extranodal lymphoma AJR Am J Roentgenol 182:1579–1586, 2004.

16. Moog F, Bangerter M, Diederichs CG, et al: Extranodal malignant lymphoma: Detection with FDG PET versus CT. Radiology 206:475–481, 1998.

17. Nakamoto Y, Chin B, Kraitchman D, et al: Effects of nonionic intravenous contrast agents at PET/CT imaging: Phantom and canine studies. Radiology 227:817–824, 2003.

18. Oehr P, Biersack HJ, Coleman RE: PET and PET/CT in Oncology. Berlin, Springer, 2004.

19. Osman M, Cohade C, Nakamoto Y, et al: Clinically significant inaccurate localization of lesions with PET CT: Frequency in 300 patients [abstract]. J Nucl Med 44(2):240–243, 2003.

20. Tai YC, Lin KP, Hoh CK, et al: Utilization of 3D elastic transformation in the registration of chest x-ray CT and whole body PET. Trans Nucl Sci 44:1606–1612, 1997.

21. Townsend D, Beyer T, Blodgett T: PET/CT scanners: A hardware approach to image fusion. Semin Nucl Med 3:193–204, 2003.

22. Wahl R: PET-CT in clinical practice: Experience in 1500 patients. Proc Jpn Soc Nucl Med, 2003.

23. Wahl RL, Quint LE, Cielak RD, et al: "Anatometabolic" tumor imaging: Fusion of FDG-PET with CT or MRI to localize foci of increased activity. J Nucl Med 34:1190, 1993.

CHEST TRAUMA

Osbert Adjei, MD, and John G. Strang, MD

CHAPTER 6

1. **What is the role of CT in blunt chest trauma?**
    Detection of aortic injury, tracheobronchial injury, pneumothorax, lung contusion, diaphragmatic rupture, and flail chest. Of these, the detection of aortic injury is the most important.

2. **What is an aortic transection?**
    An aortic transection is a traumatic tear of the aortic wall. If the tear is complete, the patient dies in seconds. Complete tear is a relatively common injury and accounts for 15% of motor vehicle accident deaths. Most tears (75–90%) are complete. If the tear is incomplete (through the intima and some but not all of the media), the patient survives as long as the tear does not extend and become complete. The patient with an incomplete tear may survive to the ambulance, to the emergency room (ER), to the CT scanner, and, if the diagnosis is made, to the OR and eventually home (Fig. 6-1).

3. **Where does aortic transection usually occur?**
    Ninety percent of aortic transections occur at the aortic isthmus at the level of the ligamentum arteriosum. One theory is that the heavy heart is mobile, whereas the aorta is fixed at the level of the ligamentum arteriosum. In a deceleration accident, the heart pulls forward while the posterior descending aorta is fixed. Another theory is that the aorta gets pinched by the compression of the chest and tears at the level of the ligamentum arteriosum. The place to look most closely on the CT is immediately under the arch.

4. **Where else can thoracic aortic injuries occur?**
    - At the ascending aorta (but such injuries are fatal and therefore not imaged)
    - At the diaphragmatic hiatus (rare)
    Concentrate on looking just under the aortic arch.

5. **Why is aortic transection the most important diagnosis you can make on chest CT?**
    - It is immediately life-threatening, with a mortality rate believed to be about 50% in 2 days (or 1% per hour).

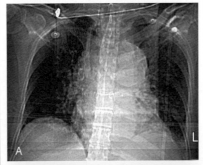
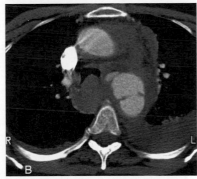

Figure 6-1. Classic presentation of aortic transection. **A,** Widened superior mediastinum on frontal projection with trachea bowed to the right. **B,** CT shows active extravasation from the proximal descending aorta at the level of the ligamentum arteriosum.

- It is surgically curable.
- It is a diagnosis that can be suspected only by chest x-ray, and the expectation has become that the diagnosis will be suspected or made by CT.

6. **What are the direct CT features of acute thoracic aortic injury?**

Signs of aortic injury may be either direct (the injury itself is seen) or indirect (hemorrhage or other effects due to the aortic injury). Direct signs include extravasation of contrast, pseudoaneurysm, and aortic transection (Fig. 6-2). More subtle direct signs include intimal flaps, pseudocoarctation, or abrupt changes in contour (Fig. 6-3). Most surgeons now operate based on direct visualization of a convincing transection on CT without waiting for confirmatory angiography. Angiography adds time and with that a risk of rupture. Some surgeons order angiography to look for carotid or other accompanying vascular injury.

Most directly visualized aortic transections are accompanied by a periaortic hematoma. In the absence of periaortic hematoma, contour irregularity and abnormalities may be due to nontraumatic etiologies, such as preexisting atherosclerosis. Of course, elderly patients

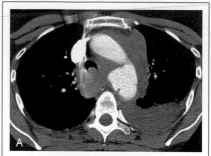
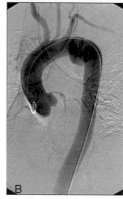

Figure 6-2. CT *(A)* and conventional angiogram *(B)* of a patient with a large traumatic aortic transection. Note the periaortic hematoma and hemothorax as well as the directly visualized traumatic pseudoaneurysm.

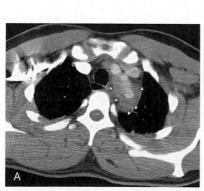
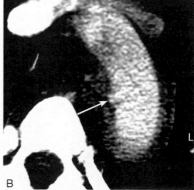

Figure 6-3. Traumatic aortic injury. *A,* Indirect sign of a periaortic hematoma *(arrowheads).* *B,* The direct injury is visible as a subtle focal contour abnormality on CT *(arrow)*—windowed for better demonstration.

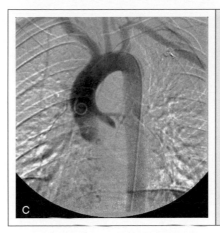

Figure 6-3.—Cond't *C,* The injury was not visible on angiography.

with atherosclerosis may also get a traumatic transection; differentiating between them can be difficult.

7. **What are the indirect CT findings of acute thoracic aortic injury?**
   A periaortic hematoma (no visible fat plane between aorta and hematoma) is the primary indirect sign of aortic transection. A conventional angiogram is indicated for patients with a periaortic hematoma on chest CT who do not have a direct sign of aortic injury, although most studies will be negative. If the hematoma is not periaortic, it is likely due to venous injury, sternal fracture, or other nonaortic injury (Figs. 6-4 and 6-5).

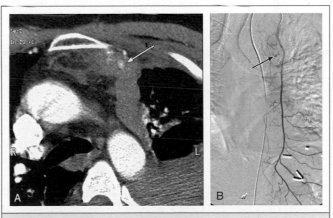

Figure 6-4. Mediastinal hematoma secondary to internal mammary artery injury. There is a large anterior mediastinal hematoma and hemothorax. *A,* The active extravasation is visible *(arrow). B,* The selective left internal mammary artery angiogram demonstrates the hemorrhage, and the vessel was embolized. Note that as the hematoma was not periaortic; there was no evidence of an aortic transection. The angiogram was for therapeutic, not diagnostic, purposes.

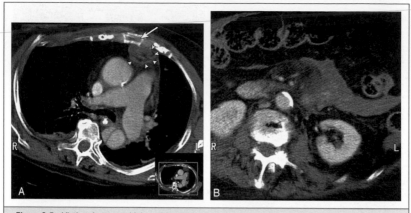

Figure 6-5. Victim of motor vehicle accident with sternal fracture *(arrow)* and aortic dissection *(A)* and mesenteric bleed *(B)*. Is the dissection acute? Note that the retrosternal hematoma *(arrowheads)* does not abut the aorta and is not a secondary sign of aortic injury.

8. **What indirect signs of thoracic aortic transection might I see on an abdominal CT?**
   Infarcts in the spleen, kidneys, bowel, and liver secondary to aortic injury, thrombus formation, and embolism (Fig. 6-6). Recommend a chest CT if you see an acute infarct (usually splenic or renal) on an abdominal CT.

9. **What is the most important single image on an abdominal CT for trauma?**
   The first! You may see a posterior mediastinal hematoma tracking down from an unsuspected aortic transection. You should add a chest CT if you see a lower thoracic posterior mediastinal hematoma (also check the spine) (Fig. 6-7).

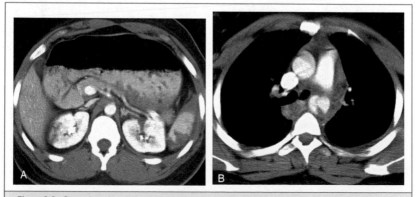

Figure 6-6. Secondary signs of aortic transection/emboli. *A,* Infarcts in the spleen and right kidney (secondary or indirect findings) from emboli secondary to the aortic injury. *B,* Transected aorta (direct finding) with periaortic hematoma. An acute traumatic aortic transection may present as a stroke or an abdominal infarct. Chest images should be added if infarcts are seen in an abdominal CT performed for trauma.

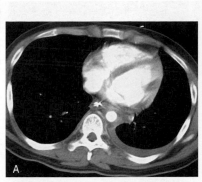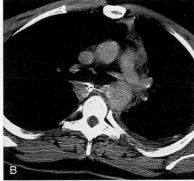

Figure 6-7. Unsuspected aortic transection presenting as a hematoma around the descending thoracic aorta on abdominal CT. **A,** First image of an abdominal CT for trauma shows the left hemothorax and periaortic hematoma. **B,** The radiologist added noncontrast thoracic images, which showed a focal posterior bulge of the proximal descending thoracic aorta. Note that the descending thoracic aorta is abnormally enlarged making it larger than the ascending thoracic aorta. This was confirmed to be an aortic transection at angiography, and the patient was successfully repaired.

10. **How does spiral CT angiography compare with conventional angiography for diagnosis of traumatic aortic transection?**
    In hemodynamically stable patients, spiral CT angiography with multidetector capability has largely replaced catheter aortography for diagnosis (Fig. 6-8). In unstable patients, transesophageal echocardiography (TEE) may be the imaging modality of choice.

11. **Does intravascular ultrasound (IVUS) have any role in evaluating patients with potential thoracic aortic injury?**
    It can distinguish ulcerated plaque from an aortic tear in older patients. IVUS requires arterial access, is not universally available, and can be time-consuming; therefore, it is a problem-solving modality.

12. **Describe the CT findings of acute pulmonary contusion and traumatic pneumatocele.**
    Pulmonary contusion presents as increased density in the lung parenchyma, due to a combination posttraumatic hemorrhage edema. Traumatic pneumatoceles are acute cystic changes in the traumatized lung parenchyma (Fig. 6-9). The mechanism of formation may be due to alveolar injury.

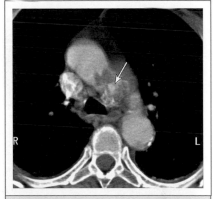

Figure 6-8. Elderly patient after motor vehicle accident. Is this a preexisting atherosclerotic ulcer *(arrow)* or a traumatic pseudoaneurysm in an atherosclerotic aorta? The patient had an intravascular ultrasound (not shown) that confirmed ulcerated plaque.

13. **How does the number of broken ribs determine the method of treatment?**
    A single rib fracture is usually treated conservatively with analgesics. Multiple rib fractures, especially if associated with hemothorax, pneumothorax, or flail chest, may have to be treated more aggressively.

14. How are the tubes for pleural effusion and pneumothorax placed?
The chest tube for effusion (chylothorax or hemothorax) is directed toward the chest base. On the other hand, the chest tube for a pneumothorax should be directed toward the apex of the hemothorax.

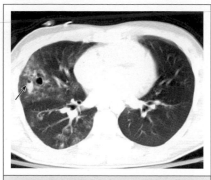

15. What are the causes of pneumothorax?
Pneumothoraces occur in 20–40% of patients with chest trauma, either from tearing by a fractured rib or from acute rise in intrathoracic pressure. In addition, spontaneous or nontraumatic pneumothorax can occur with chronic obstructive pulmonary disease (in older patients), emphysematous blebs (in tall young males), lymphangiomyomatosis (LAM), neoplasm, and pulmonary fibrosis. Up to 20% of patients who undergo lung biopsies develop pneumothorax. Thoracentesis is a less common cause of pneumothorax.

Figure 6-9. Chest CT showing pulmonary contusion and posttraumatic pneumatoceles. Note that some of the pneumatoceles are air-filled and some are blood-filled with air-fluid level *(arrow)*. A right pneumothorax and multiple rib fractures are also present in this patient (not shown).

16. Why is the plain chest x-ray not an optimal modality for pneumothorax in trauma patients?
Pleural air rises to the most nondependent part of the thorax. Because the trauma patient will be supine for a portable chest x-ray, this will be the anterior inferior portion of the chest. Small (or not so small!) pneumothoraces are easily missed in this situation (Fig. 6-10).

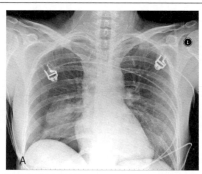
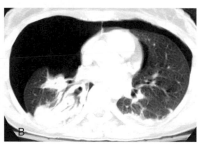

Figure 6-10. Bilateral posttraumatic pneumothoraces, right larger than left. *A,* The right pneumothorax is easily seen on the chest radiograph, but the left pneumothorax is difficult to appreciate. *B,* CT scan shows bilateral pneumothoraces.

17. What is the "deep sulcus sign" on plain x-ray?
The deep sulcus sign is a lucent costophrenic sulcus (Fig. 6-11). It represents pneumothorax in a supine patient. Other plain x-ray findings of pneumothorax in the supine patient include a relative lucency in the affected lung base and "double diaphragm sign."

18. What is the double diaphragm sign?
The double diaphragm sign is created by the interface between the ventral and dorsal portions of the pneumothorax with the anterior and posterior surfaces of the diaphragm.

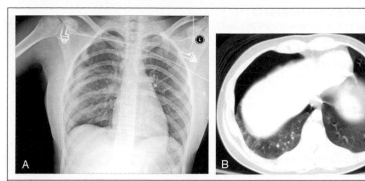

Figure 6-11. Right-sided deep sulcus sign in a patient with right pneumothorax. The pneumothorax is visible on the x-ray *(A)* as a deep right sulcus and sharp liver contour and was confirmed by CT *(B)*.

19. What is the utility of CT scan in the evaluation of pneumothorax?

Pneumothorax that is not apparent on supine plain x-rays is visible on CT in up to half of patients with blunt trauma. At the same time CT can establish the presence of other injuries in the chest, which may not be apparent on plain x-rays. CT can also reveal tension pneumothorax or hemothorax, which are surgical emergencies because they obstruct venous return (Fig. 6-12).

20. What is flail chest?

It occurs after multiple rib fractures. The affected hemithorax paradoxically contracts with inspiration and expands with expiration. Flail chest can be a surgical emergency.

21. Is chest CT needed in all patients with "normal" chest x-rays after blunt trauma?

Certain chest injuries, such as aortic lacerations, pericardial effusions, and esophageal injuries may not be apparent on a plain x-ray. These injuries are potential causes of high morbidity and mortality in trauma patients. Hence, primary routine chest CT is recommended by some for all patients with major chest trauma, even if initially asymptomatic and with a negative x-ray.

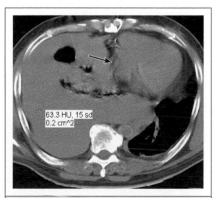

Figure 6-12. Tension hemothorax. Note the high density of the fluid and shift of the heart and compression of the right atrium *(arrow)*.

22. What is the "fallen lung" sign?

The fallen lung sign is a specific sign of tracheobronchial disruption. The lung collapses away from the hilum into a dependent position and is attached to the hilum only by its vascular pedicle. Other nonspecific signs of tracheobronchial injury include persistent pneumothorax after adequate chest tube placement and overdistention of an endotracheal tube balloon.

23. How does esophageal injury occur?

The most common scenario is Boerhaave syndrome, caused by intractable or violent retching (Fig. 6-13). Esophageal injury from penetrating trauma is less common and from blunt trauma very rare.

24. **What are the presentations of thoracic esophageal injuries?**
The most common manifestation is pleural effusion. Less common manifestations include pneumomediastinum, subcutaneous emphysema, and extravasation of enteric contrast. On CT, the site of esophageal injury presents as an area of abnormal thickening.

25. **How does the location of effusion help in localizing the level of injury in traumatic esophageal injury?**
The esophagus lies to the left at the level of the thoracic inlet and at the level of the gastroesophageal junction. Hence, injuries to the upper esophagus and gastroesophageal junction present with left effusion. The esophagus runs in the midline in the midthorax; hence midthoracic and distal esophageal injuries present with right pleural effusion.

26. **What are the causes of traumatic pneumomediastinum?**
Pneumomediastinum is usually the result of the "Macklin effect": rupture of the alveoli from sudden high pressure, with air dissecting back to the mediastinum through the pulmonary interstitium. Direct tracheobronchial injury is much less common. Other causes of pneumomediastinum include injuries to the neck, esophagus, and retroperitoneum. Usually these can be tracked to their source. Chest tube insertion in particular can lead to extensive subcutaneous emphysema, extending first into the neck and then into the mediastinum.

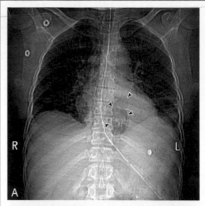

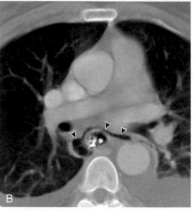

Figure 6-13. Pneumomediastinum secondary to esophageal rupture from forceful vomiting (Boerhaave syndrome). Note the mediastinal gas on the scout image (*A, arrowheads*) and the axial image (*B, arrowheads*). Esophageal lumen with nasogastric (NG) tube is marked *(asterisk)*.

27. **What is the clinical significance of the Macklin effect?**
The Macklin effect indicates severe trauma and a corresponding long intensive care stay. Also, the Macklin effect does not exclude coexisting tracheobronchial or esophageal injury.

28. **What is traumatic pseudoaneurysm of the pulmonary artery?**
It is an uncommon complication of chest trauma. It is usually associated with penetrating chest injury. Radiologically, it presents as a persistent opacity on chest x-ray. On contrast-enhanced CT the opacity shows increased enhancement.

29. **What are the CT findings in cardiac contusion?**
CT is not the primary modality for cardiac injury (even for patients who survive the initial injury). Serum levels of creatine kinase (CK)-MB and troponin 1 are used for diagnosis. CT may show pericardial effusions and anterior mediastinal hematomas. If you see a sternal fracture, suggest that the patient be evaluated for cardiac contusion.

30. **What are the manifestations of pericardial injury?**
The most common site of pericardial laceration is the left pleuropericardium. The presence of hemothorax in those patients may suggest concomitant cardiac wall injury. The second most common pericardial injury is a transverse tear along the diaphragmatic portion of the pericardium. In patients with associated diaphragmatic injury, herniation of abdominal contents into the pericardial space may occur.

KEY POINTS: CHEST TRAUMA

1. Look for traumatic pseudoaneurysms below the aortic arch, anterior to the descending thoracic aorta.

2. Do a chest CT to look for aortic injury if you see infarcts on an abdominal CT.

3. Do a chest CT to look for aortic injury if you see a periaortic hematoma at the diaphragm.

4. Some large pneumothoraces may not visible on supine, portable, trauma chest x-rays.

31. **What are the plain x-ray features of diaphragmatic injury?**
Diaphragmatic injuries are more common in penetrating than blunt injuries and are reportedly more common on the left. The specific findings on plain x-ray include herniation of hollow viscus into the thorax or an abnormal course of a nasogastric tube. Less specific x-ray findings include elevation or loss contour of the hemidiaphragm. Some of the left-sided predominance in the literature is due to older studies that made the diagnosis via plain film: It is easier to see herniated bowel on the left than herniated liver on the right.

32. **What are the CT findings of traumatic of traumatic diaphragmatic injury?**
The most common finding in traumatic diaphragmatic injury is abrupt discontinuity of the diaphragm. Complete absence of a hemidiaphragm is also possible. Other findings include herniation of abdominal contents (bowel, organs, or omentum) into the chest cavity and the "collar sign."

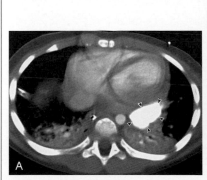
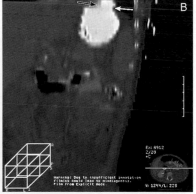

Figure 6-14. Axial and sagittal reconstructed CT of diaphragmatic injury. **A,** The axial image shows the herniated stomach behind the left ventricle *arrowheads*. It is difficult to picture the three-dimensional anatomy, however. **B,** The coronal multiplanar reformat shows the "collar sign" *(arrows)* due to constriction of the contrast-filled stomach where it passes through the diaphragmatic tear.

33. **What is the collar sign?**
The collar sign is constriction of a loop of bowel as it herniated through the torn diaphragm (Fig. 6-14).

34. **Why is it important to diagnose a diaphragmatic injury?**
An undiagnosed ruptured diaphragm with herniated bowel can become complicated by obstruction and/or strangulation—with high morbidity and mortality rates.

35. **Can there be delayed herniation of bowel through a diaphragmatic rupture?**
Yes. Because intra-abdominal pressure is higher than intrathoracic pressure, bowel may progressively herniate into the chest.

36. **What are some limitations of CT in evaluation of diaphragmatic injury?**
CT is reported to have a relative sensitivity of 70–90% for diaphragmatic tears, with a 90% specificity. However, hemoperitoneum or hemothorax may obscure the diaphragm and hence the tear. Small incidental diaphragmatic defects occur, especially in older patients, and may confuse the diagnosis. Respiratory motion (a large number of trauma patients arrive at CT already intubated!) also limits anatomic detail. The tangential relationship of the dome of the diaphragm to the CT slice makes central diaphragmatic lacerations more difficult to diagnose than peripheral lacerations. Right-sided lacerations are more difficult to diagnose than left sided—even on CT. In practice, diaphragmatic lacerations are often difficult to diagnose and require a high level of attention and suspicion.

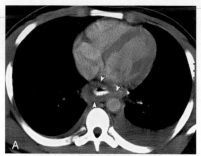

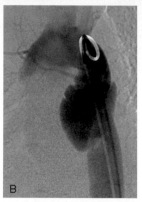

Figure 6-15. Victim of motor vehicle accident with abdominal pain and no chest symptoms. **A,** Abdominal CT showed posterior mediastinal hematoma *(arrowheads)*. **B,** Based on this result, a conventional angiogram was performed, which showed the aortic transection.

37. **Why is it necessary to include the chest bases in patients undergoing abdominal CT for trauma?**
Previously unsuspected pneumothoraces are seen on abdominal CT in about 20% of trauma patients. Up to 75% of these occult pneumothoraces ultimately require interventional management. In addition, a transected thoracic aorta may present as a periaortic hematoma at the diaphragm (Fig. 6-15).

38. **What are the most common fractures of the thoracic spine fracture?**
Anterior wedge compression fractures and burst fractures. Most fractures occur near the thoracolumbar junction. Have a high level of suspicion if you see a posterior mediastinal or prevertebral hematoma. Fractures can be quite subtle on axial images, whereas they are much more apparent on the lateral scout image. However, many trauma patients are scanned with their arms by their sides because of other injuries; this positioning obscures the spine on the lateral scout image. Coronal and sagittal reconstructions are superb with multidetector scanners and thin slices (Fig. 6-16).

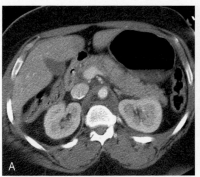
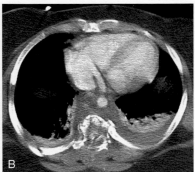
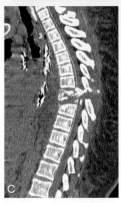

Figure 6-16. *A, B,* and *C,* Motor vehicle accident. Periaortic hematoma at the level of the crus of the diaphragm. The cause is a traumatic comminuted T8 fracture with prevertebral hematoma. Associated bilateral hemothorax and rib fractures are present. Note the beautiful sagittal reformat from the axial images on a multislice CT. This periaortic hematoma is explained and is not an indication for an angiogram.

39. **What are the CT features of traumatic thoracic vertebral body injury?**
    The injury normally presents as a compression fracture with an associated prevertebral hematoma.

40. **What does a gunshot wound to the lungs look like?**
    There will be hemorrhage and laceration along the bullet track. After the hemorrhage clears, there will usually be pneumatocele formation. There is, of course, frequently hemothorax or pneumothorax. Do not count on the bullet having passed in a straight line—bullets tumble and ricochet. A high-velocity or military bullet is much more powerful with massive tissue destruction (Fig. 6-17).

41. **What should I think about besides traumatic injuries in a trauma patient?**
    Preexisting disease. Think of every emergency department scan in two parts: a problem-oriented CT and a screening CT. The problem-oriented CT is the reason for the scan: to evaluate trauma (or bowel obstruction, paralysis, or renal colic, etc.). The screening CT is for unsuspected disease. Imagine that you are doing health screening in a mall. The most common serious screening CT diagnoses are lung cancer (high prevalence), renal cancer (slower growth, relatively easy to diagnose), aortic aneurysms, and early coronary artery calcifications. Be sure to communicate your additional findings; they are easily overshadowed and forgotten (Figs. 6-18 and 6-19).

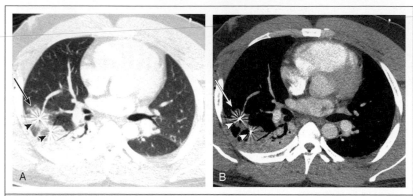

Figure 6-17. *A* and *B,* Gunshot wound to the chest. There is a path of pulmonary laceration and contusion through the lungs (direction of *large arrow*). Note the tiny bullet fragments *(arrowheads)* lying in the path. The path of tissue damage is larger than the bullet, because the bullet shock wave destroys adjacent tissue. Subacutely the hemorrhage will clear and pneumatoceles will be evident.

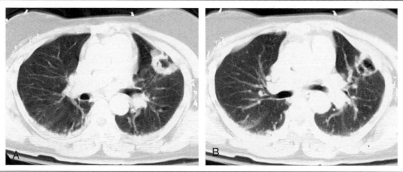

Figure 6-18. *A* and *B,* Stab wound to the left chest. CT was performed to look for pulmonary injury. There is a pleural base cavitary mass deep to the stab wound site, but no pneumothorax or pleural effusion. The appearance of the mass and the absence of other signs of pulmonary traumatic injury favor a tumor over a lung laceration/hematoma. This mass proved to be a primary lung malignancy. Note the left breast reconstruction for prior breast carcinoma.

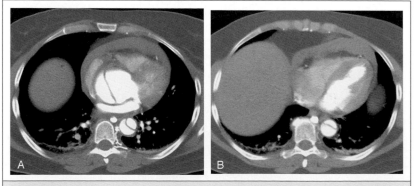

Figure 6-19. *A,* Patient in a single car accident with chest pain and widened mediastinum. Type A aortic dissection with hemopericardium and right ventricular compression due to tamponade. *B,* The aortic aneurysm predated the accident, but the precise timing of the dissection is unknown.

42. **Where is the thoracic duct? How can I diagnose an injury or obstruction to it?**
The thoracic duct runs along the spine, carrying abdominal lymphatic fluid from the abdomen to the left supraclavicular fossa, where it joins the head and neck lymphatics and enters the left subclavian vein. It lies to the right at the diaphragm, crossing to the left at approximately T5–T7. If it is injured or obstructed, chyle (lymphatic fluid from the small intestine) can leak into the pleural space and make a chylothorax. A chylothorax can be diagnosed by a fat-fluid level in a pleural effusion or a pleural effusion with a density below −17 Hounsfield units. However, a chylothorax may be present with higher density because of protein or other higher density components (Fig. 6-20).

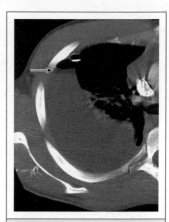

Figure 6-20. Chylothorax with fat-fluid level *(arrow)*.

BIBLIOGRAPHY

1. Ketai L, Brandt MM, Schermer C: Nonaortic mediastinal injury from blunt chest trauma. J Thorac Imag 8:120–127, 2000.

2. Muller N, Fraser R, Coleman N, Pare P (eds): Radiologic Diagnosis of Diseases of the Chest. Philadelphia, WB Saunders, 2000, p 655.

3. Naidich DP, Webb WR, Muller NL, et al: In Naidich DP, Webb WR, Muller NL, et al (eds): Computed Tomography and Magnetic Resonance of the Thorax, 3rd ed. Philadelphia, Lippincott-Raven, pp 566–569, 603–656.

4. Zinck SE, Primack SL: Radiographic and CT findings in blunt chest trauma. J Thorac Imag 4:87–96, 2000.

CHAPTER 7

CT FOR PULMONARY EMBOLISM

David John Prologo, MD, and Vikram Dogra, MD

1. **How prevalent is pulmonary embolic disease?**
   Estimated annual incidences of pulmonary embolism (PE) have been reported as 500,000 in the United States, 100,000 in France, and at least 60,000 in Italy, with an overall 3-month mortality rate of 15–17.5%. The true prevalence of PE is unknown.

2. **What is the pathophysiology of PE?**
   The most common sources of embolic thrombus are the popliteal or proximal deep veins of the leg. Less common origins of thrombus include the iliac or deep pelvic veins, renal veins, inferior vena cava, right heart, or upper extremity veins. Deep venous thrombosis and PE represent points on a continuum of disease.

3. **What are the risk factors for PE?**
   The majority of patients with PE have one or more of the risk factors in the classic triad of Virchow: stasis, hypercoagulability, and/or intimal injury. The risk increases with age.

4. **What other materials can embolize to the lung?**
   Tumor cells, air, fat, or foreign bodies, such as polymethylmethacrylate (following vertebro-plasty), talc (in intravenous drug abusers), or catheter tips, may embolize to the pulmonary vasculature. Fat embolism (after long bone fracture) causes a diffuse pattern like adult respiratory distress syndrome (ARDS).

5. **What is the clinical presentation of PE?**
   The presentation of PE is quite variable and may be subtle in patients with normal cardiac function. Clinical signs associated with PE include sudden-onset dyspnea, tachycardia, pleuritic chest pain, hemoptysis, and the presence of signs associated with deep venous thrombosis (erythema, warmth, pain, swelling, or Homans' sign [pain with dorsiflexion of the foot]).

6. **What laboratory tests are useful in the work-up of suspected PE?**
   A negative D-dimer enzyme-linked immunosorbent assay (ELISA) virtually excludes the diagnosis of PE, with reported sensitivities and negative predictive values ranging from 96–100%. Cardiac biomarkers, such as troponin and brain natriuretic peptide, are currently under investigation for their role in prognosis of patients with established PE. Arterial blood gas analysis is both insensitive and nonspecific with regard to PE.

7. **What imaging modalities other than CT are used for the diagnosis of PE?**
   - The chest radiograph is nonspecific and may be normal. Positive findings associated with PE include cardiomegaly, atelectasis, and pleural effusion.
   - Nuclear ventilation-perfusion scanning is generally reserved for patients with a contraindication to intravenous contrast because of the limited clinical utility of indeterminate or intermediate readings.
   - Lower extremity venous ultrasound, although helpful with management decisions when positive, is fairly insensitive with regard to PE (approximately 60% of patients with established PE will have a negative deep venous ultrasound exam).

- Catheter pulmonary angiography has historically been the gold standard for diagnosing PE, but it is invasive and rarely performed after the advent of multiple-row detector CT (MDCT).
- Magnetic resonance (MR) can diagnose PE but it lacks spatial resolution compared with MDCT and has not been widely studied in the setting of acute PE. Magnetic resonance imaging (MRI) is often impractical for imaging dyspneic patients.

8. **How is CT for PE performed?**
   Contrast is administered through a peripheral intravenous access site (100–150 cc) and scanning begun as the pulmonary artery is opacified, determined either through the use of an automated bolus tracker or with standardized delay times. In general, thinner collimation affords better visualization of the pulmonary arterial tree, but it is limited by scanner type and patient breath-holding capacity. Example scanning parameters are 120 kV and 250 mA, although they may be adapted to patient body habitus. Overlapping reconstruction at 50% scanning collimation is standard.

9. **How do pulmonary emboli image on CT?**
   Emboli image as partial or complete filling defects in the opacified pulmonary arteries (Fig. 7-1).

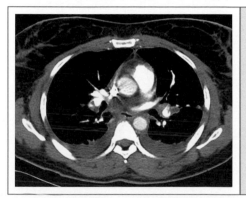

Figure 7-1. CT performed for PE in a 52-year-old woman with dyspnea and chest pain demonstrates emboli in the bilateral main pulmonary arteries, manifested as filling defects. Bilateral small pleural effusions are also present.

10. **What is the sensitivity and specificity of CT for PE? How has this compared with conventional pulmonary angiography?**
    A major early criticism of CT for PE compared with catheter angiography was its inability to visualize segmental and subsegmental pulmonary arteries. Early work done with single-slice scanners demonstrated comparable sensitivity and specificity of CT compared with ventilation-perfusion (V/Q) scanning and pulmonary angiography proximally (with values approaching 100%) but variable reported numbers (60–94%) for detection and accurate characterization of clots in the distal vasculature. The development of MDCT has significantly improved visualization of the peripheral arterial tree (Fig. 7-2). In addition, several groups have demonstrated acceptable clinical outcomes for patients ruled out for PE with CT. As a result, many consider CT to be the new gold standard for PE diagnosis.

11. **How does the multiple-row detector arrangement improve the sensitivity and specificity of CT for PE?**
    Additional detectors along the z-axis allow for imaging of greater anatomic distances per exposure when compared with single-row technology. This results in (1) improved utilization of the contrast bolus and shorter breath holds via faster scan times and (2) increased resolution of smaller objects via thinner collimation (Fig. 7-3).

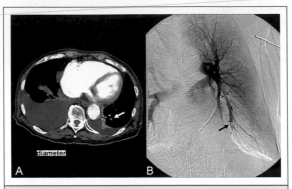

Figure 7-2. *A,* CT performed in a 63-year-old man with hypoxia and chest pain demonstrates a large right pleural effusion seen on chest x-ray and a contralateral filling defect in the distal posterior basilar segmental artery on the left *(arrow),* indicative of thromboembolism. *B,* Confirmed by conventional angiography.

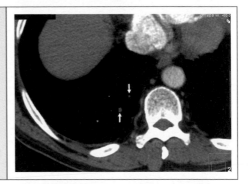

Figure 7-3. CT performed in a 67-year-old woman with hypoxia and chest pain demonstrates filling defects in segmental and subsegmental arteries to the right lower lobe, indicative of thromboemboli.

12. **What additional benefits are there to using CT in the setting of suspected acute PE?**
CT for PE affords the opportunity to interrogate the entire thorax for alternative or ancillary diagnoses (Fig. 7-4). Also, the exam itself is non-invasive and takes only minutes to perform.

13. **Can CT be used as a prognostic/risk stratification tool in patients with acute PE?**
Embolic obstruction as quantified by CT has recently been correlated with patient survival. Furthermore, indirect evidence of right heart strain (a major predictor of patient outcome in the

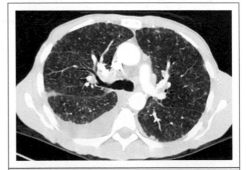

Figure 7-4. Example of the ability of CT to provide alternative or ancillary diagnoses. Selected axial image from a CT performed in a 44-year-old woman with breast cancer who presented with shortness of breath demonstrates diffuse nodular interlobular septal thickening later proven to be lymphangitic metastases.

setting of acute PE) manifests on CT as interventricular septal bowing and/or right ventricular dilatation.

14. **What are the limitations of CT for PE?**
Nondiagnostic scans most often result from inadequate opacification of the pulmonary arteries secondary to poor bolus timing, artifact from patient or respiratory motion, or noise degraded images related to patient obesity. Faster scanning with MDCT compared with single-slice spiral CT significantly reduces the number of nondiagnostic scans.

15. **What are the CT characteristics of chronic PE?**
Longstanding emboli may appear calcified or as intraluminal webs, bands, or stenoses associated with poststenotic pulmonary arterial dilatation. In addition, the presence of bronchial artery hypervascularization is often seen in the setting of chronic PE.

KEY POINTS: PULMONARY EMBOLUS

1. MDCT is a major advance for the detection of pulmonary emboli compared with single-slice CT. MDCT provides thinner images with more coverage faster, minimizing respiratory motion and bolus mistiming.

2. MDCT has become the de facto gold standard for the diagnosis of pulmonary emboli.

3. There are mimics of pulmonary emboli: mucus plugs, poor opacification of veins, partial volume averaging of air, and lymph nodes. With care, these can be distinguished from pulmonary emboli. Make sure your suspected emboli is in a pulmonary artery.

16. **What are the indications for interventional therapy for PE?**
The only indication for catheter thrombolysis or surgical embolectomy is hemodynamic instability. No other imaging or laboratory finding to date has shown strong enough correlation with poor outcome to justify the risks associated with these procedures.

17. **What are the treatment options for stable patients with PE?**
- **Anticoagulation:** Short term with intravenous unfractionated heparin and long term with vitamin K antagonists such as warfarin
- **Inferior vena cava filters:** For patients with contraindications to anticoagulation

18. **What new clinical questions have arisen related to the increased use of CT for PE?**
As smaller and smaller emboli are being imaged, both the true prevalence of PE and the risk-benefit ratios of anticoagulation are being reconsidered. Also the increasing utility of CT for PE has raised concerns about patient radiation dose and promoted the development of tube modulation devices to minimize patient radiation doses.

19. **Describe CT appearance of fat embolism.**
Trauma patients and patients undergoing orthopedic procedures are at increased risk for fat embolism. It is a type of chemical pneumonitis characterized by multiple, diffuse, bilateral opacities and interlobular septal thickening on CT 1 to 3 days after a traumatic event or intervention (Fig. 7-5). These findings often resemble pulmonary edema without pleural effusion or cardiomegaly and demonstrate a predilection for the basilar and peripheral lung regions.

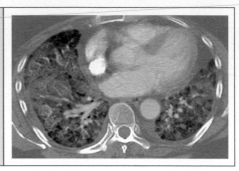

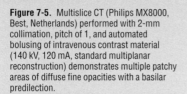

Figure 7-5. Multislice CT (Philips MX8000, Best, Netherlands) performed with 2-mm collimation, pitch of 1, and automated bolusing of intravenous contrast material (140 kV, 120 mA, standard multiplanar reconstruction) demonstrates multiple patchy areas of diffuse fine opacities with a basilar predilection.

BIBLIOGRAPHY

1. Blachere H, Latrabe V, Montaudon M, et al: Pulmonary embolism revealed on helical CT angiography: Comparison with ventilation-perfusion radionuclide lung scanning. AJR Am J Roentgenol 174:1041–1047, 2000.

2. Carson JL, Kelley MA, Duff A, et al: The clinical course of thromboembolism. N Engl J Med 326:1240–1245, 1992.

3. Choe du H, Marom EM, Ahrar K, et al: Pulmonary embolism of polymethyl methacrylate during percutaneous vertebroplasty and kyphoplasty. AJR Am J Roentgenol 183:1097–1102, 2004.

4. Donato AA, Scheirer JJ, Atwell MS, et al: Clinical outcomes in patients with suspected acute pulmonary embolism and negative helical computed tomographic results in whom anticoagulation was withheld. Arch Intern Med 17:2033–2038, 2003.

5. Goldhaber SZ: Pulmonary embolism. Lancet 363:1295–1305, 2004.

6. Goldhaber SZ, Visani L, DeRosa M: Acute pulmonary embolism: Clinical outcomes in the International Cooperative Pulmonary Embolism Registry (ICOPER). Lancet 353:1386–1389, 1999.

7. Goodman LR, Curtin JJ, Mewissen MW, et al: Detection of pulmonary embolism in patients with unresolved clinical and scintigraphic diagnosis: Helical CT versus angiography. AJR Am J Roentgenol 164:1369–1374, 1995.

8. McCollough CH, Zink FE: Performance evaluation of a multi-slice CT system. Med Phys 26:2223–2230, 1999.

9. Patel S, Kazerooni EA, Cascade PN: Pulmonary embolism: Optimization of small artery visualization at multi-detector row CT. Radiology 227:455–460, 2003.

10. Prologo JD, Dogra VS, Farag R: CT Diagnosis of fat embolism. Am J Emerg Med 22:605–606, 2004.

11. Raptopoulos V, Boiselle P: Multi-detector row spiral CT pulmonary angiography: Comparison with single-detector row spiral CT. Radiology 221:606–613, 2001.

12. Remy-Jardin M, Baghaie F, Bonnel F, et al: Thoracic helical CT: Influence of subsecond scan time and thin collimation on evaluation of peripheral pulmonary arteries. Eur Radiol 10:1297–1303, 2000.

13. Remy-Jardin M, Mastora I, Remy J: Pulmonary embolus imaging with multi-slice CT. Radiol Clin North Am 41:507–519, 2003.

14. Remy-Jardin M, Remy J, Artaud D, et al: Peripheral pulmonary arteries: Optimization of the spiral CT acquisition protocol. Radiology 204:157–163, 1997.

15. Remy-Jardin M, Remy J, Deschildre F, et al: Diagnosis of pulmonary embolism with spiral CT: Comparison with pulmonary angiography and scintigraphy. Radiology 200:699–706, 1996.

16. Schoepf UJ, Costello P: CT angiography for diagnosis of pulmonary embolism: State of the art. Radiology 230:329–337, 2004.

17. Schoepf UJ, Goldhaber SZ, Costello P: Spiral computed tomography for acute pulmonary embolism. Circulation 109:2160–2167, 2004.

18. Schoepf UJ, Holzknecht N, Helmberger TK, et al: Subsegmental pulmonary emboli: improved detection with thin-collimation multi-detector row spiral CT. Radiology 222:483–490, 2002.

19. Swensen SJ, Sheedy PF, Ryu JH, et al: Outcomes after withholding anticoagulation from patients with suspected acute pulmonary embolism and negative computed tomographic findings: A cohort study. Mayo Clin Proc 77:130–138, 2002.

20. Task Force on Pulmonary Embolism: Guidelines on diagnosis and management of pulmonary embolism. Eur Heart J 21:1314–1336, 2000.

21. Weiss K: Pulmonary thromboembolism: Epidemiology and techniques of nuclear medicine. Semin Thromb Hemost 22:27–32, 1996.

22. Wu AS, Pezzullo JA, Cronan JJ, et al: CT pulmonary angiography: Quantification of pulmonary embolus as a predictor of patient outcome—initial experience. Radiology 230:831–835, 2004.

CHAPTER 8

CHEST INFECTION

Kristina Siddall, MD, and John G. Strang, MD

1. Name six indications for chest CT in the setting of lung infection.
- Evaluate infection that has not responded to appropriate therapy, for example, approximately 4 weeks after initiation of treatment for community-acquired pneumonia.
- Clarify the specific site and appearance of a nonspecific finding on chest x-ray, especially in human immunodeficiency virus (HIV) patients.
- Evaluate symptomatic patients with a normal chest x-ray.
- Exclude bronchial obstruction by mass or foreign body as etiology of infection.
- Assess surrounding structures (i.e., pleura, mediastinum, esophagus) for complications or coexisting conditions.
- Determine therapeutic interventions for abscess and empyema.

2. How long does it take for pneumonia to resolve radiographically? Does that correspond to the clinical picture?
Half of patients with community-acquired lobar pneumonia have radiographic resolution at 3–5 weeks, and most clear within 3 months. Advanced age and comorbid illnesses increase the time to resolve. Patients subjectively note improvement in symptoms after 5 days on antibiotic therapy, long before the x-ray clears.

3. How do you distinguish between atelectasis and consolidation (pneumonia) on chest CT?
Both atelectasis and pneumonia are air-space diseases. Atelectasis causes loss of lung volume or lung collapse, whereas lung volume is maintained with infiltrate or pneumonia (Fig. 8-1).

4. Are any areas of the lung particularly prone to atelectasis?
Yes. The right middle lobe is more easily collapsed than the other lobes of the lung, because the right middle lobe bronchus is the narrowest and is surrounded by lymph nodes.

5. What is the difference in appearance between lobar pneumonia, bronchopneumonia, and interstitial pneumonia?
- **Lobar pneumonia** originates and spreads in the alveoli, sparing the bronchial tree. Lobar

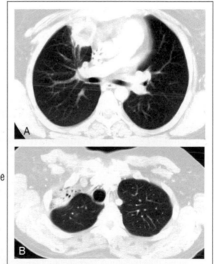

Figure 8-1. *A,* Dense consolidation in the anterior segment of the right upper lobe (RUL) secondary to pneumonia. Note that volume of the RUL is preserved. *B,* Right upper lobe atelectasis. Note that the volume of the RUL is markedly reduced as the major fissure is drawn forward *(arrowheads)* and the right lower lobe (RLL) occupies the lung apex. In both atelectasis and pneumonia, there can be air bronchograms. After intravenous (IV) contrast, atelectatic lung will enhance more than consolidated lung.

pneumonia classically produces more fluid than inflammation, appears more solid than patchy, and involves a whole lung segment or, in some cases, a whole lobe or even lung, while sparing its neighbors.

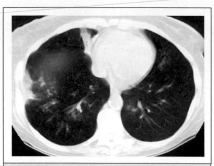

Figure 8-2. Bacterial bronchopneumonia with patchy infiltrates following the distribution of the bronchi.

- **Bronchopneumonia** originates around the bronchioles producing more inflammation than fluid. It appears patchy and is not confined by lobar anatomy (Fig. 8-2). It can become confluent when severe.
- **Interstitial pneumonias** (generally viral or *Pneumocystic carinii* pneumonia) originate in the pulmonary interstitium and can progress from diffuse reticulonodular appearance to ground-glass infiltrate to frank consolidation. Note that multilobar consolidation can be reached by any of these three pathways (alveolar, bronchial, or interstitial), and they are more distinguishable *en route* than at destination.

6. **Is the epidemiology of lobar pneumonia and bronchopneumonia similar?**
   No. Lobar pneumonia is predominantly seen in middle-aged adults with high fever. Up to 95% of cases are caused by *Streptococcus pneumoniae,* the remainder predominantly by *Legionella* and *Klebsiella*. Bronchopneumonia more commonly affects children and the elderly and is caused by multiple gram-positive organisms.

7. **What is the "bulging fissure" sign?**
   Pneumonia caused by *Klebsiella* species produces an alveolar exudate that can increase lung volume, typically the upper lobes. The bulging fissure sign describes displacement of the minor fissure by bulging lung tissue, demonstrating a convexity toward the unaffected lung. Note that although lobar expansion occurs less commonly with pneumococcal pneumonia, a patient with a bulging, infected fissure sign is more likely to be infected with *S. pneumoniae* because of the higher overall incidence of pneumococcal pneumonia.

8. **What is *Legionella* pneumonia (Legionnaires' disease)? What does it look like on CT?**
   The first known outbreak of Legionnaires' disease was at an American Legion convention hotel in Philadelphia in July, 1976 (221 cases, 34 deaths). It is currently a relatively common community-acquired pneumonia, representing approximately 6% of cases. It can also be a nosocomial pneumonia. Its demographics are typified by its original index outbreak: Legionnaires' strikes predominantly older men (the American Legion is a veterans group) and spreads primarily from contaminated water sources (e.g., evaporative cooling towers of institutional air conditioning systems in the summer), as in its index outbreak. It is usually a rapidly progressive lobar pneumonia (like pneumococcal pneumonia). There is common cavitation or abscess formation in immunocompromised patients, rarely in immunocompetent patients. Other organ involvement (gastrointestinal [GI] [diarrhea], liver, kidney) can occur.

9. **What is the classical appearance of varicella pneumonia?**
   Innumerable pulmonary nodules (5–10 mm) can coalesce into a dense consolidation over several days.

10. **How does hematogenous spread of infection appear on chest CT?**
    Septic emboli are nodules, are multiple, are peripheral with a leading pulmonary vessel, and are wedge-shaped or round. Septic emboli usually cavitate, as the dead tissue collapses (Fig. 8-3).

11. **What patients are particularly susceptible to aspiration pneumonia?**
    Remember the three As: addicts, alcoholics, and infection by anaerobes.

12. **Can atypical pneumonia present as consolidation on chest CT?**
    The traditional, atypical pneumonias, such as *Mycoplasma,* PCP, or viral pneumonia, show perihilar interstitial prominence on chest x-ray and chest CT (Fig. 8-4). There may also be associated hyperinflation and air trapping on expiratory CT. Atypical pneumonia can also appear as a consolidation.

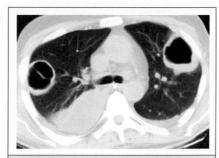

Figure 8-3. Intravenous drug user with endocarditis. Note large cavitary masses secondary to septic emboli. In most cases, the cavitary masses are 0.5–3.5 cm in diameter.

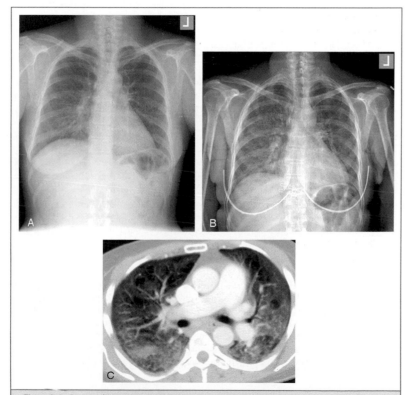

Figure 8-4. Patient with lymphoma who had recently been treated with chemotherapy develops shortness of breath. *A,* Chest x-ray was normal 2 weeks before presentation. A new perihilar air-space infiltrate has developed on chest x-ray *(B)* and CT *(C)*. This was *Pneumocystis carinii* pneumonia.

13. **What organism is notorious for superinfection of viral pneumonia? How does it appear?**
    Staphylococcus aureus. On imaging, findings are consistent with bronchopneumonia.

14. **What does foul-smelling sputum usually indicate?**
    Cavitation from an anaerobic infection. However, many anaerobic infections do not cavitate and so may not produce foul-smelling sputum.

15. **What are the similarities and differences between lung abscess and empyema?**
    Both are usually complications of pneumonia. Lung abscess occurs in the lung parenchyma and within the area of consolidation. It is usually round and irregular and vessels may go into it. It may occur due to bronchial obstruction (Fig. 8-5). Empyemas involve the pleura, are elliptical and smooth, and displace lung vessels (Fig. 8-6).

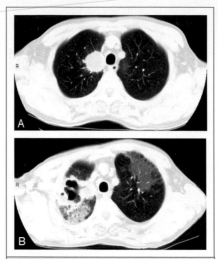

Figure 8-5. *A,* Left upper lobe lung carcinoma. *B,* Two months later, the patient presents with fever and is found to have a cavitary mass peripheral to the tumor. This mass was a postobstructive lung abscess.

16. **Why is it important to distinguish between empyema and abscess?**
    The treatment is different. Percutaneous drainage is used for empyema, whereas medical management is the first-line treatment for lung abscess to avoid spreading infection to the pleura.

17. **What is the split pleura sign?**
    An empyema occupies the virtual space between the parietal and visceral pleura. With infection, the pleura become thickened and hyperemic and enhance with intravenous contrast administration giving the appearance of a split pleura, seperated by fluid or pus.

18. **What are the CT signs of a bronchopleural fistula? What are its causes?**
    Air within an empyema suggests an abnormal connection between the lung and pleura: a bronchopleural fistula. Empyema and complications of pneumonectomy are the most common causes of bronchopleural fistula (Fig. 8-7).

19. **What are the imaging findings of primary pulmonary tuberculosis (TB)?**
    Primary pulmonary TB is the primary infection, caused by inhaling an infected droplet coughed out by an infected person. Patients with primary TB generally have respiratory symptoms. Many patients with primary TB will not have radiographic findings on either chest x-ray or CT. However, for the most part, primary TB will appear as a dense consolidation in a segment or lobe. Accompanying hilar adenopathy is common, classically (but not always) of central low density (lower than soft tissue) with peripheral enhancement.

20. **What is a Ghon tubercle?**
    A Ghon tubercle (or Ghon focus) is the pulmonary lesion of primary TB. As it heals, the infectious organisms become encapsulated by proliferative fibroblasts. Ghon tubercles often calcify and can reactivate.

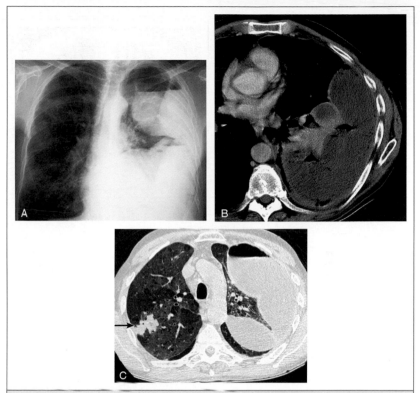

Figure 8-6. A 52-year-old smoker with dyspnea for 2 weeks and leukocytosis. **A,** Chest x-ray shows a fluid-fluid level that appears to be in the pleural space. **B,** Chest CT shows an empyema with thickened pleural rind and again with nondependent gas. **C,** Lung windows closer to the apex show layering fluid in the empyema. Did you notice the incidental right upper lobe carcinoma *(arrow)* on the initial chest x-ray? (It overlies the fifth posterior rib.)

21. What is a Ranke complex?
A Ranke complex is a Ghon tubercle in the lung plus hilar adenopathy. Both may calcify.

22. What is postprimary TB?
Postprimary TB is the reinfection of a previously exposed person. This can be from reactivation of the original latent infection or from reinfection (Fig. 8-8). Postprimary TB often has nonspecific symptoms. It has the classic TB distribution: apical and posterior segments of the upper lobes or superior segment lower lobe. It can form consolidation, cavitation, and nodules.

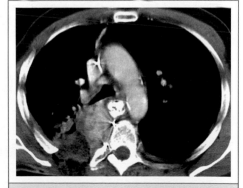

Figure 8-7. Malignant mesothelioma, after resection, with subsequent lung abscess and bronchopleural-cutaneous fistula.

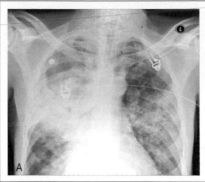
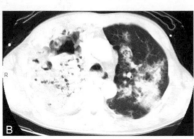

Figure 8-8. Reactivation TB in homeless man, who presented with hemoptysis. Left upper lobe cavity, consolidation, and infiltrate on chest x-ray *(A)* and CT *(B)*. Sputum was grossly positive for acid-fast bacilli (AFB). He gradually responded to multidrug antibiotic therapy.

23. **What are the radiographic findings of reactivation TB?**
    Chest CT is very helpful in identifying and characterizing reactivation TB. Cavities signify active disease and are more easily recognized on CT as opposed to plain x-ray. In addition, scarring and bronchiectasis are more easily seen on CT (Fig. 8-9).

24. **What is the appearance of miliary TB?**
    Miliary TB is TB that has spread hematogenously to form small (from 1–5 mm), usually well-circumscribed nodules (Fig. 8-10). The nodules are distributed randomly throughout the lungs. Other fungal infections

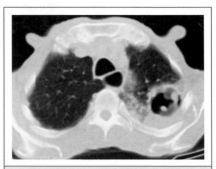

Figure 8-9. Cavitary TB. Thick, irregular cavity in posterior segment left upper lobe.

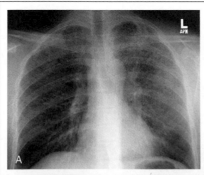
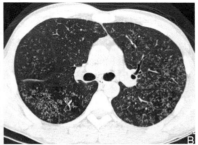

Figure 8-10. Miliary TB in a 25-year-old, previously healthy man after stab wound to chest. He was found to have innumerable small pulmonary nodules on chest x-ray *(A)* and subsequent CT *(B)*. His occupational history included "sand blasting" (road construction work involving dynamite), and silicosis was suspected. The patient left against medical advice. Cultures obtained during admission grew TB. (Sand blasting is actually using a spray of sand to knock rust and scale off ships or boilers. It is not the blowing up of sand, although drilling into rock to set explosives is an occupational exposure.)

can also have miliary spread. (Millet seeds are commonly used in birdseed mix. They are the small hard round seeds.)

25. **What is the appearance of endobronchial TB?**
Endobronchial TB is TB that has spread through the bronchi. The nodules follow the bronchi, giving a "tree-in-bud" appearance (Fig. 8-11).

26. **What are the most common organisms that cause fungal infections?**
There are fungi that predominantly attack weakened and immunocompromised patients:
- *Aspergillus* (see later)
- *Actinomyces* (normal oropharyngeal organism, can invade pleura and through chest wall)
- *Candida*
- *Nocardia*
- *Cryptococcus* (HIV patients)
- *Pneumocystis* (bat-wing infiltrates and dyspnea)

There are also fungi that infect normal patients and are usually self-limiting:
- *Histoplasma* (central United States, miliary, hematogenous spread; many tiny nodules that later calcify)
- *Coccidioides* (southwest United States, occasionally systemic and progressive)
- *Blastomyces* (central and southern United States)

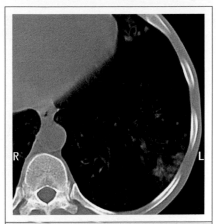

Figure 8-11. Bronchogenic TB in an HIV-positive patient. Note that the small nodules follow the bronchi with bronchial wall thickening rather than being hematogenously distributed, as with miliary TB. (This patient also had cervical cancer, but nodules from cervical cancer metastases should be hematogenously distributed.)

27. **Why do fungal infections get confused with cancer?**
Many fungal infections present as incidental nodules (which get worked up for cancer) or with insidious chronic symptoms, and patients are found to have infiltrates or masses that do not clear with antibiotics (mimicking cancer) (Fig. 8-12). The residua of fungal infections are often small nodules that are seen incidentally by CT. Because fungal organisms are ubiquitous, such nodules are extremely common and are problematic for screening for lung cancer.

28. **What are the forms of infection with *Aspergillus*?**
Aspergillus is a ubiquitous environmental fungus, with three forms of human infection:
- **Saprophytic infestation** (chronic colonization of an existing cavity or necrotic tissue): The cavity is usually secondary to TB or sarcoidosis; it commonly presents with hemoptysis.
- **Invasive** (attacking previously viable tissue, usually in an immunocompromised patient): Most commonly angioinvasive, with aggressive destruction of tissue;

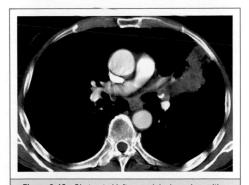

Figure 8-12. Obstructed left upper lobe bronchus with broncholith, mass, and infiltrate. Malignancy was suspected. Mixed fungal infection was found by bronchoscopy.

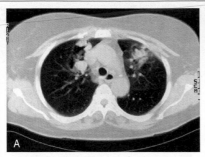

Figure 8-13. *A* and *B,* Allergic bronchopulmonary aspergillosis (ABPA) with severe central bronchiectasis and central mycetoma formation. CT shows these large lobulated masses to be contained within larger, cystic cavities, which extend to the central hilum.

it can cause lung infarction and invade pleura and chest wall. Invasive *Aspergillus* can also give a bronchopneumonia-like picture that does not respond well to antibiotics.

- **Allergic:** Usually allergic bronchopulmonary aspergillosis (ABPA). Characterized by colonization and mucoid impaction of the bronchi with development of bronchiectasis. It occurs almost exclusively in asthmatics (Fig. 8-13).

29. What is an aspergilloma? What is the air crescent sign?

An aspergilloma is a mobile mass of soft tissue density consisting of *Aspergillus* organisms. The more general term is mycetoma, for any "fungus ball." The air crescent sign is a crescent of air formed by an aspergilloma (mycetoma) in a cavity. It distinguishes an aspergilloma in a cavity from a solid mass. The mycetoma can fill the cavity completely in which case there is no air crescent sign (Fig. 8-14).

Figure 8-14. Immunocompromised patient who developed a mass before autologous bone marrow transplant (not shown). This is angioinvasive *Aspergillus* with the destruction of previously viable tissue. After bone marrow transplant, the mass cavitated and formed a central mobile aspergilloma. Note the air crescent sign.

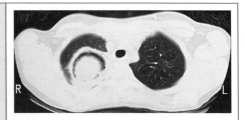

30. What are the major causes of acute mediastinitis?

Mediastinitis, a life-threatening condition, occurs in the setting of recent local surgery, penetrating mediastinal injury, traumatic intubation, esophageal rupture, or contiguous spread of infection from the lungs, pleura, oropharynx, and neck. On CT, the mediastinal fat will demonstrate inflammatory stranding and fluid collections, and, in severe cases, flecks of gas develop, indicating a more ominous course. Treatment is extensive surgical debridement (Figs. 8-15 and 8-16).

31. What lung or systemic infection classically causes massive hilar and/or mediastinal lymphadenopathy?

Pulmonary anthrax causes massive hemorrhagic mediastinal lymphadenopathy. The alert radiologist may be the first to raise the suspicion of this uncommon disease. Anthrax is attractive to bioterrorists because of its spore state, high lethal dose, and easy aerosolization (http://anthrax.radpath.org).

KEY POINTS: CHEST INFECTIONS

1. CT has a number of different roles to play in chest infection, including determining site, cause, likely infectious organisms, and complications.

2. Empyema and lung abscess must be distinguished.

3. The primary forms of tuberculous infection are primary, reactivation, miliary, endobronchial, and extrapulmonic.

4. Fungal infections often mimic cancer in their appearance (nodular masses with lymphadenopathy) and behavior when untreated (subacute indolent progression).

32. **Are diffuse small lung calcifications a sign of lung infection?**
Yes. However, they are not a sign of acute infection, but of healed lung infection, usually histoplasmosis, varicella zoster, or TB. They can also be seen in metastatic thyroid cancer.

33. **What are the cause and inheritance pattern of cystic fibrosis (CF)?**
CF is due to an autosomal recessive mutation causing abnormally thick mucus and exocrine secretions. The pancreas and the lungs are the most common sites of serious disease. In Caucasians, the incidence of the disease is 1:2000–1:3500, making it the most common inherited lethal disease in that population. CF is much less common in other populations.

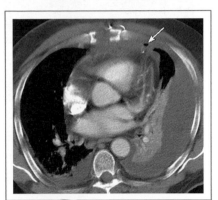

Figure 8-15. Sternal wound dehiscence after coronary artery bypass. There is a retrosternal fluid collection with a small bubble of gas within it *(arrow)*. Diagnosis can be confirmed by CT-guided aspiration.

34. **If 1 in 2500 Caucasian live births is affected by CF, what is a Caucasian's chance of being a carrier? (Assume no family history, Mendelian genetics, no new mutations, uniform mixing of the gene in the population, and no additional fetal demise.)**
If 1:2500 Caucasian children is born with CF, then in 1:625 couples, both parents are carriers (only 1 in 4 of their children would have CF). An unaffected individual's risk of being a carrier is thus the square root of 625, or 1 in 25.

The rate of carriers in the Hispanic population is 1:46; in the African-American population, 1:65; and in the Asian population, 1:90. Thus, lower risk is not trivial, particularly for interracial couples.

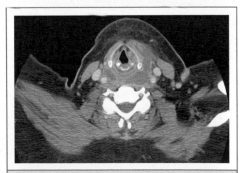

Figure 8-16. Large abscess posterior to the esophagus that originated as a retropharyngeal abscess and tracked down the posterior mediastinum.

Ninety percent of CF-causing mutations can be diagnosed by DNA probes.

35. **What are the pulmonary manifestations of CF?**
    - Symptoms and diseases are secondary to mucus impaction and poor clearance (Fig. 8-17).
    - Bronchiectasis and recurrent bacterial pneumonias occur. (Malnutrition from concomitant pancreatic disease is contributory.)
    - Pulmonary transplantation is common.

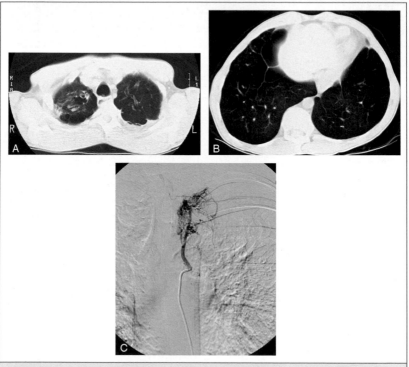

Figure 8-17. *A* and *B,* The abnormally thick mucus produced in cystic fibrosis results in chronic multiorganism lung colonization and pneumonia, bronchiectasis, air trapping, and cavity formation. Pulmonary hemorrhage can occur and is often treated by bronchial artery embolization *(C).*

BIBLIOGRAPHY

1. http://anthrax.radpath.org (radiology-oriented anthrax educational site).

2. Cassiere HA, Niederman MS: Community-acquired pneumonia. Dis Month 44:613–675, 1998.

3. Dahnert R: Radiology Review Manual, 5th ed. Philadelphia, Lippincott, Williams & Wilkins, 2003, pp 498–499.

4. Kullman JE, Fidhman EK, Teigen C: Pulmonary septic emboli: Diagnosis with CT. Radiology 174:211–213, 1990.

5. McLoud TC: Thoracic Radiology. The Requisites. St. Louis, Mosby, 1998.

6. Michigan State University DNA Diagnostic Program. Available at www.phd.msu.edu/DNA/cf_family3.html

7. Muller N, Fraser R, Colman N, Pare N: Pulmonary infection. In Muller N, Fraser R, Colman N, Pare N (eds): Radiologic Diagnosis of Diseases of the Chest. Philadelphia, W.B. Saunders, 2001, pp 141–210.

8. National Institute of Environmental Health Sciences: Review of legionnaires' disease. Available at www.niehs.nih.gov/external/faq/legion.htm

9. Webb WR: Lung disease. In Webb WR, Brant WE, Helms CA (eds): Fundamentals of Body CT, 2nd ed. Philadelphia, W.B. Saunders, 1998, pp 107–145.

10. Weissleder R, Wittenberg J, Harisinghani MG: Chest imaging. In Weissleder R, Wittenberg J, Harisinghani MG (eds): Primer of Diagnostic Imaging, 3rd ed. St. Louis, Mosby, 2003, pp 1–104.

11. Zwanger M: Pneumonia, empyema, and abscess. Emedicine.com, 2004. Available at http://www.emedicine.com/emerg/topic463.htm

CHAPTER 9

THORACIC MANIFESTATIONS OF HUMAN IMMUNODEFICIENCY VIRUS

Kristina Siddall, MD, and Margaret Ormanoski, DO

1. **When is a patient infected with human immunodeficiency virus (HIV) classified as having acquired immunodeficiency syndrome (AIDS)?**

   When the CD4+ T-cell count is < 200/µL. However, based on the Centers for Disease Control and Prevention (CDC) classification of 1993, HIV patients with CD4 counts > 200/µL may also have AIDS if they develop specific opportunistic infections or AIDS-related conditions or malignancies. One-third of the 24 AIDS-defining conditions involve the pulmonary system.

2. **What pulmonary opportunistic infection is diagnostic of AIDS in an HIV-positive patient? What are the imaging findings?**

   Pneumocystic carinii pneumonia (PCP). Thoracic CT in an AIDS patient with PCP is likely to show cysts of variable size, predominantly in the upper lobes, and perihilar parenchymal haziness or ground-glass opacities, similar to pulmonary edema (Fig. 9-1). PCP can also involve extrapulmonary organ systems, including the liver, spleen, central nervous system (CNS), sinuses, bone marrow, and mediastinal lymph nodes.

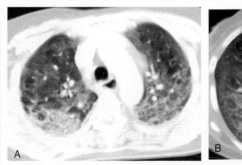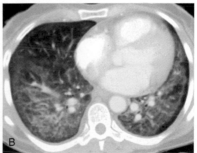

Figure 9-1. *A* and *B*, *Pneumocystis carinii* pneumonia. Ground-glass infiltrates with peripheral sparing mimicking pulmonary edema. Unlike pulmonary edema, there is not a significant pleural effusion. Lymphadenopathy is also uncommon.

3. **Can PCP be seen in patients that do not have AIDS?**

   Yes. Patients who use aerosolized medications are also at risk for infection. The upper lobes are also most commonly affected in these patients.

4. **What is a frequent complication of PCP?**

   Pneumothorax is a frequent complication.

5. **What are pneumatoceles? What is a common etiology?**

   Pneumatoceles are transient cystic changes associated with acute pneumonia or trauma. They are frequently seen in the upper lobes of patients with PCP.

6. **What is the most common fungal infection in AIDS patients?**
   Cryptococcosis, an interstitial lung disease. Cryptococcal meningitis is also common in the immunocompromised patient.

7. **Is *Aspergillus* infection common in AIDS patients?**
   No, it is infrequent. However, it is becoming more common in advanced AIDS patients, particularly invasive *Aspergillus* infection.

8. **What is the halo sign?**
   A ring of ground-glass opacity around a lung nodule or mass, thought to represent parenchymal hemorrhage (Fig. 9-2). The halo sign is most frequently due to aspergillosis and is secondary to fungal invasion into the nearby small vessels and the resulting ischemic necrosis and hemorrhage.

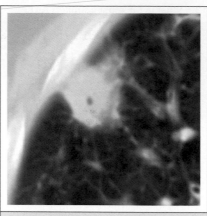

Figure 9-2. Halo sign. A dense lung mass, representing invasive *Aspergillus* infection, is shown with a characteristic halo of ground-glass opacity, representing parenchymal hemorrhage.

9. **What is the air crescent sign?**
   A "crescent" or rim of air surrounds the central solid portion (the mycetoma) in a cavitary lesion (Fig. 9-3). The air crescent is a later finding in a necrotizing process and occurs as the dead tissue retracts within the cavity. In addition to the halo sign, the air crescent sign is also commonly seen in invasive aspergillosis.

10. **What features of tuberculosis in an AIDS patient can distinguish it from infection in an immunocompetent host?**
    - The disease is more likely to be extrapulmonary, frequently spreading to the CNS.
    - Cavitation is less likely.
    - One is more likely to see a large consolidation with irregular margins.
    - Purified protein derivative (PPD) test is often negative.

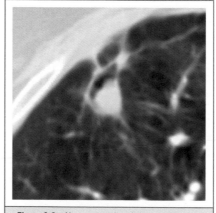

Figure 9-3. Air crescent sign. A dense lung mass, representing fungal infection, collapses within lung cavity, leaving a rim of air.

11. **Is mycobacterial infection in AIDS rare?**
    No—in fact, quite the opposite. In addition to tuberculosis, AIDS patients are affected by *Mycobacterium avium intracellulare*. This opportunistic infection causes few pulmonary symptoms and, consequently, normal imaging but may produce profuse diarrhea, malabsorption, anemia, and jaundice (Fig. 9-4).

12. **Name three causes of bilateral pulmonary nodules in AIDS patients.**
    - **Infections:** Fungal or mycobacterial
    - **Septic emboli**
    - **Neoplasms:** Lymphoma or Kaposi's sarcoma (KS)

13. **What is the most common AIDS-related neoplasm?**
    KS. The second most common is lymphoma.

14. **What neoplasm is suspected when flame-shaped pulmonary nodules are seen on CT?**
    KS. Flame-shaped pulmonary nodules are actually masses or consolidation surrounded by irregular areas of pulmonary hemorrhage, similar to findings of the halo sign (Fig. 9-5). In addition to developing red or violaceous skin lesions, patients with KS can have pulmonary symptoms, such as cough and dyspnea.

15. **What are the CT findings of KS in the lung?**
    CT of the chest demonstrates confluent lung nodules, pleural effusions, and lymphadenopathy (Figs. 9-6 and 9-7).

16. **What radiologic examination can help differentiate KS from the other causes of pulmonary nodules?**
    Nuclear medicine gallium scan. Infections and lymphoma demonstrate increased gallium radiotracer uptake, whereas KS lesions show no radiotracer uptake.

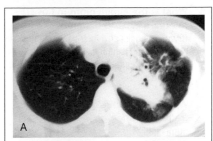

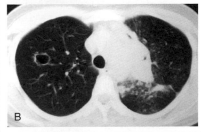

Figure 9-4. *Mycobacterium avium* complex infection, with contralateral post-PCP pneumatoceles. *A,* There is extensive consolidation with cavitation in the left upper lobe as well as obstruction of the apical segment bronchus of the left upper lobe. *B,* Thin-walled, lucent cavities are identified within the right upper lobe, which are pneumatoceles after PCP infection.

17. **Name three causes of diffuse lung infiltrates in immunocompromised patients.**
    - PCP
    - KS
    - Lymphocytic interstitial pneumonia (LIP)

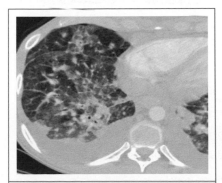

Figure 9-5. Kaposi's sarcoma. Flame-shaped nodules and tumor surrounded by rim of pulmonary hemorrhage.

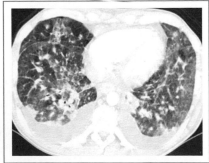

Figure 9-6. Kaposi's sarcoma. Nonspecific findings of diffuse lung nodules and bilateral pleural effusions with antecedent mucocutaneous lesions lead to the diagnosis of KS.

18. **What subtype of lymphoma occurs in AIDS patients?**
AIDS-related lymphoma (ARL) is most commonly derived from B cells. Epstein-Barr virus (EBV), a pathogen also associated with mononucleosis, is usually the culprit.

19. **What lymph-node groups are most frequently affected in ARL?**
Surprisingly, 30–90% of ARL cases are extranodal and are typically in the gastrointestinal tract, liver, bone marrow, and CNS. Twenty-five percent of cases are intrathoracic and affect both the lung parenchyma and pleura (National Cancer Institute).

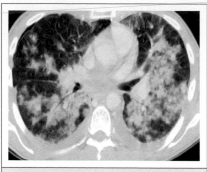

Figure 9-7. Kaposi's sarcoma. Confluent nodules appear similar to patchy consolidation. Also note hilar lymphadenopathy.

20. **What interstitial pneumonia is seen in immunocompromised patients?**
LIP is an uncommon condition that is prelymphomatous. LIP occurs in patients with HIV, particularly children, and in patients with autoimmune disorders, such as rheumatoid arthritis.

21. **A patient with HIV presents with diffuse vesiculopustular eruption, cough, and bilateral pulmonary nodules. What illness should be first in your differential diagnosis?**
Chickenpox caused by varicella zoster virus (VZV). Fifteen percent of immunocompetent patients with chickenpox will develop pneumonia; patients with immunodeficiency are at an even greater risk. Findings of VZV pneumonia are nonspecific, but commonly, scattered, poorly-defined lung nodules are visualized.

KEY POINTS: SELECTED AIDS-DEFINING CONDITIONS IN HIV PATIENTS WITH CD4 COUNT > 200/μL

1. Candidiasis of bronchi, trachea, or lungs

2. Candidiasis, esophageal

3. Coccidioidomycosis, disseminated or extrapulmonary

4. Histoplasmosis, disseminated or extrapulmonary

5. Kaposi's sarcoma

6. Lymphoma, Burkitt's (or equivalent term)

7. Lymphoma, immunoblastic (or equivalent term)

8. *Mycobacterium avium* complex or *Mycobacterium kansasii,* disseminated or extrapulmonary

9. *Mycobacterium tuberculosis,* any site (pulmonary or extrapulmonary)

10. *Mycobacterium,* other species or unidentified species, disseminated or extrapulmonary

11. *Pneumocystis carinii* pneumonia

12. Pneumonia, recurrent

BIBLIOGRAPHY

1. Abramson S: The air crescent sign. Radiology 218:230–232, 2001.

2. AIDS Defining Conditions. Available at
   http://www.thewellproject.org/Diseases_and_Conditions/Opportunistic_Infections/
   AIDS_Defining_Conditions.jsp

3. AIDS Map. Available at www.aidsmap.com/en/docs/83B51ACD-6225-477E-9308-7CE110FD0442.asp

4. Castañer E, Gallardo X, Mata JM, Esteba L: Radiologic approach to the diagnosis of infectious pulmonary
   diseases in patients infected with the human immunodeficiency virus. European Journal of Radiology
   51:114–129, 2004.

5. Centers for Disease Control and Prevention: Definition of AIDS and general discussion. Available at
   www.cdc.gov/mmwr/preview/mmwrhtml/00018871.htm

6. Fauci AS, Lane HC: HIV disease: AIDS and related disorders. In Braunwald E, Fauci AS, Kasper DL, Hauser SL,
   Longo DL, Jameson JL (eds): Harrison's Principles of Internal Medicine, 15th ed. New York, McGraw-Hill, 2001,
   pp 1852–1911, 2001.

7. Fraser RS, Muller NL, Coleman N, Pare PD: Fraser and Pare's Diagnosis of Diseases of the Chest, 4th ed.
   Philadelphia, W.B. Saunders, 1999.

8. Fraser RS, Pare PD: Synopsis of Diseases of the Chest, 2nd ed. Philadelphia, W.B. Saunders, 1994, pp 296–300,
   513–514, 369–372, 315–329.

9. Harley WB: Mycobacterium avium intracellulare. Emedicine.com, 2004. Available at
   http://www.emedicine.com/med/topic1532.htm

10. McLoud TC: Thoracic Radiology. The Requisites. St. Louis, Mosby, 1998.

11. Suakkonen JJ: Lymphocytic interstitial pneumonia. Emedicine.com, 2001. Available at
    http://www.emedicine.com/med/topic1353.htm

12. Webb WR: Lung disease. In Webb WR, Brant WE, Helms CA (eds): Fundamentals of Body CT, 2nd ed.
    Philadelphia, W.B. Saunders, 1998, pp 107–145.

CHAPTER 10

HIGH-RESOLUTION CT

Kristina Siddall, MD

1. **What are the indications for high-resolution computed tomography (HRCT)?**
   - Diagnose and characterize diffuse interstitial disease, small airways disease, and bronchiectasis.
   - Detect occult lung disease in patients with otherwise normal chest imaging.
   - Determine high yield location for open lung biopsy.
   - Follow acute lung disease response to therapy.

2. **How is HRCT performed?**
   HRCT arose in the pre-helical CT, pre-picture archiving and communication systems (PACS) era. HRCT was very different from routine chest CT at that time. Fundamentally, HRCT sampled the lung at high resolution for diffuse disease, whereas routine CT evaluated the entire lung, mediastinum, and chest wall for focal diseases. With the addition of spiral scanning, it became practical to add a series of routine contiguous sections to the HRCT. Typically, an HRCT included the following:
   - No intravenous (IV) contrast (not necessary)
   - Thin (1–2 mm) images in inspiration
   - Noncontiguous images 1–2 cm apart (the entire lungs were not scanned, only sampled for diffuse disease)
   - Several thin noncontiguous expiratory images
   - Reconstruction using high spatial frequency algorithm
   - Sometimes prone images (to distinguish dependent density from posterior fibrosis)
   - Filming with large image size, sometimes lung windows only

3. **Why are expiratory images performed?**
   To exclude air trapping, a phenomenon seen in obstructive lung diseases. Abnormal regions of the lung will remain lucent or air-filled, failing to normally increase in attenuation during exhalation (Fig. 10-1).

4. **What is another reason that expiration images are obtained?**
   To help distinguish mosaic perfusion from air trapping. Mosaic perfusion occurs when a regional decrease in ventilation, such as in small airways disease, causes a corresponding decrease in perfusion. In some cases, the vessels in the better-ventilated, higher-attenuation lung areas will appear larger in caliber (Fig. 10-2).

5. **Is IV contrast used in HRCT?**
   No. However, HRCT can be performed in conjunction with contrast-enhanced chest CT.

6. **Does HRCT become irrelevant with multidetector scanners and PACS?**
   With multidetector CT (MDCT), it is practical to get thin (1–2 mm) contiguous slices on every patient. It is also possible to apply edge-enhancing filters on a PACS work station rather than having to reconstruct with different algorithms and film the study. So every routine chest CT can become a HRCT using the same data!
   So does HRCT become irrelevant? On the contrary—because HRCT will probably merge into routine chest CT protocols, HRCT interpretive skills will become more important because every chest CT will include HRCT images.

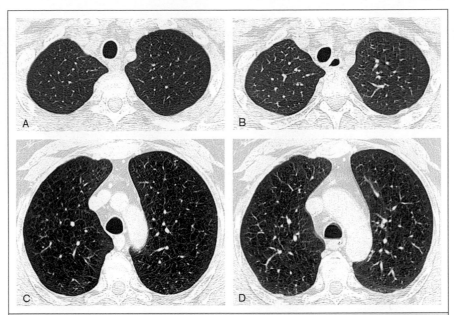

Figure 10-1. *A,* Normal inspiration. *B,* Normal expiration. Note how the lungs increase in density after exhalation. *C,* Inspiration in a patient with emphysema. Note overall parenchymal lucency. *D,* Expiration in emphysematous lung. Note persistent diffuse lucency in lung after expiration. Air is trapped.

7. **What is the effective difference between HRCT and a standard 5- or 7-mm thick thoracic CT?**
   Thicker slices have much more partial volume averaging. For example, a nodule seen on standard CT may represent the superimposition of multiple processes (e.g., atelectasis and normal lung); it may subsequently disappear on thin-slice HRCT. A true small nodule or septal wall will disappear when averaged with adjacent air (Fig. 10-3).

8. **Why does HRCT look grainy compared with conventional CT?**
   The thin slices and edge-enhancing algorithm or data filter for HRCT sharpen detail, but at the cost of increased noise relative to image contrast. In the lung,

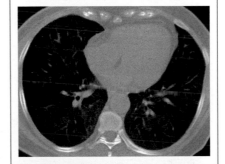

Figure 10-2. Mosaic perfusion on expiration. Hyperlucent areas of lung parenchyma contain vessels of thinner caliber in contrast to parenchyma with normal vascularity.

however, the difference in density between aerated lung and everything else is so great that there is sufficient contrast relative to noise. Partial volume effects with thicker slices are more problematic than the additional noise with thin slices.

9. **Why isn't HRCT used for all parts of the body?**
   Because you need a high difference in contrast to overcome the increased noise. Thin slices are most useful in bone (trabeculae versus marrow), angiography (contrast-filled vessel versus surrounding fat), and lung (structures versus air) and not so useful in organs in which the density difference is subtle.

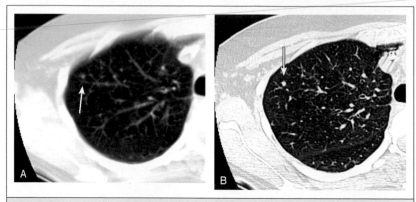

Figure 10-3. *A,* Standard thoracic CT demonstrates a subtle nodular density within the right upper lobe, which could be mistaken for a pulmonary vessel on end. *B,* HRCT shows the same nodule more sharply, because there is less volume averaging. The nodule in A appears hazy, because of volume averaging of the aerated lung parenchyma around the nodule and the nodule itself.

10. **How can HRCT help decide where to biopsy?**

HRCT is most helpful in determining thoracoscopic or open biopsy location for patchy but diffuse disease by identifying areas of ground-glass abnormality. This ensures that the biopsy is done in an area of active disease—not an area that is spared or an area that is end stage and fibrotic.

HRCT can also help with biopsy. For example, a lesion seen on conventional chest CT may be a product of volume averaging (*see* previous discussion) and not be visualized on HRCT, obviating the need for biopsy. A nodule may appear noncalcified on conventional CT due to partial volume averaging, but on HRCT it demonstrates benign calcification (Fig. 10-4).

11. **What is the smallest object size that can be resolved on a high-resolution chest CT?**

The smallest object size is 100–400 microns, similar to the resolution of a gross pathology specimen.

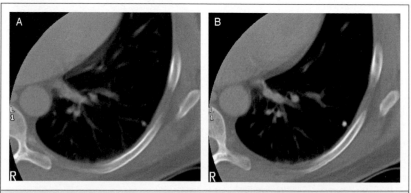

Figure 10-4. *A,* The subpleural nodule measures soft tissue density. *B,* Similar to the loss of volume averaging in Fig. 10-3B, the pulmonary nodule appears to change character with high resolution; in this case, it is not actually soft tissue density but calcium and assumed to be more benign in nature.

12. What is the cause of star artifact?

Pulsation of the heart adjacent to the left lung base causes thin streaks to radiate from pulmonary vessels' edges and linear structures in the lung to appear double (Fig. 10-5).

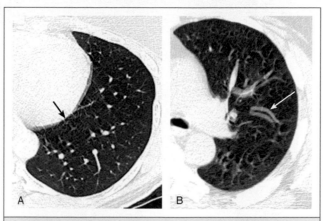

Figure 10-5. *A,* The artifact caused by cardiac motion gives the appearance of a double left-heart border *(arrow)* or "star artifact." *B,* The star artifact can produce the appearance of duplicated pulmonary vessels *(arrow)* and even mimic the appearance of bronchiectasis with parallel thickened walls. In this instance, the artifact is sometimes termed "pseudobronchiectasis."

13. What is the smallest anatomic unit of the lung seen on HRCT?

The secondary pulmonary lobule contains the bronchiole and pulmonary artery. It is outlined by the interlobular septa, which encase the pulmonary veins and lymphatic system. A normal lobule is polygonal in shape and is about 2 cm in diameter (Fig. 10-6).

14. What are "parenchymal bands" or "long lines"?

They are 2.5-cm, thickened septal lines spanning across more than one lobule.

15. How do Kerley B lines appear on HRCT?

Kerley B lines (or septal lines) are pathognomonic for interstitial disease on chest radiograph and are often secondary to pulmonary edema. These lines are thickened interlobular septa secondary to distention or abnormality in the pulmonary veins and/or lymph channels. Cascading polygons and short lines perpendicular to subpleural surface are seen on HRCT (Fig. 10-7).

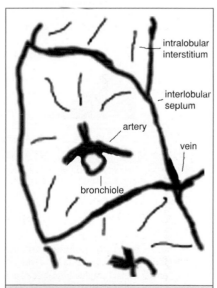

Figure 10-6. Secondary pulmonary lobule. The diameter of both the pulmonary artery and central bronchiole is about equal. However, in the peripheral third of the lung, the bronchiole is not well visualized, similar to the lack of pulmonary markings in the peripheral third of the lung on a normal chest x-ray.

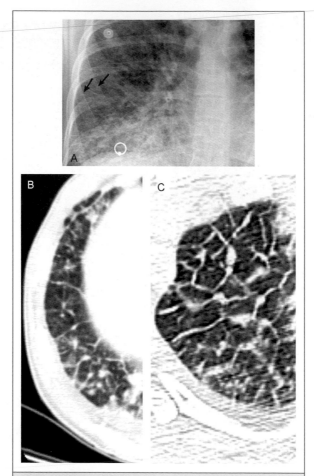

Figure 10-7. *A,* Kerley B lines seen in acute pulmonary edema. Note the extension of the interstitial markings to the periphery, perpendicular to the pleura on plain x-ray. *B* and *C,* High-resolution CT appearance of Kerley B lines, or septal lines. Cascading polygons correspond to thickened interlobular septa surrounding the secondary pulmonary lobule.

16. **Name the four most common entities that demonstrate septal lines on HRCT.**
    Interstitial pulmonary edema and **alveolar proteinosis** will show smooth thickening of the interlobular septa. **Lymphangitic spread of tumor** may have smooth or nodular septal lines on the background of normal lung architecture. **Sarcoidosis** can have a variable appearance but will show a nodular pattern of interlobular septal thickening when the disease is active.

17. **What is bronchiectasis? Is it related to atelectasis?**
    Bronchiectasis is irreversible bronchial dilatation. Acute atelectasis is focal alveolar collapse and is typically reversible. Chronic atelectasis, however, can lead to scarring and bronchiectasis.

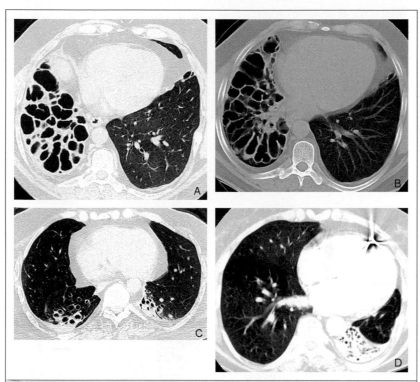

Figure 10-8. *A* and *B,* Cystic bronchiectasis. Marked bronchial dilatation with obliteration of normal lung parenchyma in a patient with chronic bronchitis and necrotizing *Klebsiella* infection, respectively. *C,* Cylindrical bronchiectasis. Mild dilatation of the bronchi in the bilateral lower lobes. *D,* Another example of cylindrical bronchiectasis in a patient with a history of tuberculosis.

18. **What are the different types of bronchiectasis? Do they differ in the degree of severity?**
    - **Cylindrical bronchiectasis** is the mildest form, showing minimal dilation of the bronchi with straight, regular wall thickening.
    - **Varicose bronchiectasis**, similar in severity to the cylindrical type, appears more irregular and is usually secondary to a postobstructive process.
    - **Cystic or saccular bronchiectasis** is the most severe form, secondary to ulceration and can demonstrate air-fluid levels.
    See Fig. 10-8.

19. **What are the causes of bronchiectasis?**
    - Congenital conditions, such as Kartagener's syndrome, in which impaired ciliary function leads to growth arrest of the bronchi
    - Chronic or prolonged infection
    - Obstruction, such as after repeated foreign body aspiration or instrumentation

20. **What is the signet ring sign?**
    A thick-walled bronchus larger in diameter than the adjacent pulmonary artery branch. The signet ring sign is pathognomonic for bronchiectasis (Fig. 10-9).

21. **What is honeycombing? What is its pathologic origin? What is its significance?**
Thick-walled air-containing spaces replace normal alveoli. These spaces are usually less than 1 cm in diameter and frequently are layered in a peripheral or subpleural location. Honeycombing signifies chronic lung disease and nearly all patients with end-stage pulmonary fibrosis will have honeycombing on HRCT (Fig. 10-10).

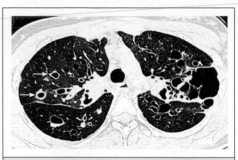

Figure 10-9. The signet ring sign *(arrows)* in a patient with bronchiectasis, particularly in the right lower lobe. The thickened bronchial wall in cross section makes up the band of the ring. The relatively small pulmonary artery, in comparison to the accompanying bronchiole's diameter, corresponds to the signet or a gemstone. Normally, the diameters of the bronchiole and the pulmonary artery are the same.

22. **Why does bronchiolar dilatation give a "tree-in-bud" appearance on HRCT?**
The dilated centrilobular bronchiole fills with mucus or pus (Fig. 10-11).

23. **What is "ground-glass" opacity? Is it a specific to a certain disease? Why is it important?**
Homogeneous granular haziness or increase in lung parenchyma density that resembles the appearance of ground glass. Vessels remain visible in the area. Ground-glass opacity is a nonspecific finding on CT; however, its presence should prompt quick patient evaluation and treatment because ground glass is seen in the majority of acute, reversible, interstitial diseases (Fig. 10-12).

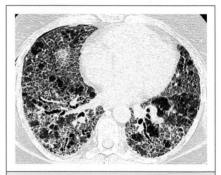

Figure 10-10. Honeycombing. Thick-walled, air-filled cysts of variable diameter, usually less than 1 cm.

24. **What is "dependent density"?**
Dependent density is a normal finding. It is a band of ground-glass opacity abutting the posterior pleura in a supine patient, which corresponds to partial atelectasis of the dependent lung. This resolves on prone imaging. Interstitial fibrosis does not resolve with positional changes.

25. **How can you best distinguish ground-glass opacity from consolidation?**
Consolidation obscures the pulmonary vessels. Air bronchograms (air in bronchi surrounding by consolidated lung) are usually present in consolidative processes (Fig. 10-13).

26. **Define pulmonary nodule.**
A pulmonary nodule is a spherical lung lesion ranging from 1 mm to 3 cm in diameter.

27. **What are the most common distributions of pulmonary nodules associated with *systemic* disease?**
They are random, perilymphatic, and centrilobular.

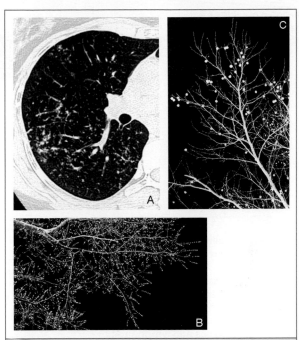

Figure 10-11. *A,* High-resolution CT of a patient with endobronchial tuberculosis demonstrates dilated fluid-filled bronchioles in the pattern of a "tree-in-bud." *B,* A photograph of a botanical tree "in bud," printed in reverse. Each bud contains the leaf and flower for the coming season. The tree is "in bud" in the early spring when the buds start to swell before opening. *C,* Note the difference between the photographs of tree-in-bud and a different botanical tree-in-fruit. The fruit are on twigs and so have a variable relationship to the branches on this projection image. The tree-in-fruit is equivalent to metastases, which have a variable relationship to the bronchioles. (Figures *B* and *C* courtesy of Kathryn Strang.)

KEY POINTS: ENTITIES WITH A "TREE-IN-BUD" APPEARANCE ON HRCT

1. Endobronchial *Mycobacterium tuberculosis*

2. Atypical mycobacterial infection (e.g., *Mycobacterium avium*)

3. Cystic fibrosis

4. Bronchopneumonia

5. Panbronchiolitis

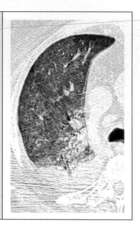

Figure 10-12. Diffuse ground-glass opacity indicating a reversible condition; in this case, congestive heart failure.

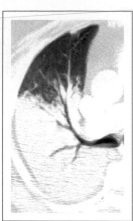

Figure 10-13. Diffuse haziness in the anterior right upper lobe—ground-glass opacity in pulmonary edema. Note visualization of the vessels through the abnormal lung. In contrast, the posterior right upper lobe is consolidated. Note nonvisualization of the vessels, but air bronchograms are present. There is not volume loss, distinguishing this case with air-space filling (consolidation) from cases with air- loss (atelectasis).

28. **Calcified multifocal pulmonary nodules are most commonly associated with what group of diseases?**
   They are most commonly associated with granulomatous diseases, such as tuberculosis or sarcoidosis.

29. **Can you reliably distinguish between hematogenous metastases and lymphangitic spread of tumor on HRCT?**
   No. However, each has specific characteristics, which can help to differentiate them. Lymphangitic metastases typically have interlobular thickening, are more commonly unilateral, and are sometimes associated with lymphadenopathy and a unilateral pleural effusion. Hematogenous metastases are usually bilateral, diffuse to peripheral, and nodular without significant interlobular thickening.

30. **Is bronchioloalveolar carcinoma primarily seen as consolidation or nodules? What is its distribution?**
   It can be seen as both a diffuse, patchy, or multifocal consolidation or ill-defined centrilobular nodules or a mixture of both.

31. **What is the typical presentation of the idiopathic interstitial pneumonias?**
   Chronic interstitial pneumonia commonly presents in a 40- to 60-year-old patient with dyspnea and idiopathic cough.

32. **Are usual interstitial pneumonia (UIP) and desquamative interstitial pneumonia (DIP) part of the same disease continuum?**
   No. However, both UIP and DIP are classified as idiopathic interstitial pneumonias (IIPs). UIP has a gradual, deteriorating course and is less responsive to treatment. UIP progresses to IPF, an end-stage lung disease, with an average survival of 3 years after diagnosis. DIP, on the other hand, is more insidious, is responsive to corticosteroids, and has a median survival of about 12 years. DIP is also a more diffuse process (Fig. 10-14).

33. **Describe four classic findings of IPF.**
   - *Intralobular* and *interlobular* interstitial thickening
   - Subpleural and peripheral honeycombing and bronchiectasis

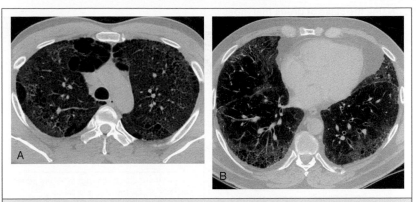

Figure 10-14. *A,* A smoker with emphysema and desquamative interstitial pneumonia, a potentially reversible condition, showing bilateral ground-glass opacities. *B,* Subpleural honeycombing in a patient with usual interstitial pneumonia. Note the lower lobe involvement. (Figures courtesy of Robert White, MD.)

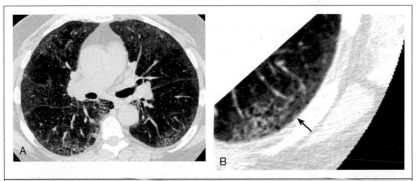

Figure 10-15. *A,* Early changes of IPF. Note patchy, asymmetric distribution, interlobular thickening (nicely seen along fissures), and honeycombing. *B,* Fine, subpleural, reticular pattern consistent with intralobular interstitial thickening.

- Basal lung predominance
- Eventual volume loss

See Fig. 10-15.

34. **How do the pulmonary manifestations of collagen vascular disease resemble those of IPF?**
    Rheumatoid arthritis, scleroderma, and mixed connective tissue disease have the same distribution and abnormalities as IPF, and they may also demonstrate pleural thickening (Fig. 10-16).

35. **What interstitial pneumonia is seen in immunocompromised patients?**
    Lymphocytic interstitial pneumonia (LIP), an uncommon interstitial lung disease that is prelymphomatous. Up to 70% of children with human immunodeficiency virus (HIV) will have LIP.

36. **What is the most common interstitial disease seen in children?**
    Frequencies of the types of interstitial lung disease in children are as follows: 25% idiopathic, 20% interstitial pneumonias, such as LIP, 10% infection, 10% environmental, and 10% lymphoproliferative disorders.

37. **Name the class of drugs that most frequently causes pulmonary fibrosis.**

Chemotherapeutic agents. Particularly, methotrexate, bleomycin, cyclophosphamide, and busulfan. Antibiotics, such as nitrofurantoin, are the second most common class.

38. **What lung findings suggest toxicity from the antiarrhythmic drug amiodarone?**

High-attenuation nodules, masses, or consolidation without the presence of calcification. (Amiodarone is high attenuation because it contains iodine.) The finding of increased density in the liver from the drug-laden macrophages is also helpful in making the diagnosis.

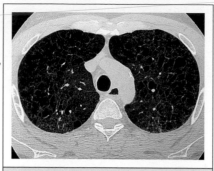

Figure 10-16. Similar findings to IPF in a patient with progressive systemic sclerosis. Cystic transformation of lung parenchyma leading to diffuse interstitial fibrosis. Note also the air-fluid level in the dilated esophagus, typical of scleroderma. (Figure courtesy of Robert White, MD.)

39. **What is the threshold of exposure for the development of radiation pneumonitis?**

The exposure threshold is 30–40 Gray, the equivalent skin dose of 32,000 posteroanterior (PA) chest radiographs.

40. **What is the distribution of radiation injury to the lung?**

Radiation injury is usually confined to radiation port, typically the upper lungs and adjacent to the mediastinum, and occurs approximately 3 weeks following treatment. Acute pneumonitis will appear as ground-glass consolidation and progresses to radiation fibrosis, bronchiectasis, and dense consolidation over the next 6 months to a year (Fig. 10-17).

41. **What does BOOP stand for?**

BOOP stands for bronchiolitis obliterans organizing pneumonia, caused by connective tissue masses filling the terminal bronchioles and alveoli. Radiologically, unilateral or bilateral consolidations can be seen.

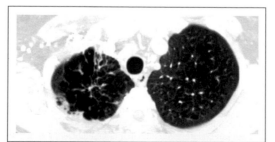

Figure 10-17. Radiation injury. Right upper lobe disease after remote radiotherapy to the right mediastinum for metastatic adrenal carcinoma. Note the overall volume loss, streaky opacities medially, and pleural thickening and consolidative changes peripherally. The left upper lobe is normal.

42. **How do you distinguish cysts from honeycombing?**
A cyst is an air-containing lesion with a diameter of greater than 1 cm and a wall thickness of less than 2 mm. Honeycomb lesions also contain air but are smaller in diameter and have a wall thickness greater than 2 mm.

43. **What is the difference between a bulla and a bleb? Why is this clinically significant?**
Both are air spaces. A bulla is an intra-parenchymal epithelial-lined air space, greater than 1 cm in diameter with a 1-mm thick wall. A bleb is an air collection within the layers of the pleura that does not have an epithelial lining and is usually seen at the lung apex. The difference is largely semantic, and *bulla* is the generally preferred term. However, subpleural blebs can cause spontaneous pneumothorax (Fig. 10-18).

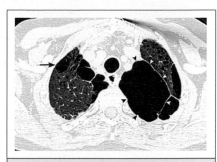

Figure 10-18. Large bilateral upper lobe bullae *(arrowheads)* and blebs *(arrow)*. Bullae are epithelial-lined spaces, and blebs are air collections between the layers of the pleura.

44. **Is emphysema permanent?**
Yes. The abnormal enlargement of air-spaces and destruction of air-space walls is caused by an imbalance of proteases and antiproteases and is permanent.

45. **Which type of emphysema is most common? Which is most frequently seen in smokers?**
Small air-space lucencies in the upper lungs characterize centrilobular emphysema, the subtype most frequently seen in the general population and in smokers.

46. **How can emphysema be distinguished from cystic lung disease?**
Emphysema on HRCT demonstrates lucent areas *without* discernible walls.

47. **What are the most frequently seen cystic lung diseases?**
IPF, lymphangiomyomatosis (LAM), and Langerhans' cell histiocytosis or eosinophilic granu-loma (EG) are the most frequent cystic lung diseases.

48. **What is LAM?**
LAM is an uncommon condition that occurs almost exclusively in women of childbearing age. They present with dyspnea and spontaneous pneumothorax. Imaging shows cysts produced by the growth of immature smooth muscle around bronchioles and lymphatics. The cysts are uniformly distributed and meas-ure 2 mm to 5 cm in diameter (Fig. 10-19). Large, recurrent, chylous (triglyceride-containing) pleural effusions are also seen. Chylous effusions can be fat density but are often indistinguishable in attenuation from other types of pleural effusions.

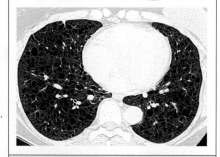

Figure 10-19. Lymphangiomyomatosis. Diffuse bilateral symmetric cysts, approximately 1 cm in size.

49. **What nonneoplastic lung diseases affect smokers more frequently than nonsmokers?**
    - **Centrilobular emphysema is more frequent.**
    - **EG:** 90% of patients diagnosed are young or middle-aged smokers. This cystic lung disease affects the upper lobes and spares the costophrenic angles.
    - **DIP:** 90% of patients are smokers.
    - **Giant bullous emphysema:** Most patients are young male smokers. It affects the upper lobes and can involve a large volume of the hemithorax.

50. **How does sarcoidosis typically present?**
    At least 50% of patients are asymptomatic. If symptomatic, the patient will often present with flu-like symptoms. Patients are typically 20–40 years of age.

51. **What is the etiology of sarcoidosis?**
    Noncaseating granulomas are found in sarcoidosis.

52. **Describe three different HRCT appearances of sarcoidosis.**
    - Small, perilymphatic nodules from the hila to pleura
    - Large nodules with consolidation
    - Large fibrous tissue masses with bronchiectasis, particularly in upper lobes and associated with volume loss (Fig. 10-20)

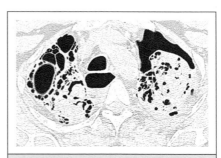

Figure 10-20. End-stage sarcoidosis. Bi-apical bronchiectasis and large areas of lung fibrosis with associated volume loss. Note left pneumothorax.

53. **What fraction of patients affected by sarcoidosis have lymphadenopathy?**
    At least 75% will have mediastinal or hilar lymphadenopathy during the disease course.

54. **What chronic granulomatous disease has nearly identical findings and histology to sarcoidosis?**
    Berylliosis, caused by inhalation of beryllium particles, also demonstrates ground-glass opacity, parenchymal nodules, and septal lines. Workers employed in aviation, electronics, the oil industry, and nuclear production are particularly at risk.

55. **What is "crazy paving"? In which lung disease is it characteristically visualized?**
    Geographic (well-delineated from normal tissue) ground-glass opacity with localized interlobular septal thickening. Pulmonary alveolar proteinosis causes bilateral, symmetric filling of alveoli with lipid-rich proteinaceous material. The majority of cases arise in smokers.

56. **How does crazy paving differ from mosaic perfusion?**
    The major difference is that thick walls delineate the regional abnormalities in a crazy paving pattern. Mosaic perfusion does not show this interlobular thickening (Fig. 10-21).

57. **What is the role of HRCT in detection of occupational lung disease?**
    HRCT is helpful in finding evidence of disease in the symptomatic patient with a clinical history of exposure but with a normal chest x-ray.

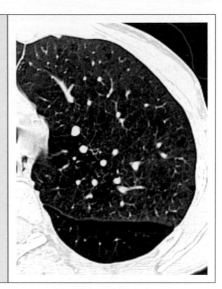

Figure 10-21. Differential, or "mosaic," perfusion in a patient with α_1-antitrypsin deficiency. This genetic disorder causes emphysematous changes in young and middle-aged white adults. The bases are more severely affected in α_1-antitripsyn deficiency, as opposed to the apices in tobacco-related emphysema. The oligemic area of thinned vessels and parenchymal hyperlucency in the left lower lobe is sharply demarcated from the better-vascularized, less diseased upper lobe.

58. How common are subpleural nodules in occupational lung disease?
They are seen in 80% of patients with silicosis or pneumoconiosis.

59. What causes coal worker's pneumoconiosis (CWP)?
Coal dust alone causes simple CWP. On HRCT, small nodules (< 7 mm in diameter) or areas of fibrosis development into focal emphysema. Lamellar, or "eggshell," calcification is seen in the mediastinal and hilar lymph nodes. Complicated CWP or progressive massive fibrosis (PMF) is caused by coincident silica and coal dust exposure. Large fibrous tissue masses form from the upper lung periphery toward the hila, cavitate, and necrose leaving residual large bullae.

60. How does silicosis appear on HRCT?
Silicosis appears as 1- to 10-mm variably calcified nodules in upper lungs.

61. Why is it best to perform an HRCT scan of a patient with suspected asbestosis in a prone position?
Asbestosis affects the posterior lung, which is not well evaluated with the patient in the supine position when the dependent lung tends to collapse. Subpleural and interstitial septal lines, parenchymal bands, parietal pleural thickening, and honeycombing are common findings.

62. How can hypercalcemia present on HRCT?
Interstitial calcifications present in the lung parenchyma. It can be seen in chronic renal failure and secondary hyperparathyroidism.

BIBLIOGRAPHY

1. American Thoracic Society: American Thoracic Society/European Respiratory Society International Multidisciplinary Consensus Classification of the Idiopathic Interstitial Pneumonias. Am J Respir Crit Care Med 165:277–304, 2002.

2. Boiselle PM, McLoud TC: Thoracic Imaging: Case Review St. Louis, Mosby, 1999, pp. 45–46, 55–58, 121–124.

3. Demedts M, Wells AU, Anto JM, et al: Interstitial lung disease: An epidemiological overview. Eur Resp J 18:2S–16S, 2001.

4. Gavin JR, D'Alessandro MP: Normal anatomy and the secondary lobule. In Diagnosis of Diffuse Lung Disease. Virtual Hospital. Mosby, 2004. Available at http://www.rh.org/adult/provider/radiology/DiffuseLung/DiffuseLung.html

5. Hagood JS: Interstitial lung disease in children. E-medicine.com, 2002. Available at http://www.emedicine.com/ped/topic1950.htm

6. Hansell DM: High-resolution computed tomography of the lung. In Armstrong P, Wilson AG, Dee P, Hansell DM (eds): Imaging of Diseases of the Chest, 3rd ed. St. Louis, Mosby, 2000, pp 133–161.

7. Hayton AS, Klein JS: Interstitial lung disease. In Brant WE, Helms CA: Fundamentals of Diagnostic Radiology, 2nd ed. Philadelphia, Lippincott, Williams & Wilkins, 1999, pp 415–455.

8. Mayberry JP, Primack SL, Müller NL: Thoracic Manifestations of Systemic Autoimmune Diseases: Radiographic and High-Resolution CT Findings. RadioGraphics 20:1623–1635, 2000.

9. McLoud TC: Thoracic Radiology: The Requisites. St. Louis, Mosby, 1998.

10. Muller NL: Differential diagnosis of chronic diffuse infiltrative lung disease on high resolution computed tomography. Semin Roentgenol 26:132–142, 1991.

11. Pallisa E, Roman A, Majo J, et al: Lymphangioleiomyomatosis: Pulmonary and abdominal findings with pathologic correlation. Radiographics 22:S185–S198, 2002.

12. Raghu G, Brown KK: Interstitial lung disease: clinical evaluation and keys to an accurate diagnosis. Clin Chest Med 25:409–419, 2004.

13. Ryu JH, Myers JL, Swensen SJ: Bronchiolar disorders. Am J Resp Crit Care Med 168:1277–1292, 2003.

14. University of Virginia: On-line high-resolution CT tutorial: www.med-ed.virginia.edu/courses/rad/hrct

15. Webb WR: Lung disease. In Webb WR, Brant WE, Helms CA (eds): Fundamentals of Body CT, 2nd ed. Philadelphia, W.B. Saunders, 1998, pp 107–145.

16. Webb WR, Muller NL, Naidich DP: High-resolution CT of the Lung, 2nd ed. Philadelphia, Lippincott-Raven, 1996.

17. Weissleder R, Wittenberg J, Harisinghani MG: Chest imaging. In Weissleder R, Wittenberg J, Harisinghani MG (eds): Primer of Diagnostic Imaging, 3rd ed. St. Louis, Mosby, 2003, pp 1–104.

PNEUMOCONIOSES

Andrea Zynda-Weiss, MD

CHAPTER 11

1. What are the pneumoconioses?
Pneumoconioses are a diverse group of occupationally acquired respiratory disorders secondary to inhalation of various particles. They are characterized by a tissue reaction to the presence of inhaled dust in the lungs. The most common are silicosis, coal workers' pneumoconiosis (CWP), siderosis, and asbestos-related disease.

2. Describe the clinical presentation and prognosis of the pneumoconiosis.
Because the pneumonoconioses are a group of diseases, they present with a wide spectrum of clinical symptoms. The prognosis depends on the specific particle inhaled and the duration and degree of exposure.

3. What is the pathology of pneumoconiosis?
One form of pneumoconiosis is characterized by fibrosis, which can be focal nodular or diffuse. Examples includes silicosis (focal nodular) and asbestosis (diffuse). This can lead to significant functional impairment. Another form of pneumoconiosis is due to particle-laden macrophages with little or no fibrosis, such as seen with iron, tin, or barium. This form results in little, if any, functional impairment.

4. What is the International Labour Organization Classification of Pneumoconioses?
The International Labour Organization Classification of Pneumoconioses (Table 11-1) is designed to standardize the description of pneumoconioses findings on chest radiographs in a reproducible manner. It includes descriptions of opacities, zones, and profusion (severity).

5. What is silicosis?
Silicosis is a fibrotic lung disease due to the inhalation of silicon dioxide or free crystalline silica dust found in quartz.

6. What occupations are associated with silicosis?
Workers are exposed to silica in any mining, quarrying, and tunneling occupation because silica is a primary constituent of rock. Silicosis is seen in stonecutting, polishing, and cleaning monumental masonry. Sandblasting, which is the firing of sand particles to resurface metal, exposes workers to large quantities of silica dust. Glass manufacturing, ceramic manufacturing, porcelain and pottery manufacturing, brick lining, boiler scaling, and vitreous enameling all have occupational exposure. Coal workers are exposed to dust containing silica in addition to coal and other minerals.

7. What are the forms of silicosis?
There are three forms of silicosis: chronic simple, complicated, and acute silicoproteinosis.

8. What are the histologic findings in silicosis?
Silicotic nodules consist of discrete, whorled, hyalinized, fibrotic nodules sharply separated from the surrounding lung tissue. They occur primarily in the peribronchiolar regions and in the paraseptal and subpleural tissues.

TABLE 11-1. INTERNATIONAL LABOUR ORGANIZATION CLASSIFICATION OF PNEUMOCONIOSES

Feature	Classification
Small round opacities	P: Up to 1.5 mm Q: 1.5–3 mm R: 3–10 mm
Small irregular opacities	S: Fine T: Medium U: Coarse
Large opacities	A: 1–5 cm B: >5 cm but less than equivalent of right upper lung zone C: Larger than equivalent of right upper lung zone
Profusion (severity)	0: Small opacities absent or minimal 1: Few small opacities present with normal lung markings seen 2: Numerous opacities with partial obscuration of normal lung markings 3: Innumerable small opacities with total obscuration of normal lung markings
Pleural thickening	Diffuse Circumscribed
Zones	Upper Middle Lower

9. **What is simple chronic silicosis?**

   Chronic simple silicosis is seen 10–20 years after exposure to silica dust and is characterized by fibrotic nodules. There are no significant changes in pulmonary function.

10. **What diseases are associated with silicosis?**

    Silicosis is associated with an increased prevalence of connective tissue diseases including progressive systemic sclerosis, rheumatoid arthritis, Caplan's syndrome, and systemic lupus erythematosus.

11. **What are the imaging features of simple silicosis?**

    Simple silicosis is characterized by small, well-circumscribed 1- to 10-mm nodules predominately involving the upper and posterior lung zones. The right upper lung zone is particularly involved due to regional differences in lymphatic flow. Nodules may be centrilobular in location. Subpleural nodules may aggregate to form pseudoplaque.

    The nodules may calcify centrally. Hilar and mediastinal adenopathy with eggshell calcifications may be present (Fig. 11-1).

12. **What are the characteristics of complicated silicosis? What is progressive massive fibrosis?**

    The appearance of large, conglomerate masses of confluent areas of fibrosis characterizes complicated silicosis, also known as progressive massive fibrosis. Clinical symptoms of cough and dyspnea appear. Tuberculosis (TB) may be superimposed.

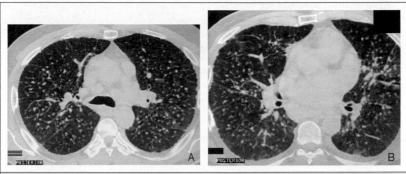

Figure 11-1. *A* and *B,* Multiple discrete small nodules of silicosis. (Courtesy of Richard White, MD.)

13. **What are the imaging features of complicated silicosis?**

   CT demonstrates confluent opacities (>1 cm) especially in the mid to upper lung zones and extending to the hilum. Overinflated emphysematous lung tissue is seen in the surrounding lung, especially at the bases and between the mass and pleura. Cavitation may occur due to ischemic necrosis. The masses can be bilateral, symmetric, and calcified. Hilar and mediastinal adenopathy with eggshell calcifications may also be present (Fig. 11-2).

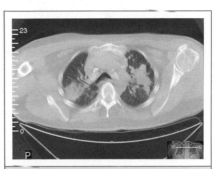

Figure 11-2. Conglomerate masses in silicosis. (Courtesy of Richard White, MD.)

14. **What is acute silicoproteinosis?**

   Silicoproteinosis occurs after heavy exposure to free silica in enclosed spaces in a short period of time, in as little as a few weeks. It is rapidly progressive with death due to respiratory failure. Pathologically it is characterized by proliferation of type II pneumocytes and alveoli filled with eosinophilic, periodic acid–Schiff (PAS)-positive lipid-rich exudates.

15. **What is the radiographic appearance of acute silicosis?**

   High-resolution CT (HRCT) demonstrates diffuse ground-glass opacities and air space consolidation. There may be a perihilar distribution. A "crazy paving" pattern may be present with patchy areas of ground-glass opacities with fine intralobular reticulations. The findings are identical to alveolar proteinosis. Acute silicosis can be complicated by TB and atypical mycobacterial infection.

16. **Is HRCT superior to conventional CT in evaluating silicosis?**

   HRCT has been shown to be superior to conventional CT and chest radiographs in evaluating silicosis. HRCT can provide information about the stage of the disease by demonstrating coalescence of nodules before they are apparent on chest radiographs. Functional impairment corresponds to the severity of emphysema rather than the severity of nodular opacities. HRCT can also help detect superimposed conditions such as bronchogenic carcinoma or TB.

17. **What is coal workers pneumoconiosis (CWP)?**

   CWP is due to inhalation of coal dust by underground miners.

18. **What are the forms of CWP?**
    There are two forms: simple and complicated.

19. **What are the histologic findings in CWP?**
    The basic lesion of simple CWP is the coal macule, which is similar to a silicotic nodule without a hyaline center and laminated collagen. Bronchioles are distended causing focal emphysema. In complicated CWP, there are large opacities consisting of collagen, free pigment, pigment-laden macrophages, proteinaceous material, and calcium phosphates. There may be central necrosis due to ischemia.

20. **What are the imaging findings in simple CWP?**
    The findings are very similar to simple silicosis. There are small pulmonary nodules with an upper lung zone predominance. The pulmonary nodules may be less well defined than those in silicosis, but this is not always the case. The nodules may form subpleural aggregates. There may be hilar and mediastinal adenopathy with eggshell calcifications.

21. **What is complicated CWP?**
    Complicated CWP is characterized by progressive massive fibrosis and may occur due to concurrent exposure to silica. It is associated with respiratory impairment and premature death.

22. **What are the imaging findings of complicated CWP?**
    Complicated CWP is identical to complicated silicosis radiologically. Masses with irregular borders, distortion of the pulmonary parenchyma, and cicatricial emphysematous changes are seen. Masses are >1 cm with upper and posterior lung predominance. Interstitial pulmonary fibrosis is not a prominent feature of CWP. Cavitation may occur and can be complicated by infections including TB and aspergillosis.

23. **What other conditions may develop in coal workers?**
    Coal miners develop emphysema, with centrilobular emphysema being the most common type. Scar emphysema may develop around progressive massive fibrosis lesions.

24. **What is Caplan's syndrome?**
    Caplan's syndrome is a form of rheumatoid lung disease in which rheumatoid nodules are superimposed on simple silicosis or CWP. It is more common in CWP. The pulmonary findings may precede the development of arthritis.

25. **What are the radiologic findings in Caplan's syndrome?**
    Large nodules ranging from 0.5–5 cm are seen, especially in the upper lobes and periphery. These may calcify and cavitate.

26. **What is siderosis?**
    Siderosis is pneumoconiosis due to the inhalation of dust containing a large amount of iron. Fibrosis and functional impairment are not seen, unless the iron is mixed with a large amount of silica.

27. **What occupations are associated with siderosis?**
    The following occupations are associated with siderosis: arc welders, workers who cut/burn steel, workers who mine and process iron ore, iron and steel rolling mill workers, foundry workers, and silver polishers.

28. **What are the imaging findings in siderosis?**
    Pure siderosis is characterized by diffuse fine reticulonodular opacities that are less dense and less profuse than in silicosis. The nodules are centrilobular, widespread, and poorly defined with

branching linear structures. There can be extensive ground-glass attenuation without a zonal predominance. There is no fibrosis and no hilar adenopathy. The findings may completely resolve after the exposure is discontinued.

29. **What is chronic berylliosis?**
Berylliosis is a chronic granulomatous disorder due to exposure to dust, fumes, or aerosols of beryllium metal or its salts. It primarily involves the lungs but may also involve the liver, spleen, lymph nodes, bone marrow, and skin. Pathologically it is characterized by noncaseating granulomas indistinguishable from those of sarcoidosis.

30. **What occupations are associated with berylliosis?**
Beryllium is like aluminum and makes alloys with high heat resistance and improved hardness and stiffness. Exposure to beryllium can occur in manufacture of aircraft parts, electronics, undersea communication cables, fluorescent lamps, household appliances, air conditioners, electric ranges, and x-ray tubes. Beryllium is used to make the windows of x-ray tubes because it does not absorb x-rays.

31. **What are the imaging characteristics of chronic berylliosis?**
The findings closely resemble those of sarcoidosis. Most commonly there are small nodules or reticulonodular opacities involving all lung zones. The nodules may be very small (<2 mm) producing a granular appearance. There may be prominent thickening of the bronchovascular bundles with thin- and thick-walled cysts and traction bronchiectasis. Conglomerate masses may develop. Hilar adenopathy is common. Pulmonary fibrosis and emphysematous bullae may develop in long-standing disease.

32. **What is acute berylliosis?**
Acute berylliosis is characterized by pulmonary edema due to a chemical pneumonitis after a brief overwhelming exposure.

33. **What is asbestos?**
Asbestos is a material with high heat and acid resistance that was widely used as a durable, fireproof material in various industries and construction. The fire-resistant qualities of asbestos were known even in the 13th century. However, Europeans believed the fibers came from a salamander that lived in fire. During his travels in China, Marco Polo learned that the fibers were a mineral mined in China and used to make fireproof cloth. Asbestos continued to be used in numerous ways large and small (the burning broom in *The Wizard of Oz*) until the last portion of the 20th century when its carcinogenic effects were fully recognized. There are many private legal web sites with information on the history of asbestos.

34. **What occupations are associated with asbestos-related disease?**
The two major sources of exposure are primary occupations of asbestos mining and processing and secondary occupations such as insulation manufacturing, textile manufacturing, construction, shipbuilding, and manufacture and repair of gaskets and brake linings.

35. **What are the forms of asbestos-related disease?**
Asbestos-related diseases can be divided into pleural and parenchymal disease. Pleural manifestations include benign pleural disease and malignant mesothelioma. Parenchymal manifestations include asbestosis, rounded atelectasis, and bronchogenic carcinoma. There is a 20-year latency between the initial exposure and the development of asbestos-related disease.

36. **What are the benign pleural manifestations of asbestos-related disease?**
The most common manifestations of asbestos exposure are asymptomatic pleural plaques. They appear as bilateral, focal irregular areas of pleural thickening along the parietal pleura and

fissures. The posterolateral and diaphragmatic contours are most often involved with sparing of the apices. Calcification begins in the parietal pleural and may form within the center of plaques. Dense lines paralleling the chest wall, mediastinum, pericardium, and diaphragm are seen. Bilateral diaphragmatic calcifications with clear costophrenic angles are pathognomonic for asbestos-related disease. Pleural calcifications occur in more than 20% of asbestos-related disease after 20 years and in 40% after 40 years (Fig. 11-3).

Diffuse pleural thickening occurs less frequently. It appears as smooth, homogeneous, uninterrupted pleural density extending over one fourth of the chest wall, which may obliterate the costophrenic angles. Calcification is rare and extensive calcifications suggest other etiologies such as previous TB, empyema, or hemothorax. On CT, diffuse pleural thickening appears as a continuous area of pleural thickening greater than 3 cm thick, extending for more than 8 cm craniocaudal and 5 cm around the perimeter of the hemithorax. Diffuse pleural thickening is often symptomatic. This is a less specific finding for asbestos exposure because pleural thickening can be seen in many conditions including previous infection, connective tissue disease, hemothorax, pleural metastases, and other conditions. Subcostal fat may mimic pleural thickening on chest radiographs, but CT can easily differentiate them based on their densities.

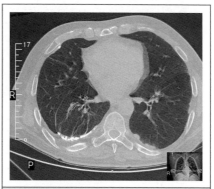

Figure 11-3. Asbestos-related pleural plaques. Note the calcified and noncalcified plaques, less than 1 cm in thickness. (Courtesy of Richard White, MD.)

Diffuse exudative pleural effusions can also be seen following asbestos exposure and may occur earlier than other manifestations of asbestos-related disease. They may be unilateral or bilateral.

37. What is asbestosis?

Asbestosis is pulmonary fibrosis that occurs in asbestos workers. Most workers have been exposed to high levels of dust for a prolonged period of time. There is a dose-effect relationship. A latency period of at least 20 years is seen. Asbestosis is symptomatic and associated with functional impairment.

38. What are the pathologic findings in asbestosis?

Pulmonary fibrosis begins in and around the respiratory bronchioles of the lower lobes adjacent to the visceral pleura. There may be diffuse interstitial fibrosis and honeycombing with destruction of the alveolar architecture. An intra-alveolar reaction similar to desquamative interstitial fibrosis occurs.

39. What are the radiographic findings in asbestosis?

Small linear or reticular opacities are seen at the lung bases. These can progress to honeycombing. The heart border is obscured by pleural and parenchymal changes ("shaggy" heart sign). Pleural plaques or thickening are often present. Hilar adenopathy is absent. The findings are similar to idiopathic pulmonary fibrosis.

40. What are the CT findings in asbestosis?

CT is superior to standard chest radiographs in the characterization of parenchymal abnormalities and evaluation of early disease. Parenchymal abnormalities include curvilinear subpleural lines, thickened interstitial short lines, subpleural dependent densities, parenchymal bands, and honeycombing. Curvilinear subpleural lines are parallel to and within 1 cm of the chest wall. Thickened interlobular septa consist of lines 1–2 cm in length in the peripheral lung extending to the pleura. Subpleural dependent densities border the dependent pleura. Parenchymal bands are linear densities less than 5 cm long running through the parenchyma extending to the pleura. Honeycombing occurs in advanced disease. Ground-glass opacities can occur. Even in the presence of pleural plaques, the findings on HRCT are nonspecific and can be seen with other disease processes.

41. How is the diagnosis of asbestosis made?
Because the radiologic findings are nonspecific, the diagnosis is based on the combination of clinical, physiologic, and radiologic information in a patient with a history of asbestos exposure. Physical findings include bibasilar crackles and restrictive pulmonary function tests.

42. What are additional benign parenchymal lesions in asbestos-related disease?
Additional benign lesions are rounded atelectasis, benign fibrotic masses, and transpulmonary bands.

43. What is rounded atelectasis?
Rounded atelectasis is peripheral collapse in patients with pleural disease. It is also known as "atelectatic asbestos pseudotumor." The most common location is subpleural, posterior, or basal regions of the lower lobes. It is frequently bilateral. It appears as a 2.5- to 8-cm focal pleural mass abutting a region of pleural thickening. The mass has a curvilinear tail known as the "comet tail sign," which is produced by the crowding of the bronchovascular bundle producing a whorled appearance. There is always associated volume loss in the affected lobe. There may be partial interposition of the lung between the pleura and mass. The mass can also be wedge-shaped, lentiform, or irregular. The size remains stable or may decrease on serial examinations (Fig. 11-4).

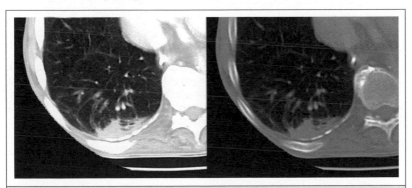

Figure 11-4. Round atelectasis is often associated with pleural thickening or pleural calcifications. The comet-tail sign is again seen.

44. What malignancies are associated with asbestos exposure?
Approximately 25% of heavily exposed asbestos workers will develop bronchogenic carcinoma. Asbestos exposure in smokers is associated with an 80–100 times increased risk of bronchogenic carcinoma compared with nonsmoking, nonexposed populations. Malignant mesothelioma is a rare tumor that occurs almost exclusively in asbestos workers. About 10% of asbestos workers will develop malignant mesothelioma, which has a latency of 20–40 years after asbestos exposure. There is also an increased incidence of gastric carcinoma in these patients.

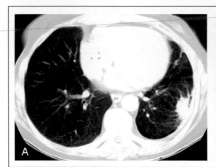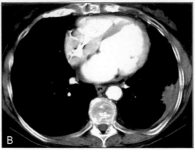

Figure 11-5. *A,* Asbestos exposure with pleural plaques. *B,* Rounded atelectasis. Note the vessels converging on the mass and the adjacent pleural thickening. The mass is formed by the thickened infolded pleura and pulls pulmonary parenchyma together. Differentiation from a lung carcinoma can be difficult. (Courtesy of Richard White, MD.)

45. **Are there distinguishing features of asbestos-related lung cancer?**
    Bronchogenic carcinoma related to asbestos exposure frequently occurs in the peripheral aspect of the lower lobes. However, it can occur in any location when associated with smoking. The lung cancer may occur in the setting of preexisting interstitial disease (Fig. 11-5).

46. **What is malignant mesothelioma?**
    Malignant mesothelioma is a rare tumor of the serosal lining of the pleural cavity, peritoneum, or both that occurs almost exclusively in asbestos workers. Family members of asbestos workers and people who reside near asbestos mines and plants are at increased risk of developing malignant mesothelioma from asbestos exposure. In addition to asbestos exposure, other risk factors for malignant mesothelioma include chronic inflammation, such as from TB or empyema, and irradiation. Benign mesothelioma is not associated with asbestos exposure.

47. **What are the radiologic findings of malignant mesothelioma?**
    Initial chest radiograph often demonstrates a unilateral pleural effusion. CT demonstrates thick (>1 cm), nodular, circumferential pleural thickening and mediastinal pleural involvement. The masses are typically greater than 5 cm thick, irregular, and lobulated. It can also present as a single, discrete pleural mass. Associated pleural plaques are seen in 50% of cases. Pleural calcifications are present in 20%. Tumor may extend into interlobular fissures and septa. Pleural effusion is seen in approximately 75%. Advanced cases demonstrate rib destruction and invasion of the chest wall, pericardium, diaphragm, and abdomen. Ascites can be present; the peritoneum is involved in 35% (Figs. 11-6 and 11-7).

48. **What is the differential diagnosis for malignant mesothelioma?**
    Pleural fibrosis from infection (e.g., TB, fungal infection, or actinomycosis), fibrothorax, empyema, and metastatic adenocarcinoma can have a similar appearance.

49. **What is stannosis?**
    Stannosis is a pneumoconiosis caused by inhalation of tin. Radiologic findings include high-density, small (1-mm) nodules distributed evenly throughout the lungs. The condition shows no functional impairment.

50. **What is barytosis?**
    Barytosis is pulmonary disease that develops secondary to exposure to barium dust and its salts. It produces extremely opaque discrete nodular densities in the mid lung zones, sparing the

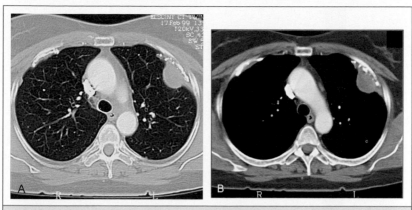

Figure 11-6. Focal malignant mesothelioma on lung *(A)* and soft tissue *(B)* windows. Differentiation from a pleural plaque is not easy. Most benign pleural plaques are less than 1 cm in thickness. (Courtesy Richard White, MD.)

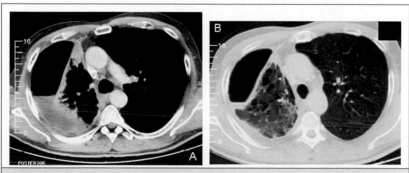

Figure 11-7. *A*, Irregular pleural thickening and loculated effusion in asbestos-exposed patient: malignant mesothelioma. *B*, Procedure-related pneumothorax. Differentiation from diffuse benign pleural plaques with effusion can sometimes be difficult and is an indication for pleural biopsy. The mediastinum does not shift away from the mass and effusion due to the retractile nature of the tumor. (Courtesy of Richard White, MD.)

apices and bases. The findings often regress after the worker is removed from the dust-filled environment.

51. What is hard metal pneumoconiosis?

Hard metal refers to an alloy of tungsten, carbon, cobalt, and other metals. Exposure to the dust occurs in the manufacture or use of the metal. Hard metal pneumoconiosis can cause interstitial pneumonia, desquamative interstitial pneumonia, or giant cell interstitial pneumonia. Giant cell interstitial pneumonia is almost pathognomonic for hard metal pneumoconiosis. The radiographic findings include diffuse micronodular and reticular disease. Lymph node enlargement may be seen. Small cystic spaces may be seen in advanced disease. Areas of ground-glass attenuation, consolidation, reticular hyperattenuating areas, and traction bronchiectasis are seen on HRCT (*see* Table 11-2).

TABLE 11-2. SUMMARY OF PNEUMOCONIOSES

Disease	Occupations	Lung Zones	Pattern	Adenopathy	Functional Impairment
Simple silicosis	Mining, coal workers, sand blasting, glass makers	Upper posterior	Small nodules	Eggshell calcifications	No
Progressive massive fibrosis	Mining, coal workers, sand blasting, glass makers	Mid to upper; hilar	Large conglomerate masses	Eggshell calcifications	Yes
Acute silicoproteinosis	Mining, coal workers, sand blasting, glass makers	Perihilar	Crazy paving and ground-glass opacities	No	Yes—often fatal
Coal workers' pneumoconiosis	Coal miners	Upper posterior	Small nodules	Eggshell calcifications	No
Siderosis	Iron workers	Centrilobular	Diffuse fine reticulonodular	No	No
Chronic berylliosis	Aircraft parts, x-ray tubes, electronics manufacturing	All	Reticulonodular; small nodules	Hilar, calcified	Yes—may involve spleen, liver, nodes, marrow
Acute berylliosis	Aircraft parts, x-ray tubes, electronics manufacturing	All	Pulmonary edema		Yes
Stannosis	Tin workers	All	High-density 1-mm nodules	No	No

Barytosis	Barium	Mid lung	Very dense nodules		No
Hard metal pneumoconiosis	Hard metal manufacturing	Diffuse	Interstitial pneumonia; ground-glass opacities	Yes	Yes
Asbestos-related pleural plaques	Asbestos mining, construction, ship builders	Posterolateral parietal pleura, especially diaphragms	Pleural thickening and calcifications	No	No
Asbestos-related diffuse pleural thickening	Asbestos mining, construction, ship builders	Posteromedial lower lobes; costophrenic angles	Smooth uninterrupted thickening along chest wall	No	Yes
Asbestosis	Asbestos mining, construction, ship builders	Bases	Parenchymal bands, curvilinear subpleural lines, honeycombing, reticulonodular opacities	No	Yes
Malignant mesothelioma	Asbestos mining, construction, ship builders	Mediastinal pleura	Pleural thickening with mediastinal involvement, thick masses, pleural effusion		Yes

KEY POINTS: PNEUMOCONIOSES

1. Pneumoconioses are occupationally acquired diseases due to particulate inhalation. The fact that they are occupationally acquired leads to a high political and legal profile.

2. There is an International Labour Organization grading of pulmonary findings in pneumoconioses.

3. CWP, silicosis, and asbestos-related diseases are the most important pneumoconiosis.

4. Asbestos causes a range of pulmonary diseases including calcified pleural plaques (asbestos exposure), rounded atelectasis, asbestosis, and malignant mesothelioma and is a major risk factor for lung cancer.

BIBLIOGRAPHY

1. Dahnert W: Radiology Review Manual, 4th ed. Philadelphia, Lippincott, 2000.
2. Edwards M: Marco Polo in China. National Geographic June 2001, pp 20–45.
3. Kim KI, Kim CW, Lee MK, et al: Imaging of occupational lung disease. Radiographics 21:1371–1391, 2001.
4. McLoud T: The pneumoconioses. In Thoracic Radiology: The Requisites. St. Louis, Mosby, 1998, pp 227–247.
5. Oikonomou A, Muller NL: Imaging of pneumoconiosis. Imaging 15:11–22, 2003.

CHAPTER 12

CT OF MISCELLANEOUS THORACIC INFLAMMATORY CONDITIONS

Kalpesh Patel, MD, and John G. Strang, MD

1. **What are the components of the pulmonary interstitium?**
   - Axial compartment
   - Interlobar septa
   - Subpleural space
   - Alveolar walls

   Involvement of any one of these compartments by disease processes will give radiographic findings.

2. **What are the four general categories of CT appearance of lung diseases?**
   - Reticular opacities
   - Nodules and nodular opacities
   - Increased lung opacity
   - Decreased lung opacity

3. **What are the five pleuropulmonary abnormalities associated with rheumatoid disease?**
   - Pleurisy with or without effusion
   - Diffuse interstitial pneumonitis or fibrosis
   - Pulmonary (necrobiotic) nodules
   - Caplan's syndrome (pneumoconiotic nodules)
   - Pulmonary hypertension secondary to rheumatoid vasculitis

4. **What is the most common thoracic manifestation of rheumatoid disease?**
   Pleural involvement—pleurisy is the most common thoracic manifestation.

5. **What type of immunologic reaction is common in rheumatoid lung disease?**
   The most common immunologic reaction in rheumatoid lung disease is Type 3 immune complexes.

6. **What are the classic symptoms and signs of interstitium rheumatoid disease?**
   Progressive dyspnea. Pulmonary function tests show features of restrictive ventilatory impairment.

7. **Describe the typical interstitial lung pattern in rheumatoid lung.**
   - **Early stages:** Irregular linear hyperattenuating areas in a fine reticular pattern, usually involving the lower lung zones
   - **Later stages:** Reticular pattern becomes more coarse and diffuse, with eventual honeycombing

8. **True or false: The chest x-ray is normal in more than half of patients with rheumatoid lung.**
   The statement is true.

9. **What are the two most common conditions associated with interstitial fibrosis?**
   - Rheumatoid arthritis
   - Progressive systemic sclerosis (scleroderma)

10. **What musculoskeletal changes may be seen with rheumatoid arthritis?**
    - Resorption of the distal clavicles
    - Erosive arthritic changes

11. **What are the common findings on radiographs?**
    Lymph node enlargement, parenchymal abnormalities (sarcoid granulomas as nodules, fibrosis, bronchiectasis), or a combination of the two (Fig. 12-1) are common.

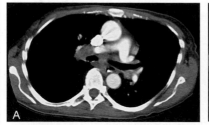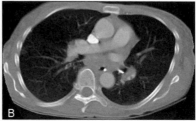

Figure 12-1. *A* and *B*, Sarcoidosis with mediastinal and hilar lymphadenopathy and innumerable small pulmonary nodules.

12. **What is the most frequent finding on chest x-ray?**
    The most frequent finding is bilateral hilar adenopathy (98%).

13. **Where are sarcoid granulomas located?**
    They are distributed primarily along the lymphatics. Therefore, they lie along the peribron-chovascular interstitium, the interlobular septa, and the subpleural interstitium. They can cavitate (Fig.12-2).

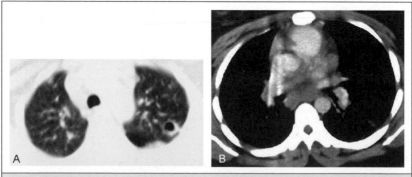

Figure 12-2. *A* and *B*, Chest CT shows multiple nodular opacities throughout the lungs, some of which have cavitated. Also present are mediastinal and hilar adenopathy.

14. **What is the characteristic distribution of fibrosis in late stage sarcoid?**
    The distribution is pronounced in the apical and posterior portions of the upper lobes and the superior segments of the lower lobes (Fig. 12-3).

15. **True or false: Sarcoidosis is unique in that it causes upper lobe bullous/fibrobullous disease.**
False. Other entities include ankylosing spondylitis, progressive massive fibrosis of silicosis, and emphysema.

16. **What are the stages of sarcoid on plain film?**
- **Stage 0:** Normal film (10%)
- **Stage 1:** Adenopathy (50%)
- **Stage 2:** Adenopathy with pulmonary opacities (30%)
- **Stage 3:** Pulmonary opacities without hilar adenopathy (10%)
- **Stage 4:** Pulmonary fibrosis, upper lobes with bullae

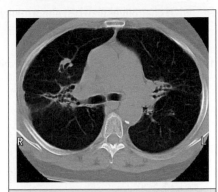

Figure 12-3. Sarcoidosis with hilar retraction and central traction bronchiectasis.

17. **What is the syndrome called when sarcoid is associated with fever and large joint arthralgia?**
This is called Lofgren syndrome.

18. **What tests can be used to assess sarcoid activity?**
- **Angiotensin-1 converting enzyme (ACE) titer**
- **Bronchopulmonary lavage:** Evaluating the number of T-suppressor lymphocytes
- **Gallium scan:** Indicator of macrophage activity

19. **True or false: The lung volumes are normal in sarcoid.**
True, in the early part of the disease. This may help narrow down the differential diagnosis. However, in the late stages the volume is decreased due to fibrosis.

20. **What is the most common radiographic manifestation of systemic lupus erythematosus (SLE)?**
The most common radiographic manifestation is unilateral or bilateral pleural effusions, frequently also with pericardial effusion.

21. **How would you differentiate SLE from rheumatoid disease or scleroderma?**
Pulmonary fibrosis is less common in SLE.

22. **What are the other radiographic clues for SLE?**
- Loss of lung volume secondary to diaphragmatic dysfunction
- Musculoskeletal changes related to renal failure and steroid therapy
- Tumoral calcinosis

23. **What are the most common symptoms with scleroderma?**
Dyspnea and dry, nonproductive cough are the most common symptoms.

24. **What is the most common CT finding of SLE?**
Pulmonary fibrosis (20–65%), usually with basilar predominance. Initially it appears as a fine reticular pattern that progresses to coarse reticulation and honeycombing.

25. **Is the prevalence of lung cancer increased with scleroderma?**
Yes, it is increased, particularly in scleroderma with pulmonary fibrosis.

26. What gastrointestinal (GI) abnormality do these patients have?
They have dilated esophagus, which may lead to aspiration (Fig. 12-4).

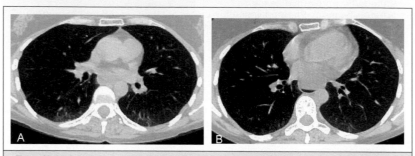

Figure 12-4. *A* and *B*, Posterior pulmonary fibrosis, with esophageal stricture. Also note the dilated esophagus secondary to systemic sclerosis.

27. What are the characteristics of Wegener's granulomatosis?
Characteristics of Wegener's granulomatosis are the disease triad of necrotizing vasculitis that involves the upper respiratory tract, the lungs, and the renal glomeruli.

28. What should come to mind when a middle-aged woman presents with hemoptysis and sinus disease?
Think Wegener's granulomatosis until proven otherwise.

29. What is the most frequent lung pattern in Wegener's granulomatosis?
Multiple rounded nodules or masses, generally well-defined, of various sizes. They may cavitate and are commonly bilateral and multiple (Fig. 12-5).

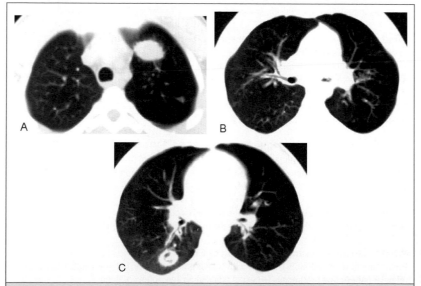

Figure 12-5. Cavitary sarcoidosis. CT shows multiple parenchymal masses. *A,* Cut-off of the left upper lobe bronchus. *B,* Thickening and irregularity of the left main stem bronchus and hyperlucency of the left lung due to air trapping. *C,* The right lower lobe mass is cavitated.

30. **What laboratory test can be useful to suggest Wegener's granulomatosis?**
    Antineutrophilic cytoplasmic antibody (c-ANCA) is useful.

31. **What is the most common vasculitis that produces a saddle-nose deformity?**
    Wegener's granulomatosis. Inflammation destroys the cartilage of the nose.

32. **What is the differential diagnosis for cystic lung disease?**
    - Lymphangioleiomyomatosis (LAM)
    - Tuberous sclerosis of the lung
    - Histocytosis X
    - Juvenile laryngotracheobronchial papillomatosis

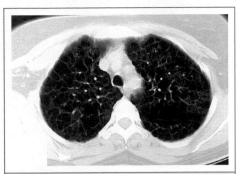

33. **What is the pathophysiology of LAM?**
    LAM is characterized by progressive proliferation of smooth muscle in the airways, arterioles, venules, and lymphatics of the lung, leading to progressive shortness of breath, lung cysts, pneumothorax, hemoptysis, and chylous effusion (Fig. 12-6).

Figure 12-6. Lymphangiomyomatosis. Diffuse, innumerable thin-walled cysts of various sizes scattered throughout all lung zones.

34. **What other pathologic disease has similar characteristics to LAM?**
    Tuberous sclerosis has similar characteristics.

35. **Do you see lung nodules in LAM?**
    No. The absence of lung nodules distinguishes LAM from eosinophilic granuloma of the lung.

36. **What is the most common complication of LAM?**
    Pneumothorax is the most common complication.

37. **What are the three types of histocytosis X?**
    - Letter-Siwe syndrome
    - Hand-Schüller-Christian syndrome
    - Eosinophilic granuloma (most commonly affects lungs)

38. **What is the characteristic appearance of cysts in the lung in histiocytosis X?**
    The cysts are usually less than 10 mm in diameter. They can attain bizarre and unusual shapes caused by paracicatricial emphysema. As in LAM, the interstitial patterns that appear on chest radiographs are actually innumerable overlapping lung cysts. In histiocytosis X, the cysts are usually absent in the lower lobes, whereas cysts are seen in the lower lobes with LAM.

39. **What are the common presenting complaints in patients with histocytosis X?**
    - Cough and dyspnea
    - Hemoptysis (5%)

40. **What toxic effect can amiodarone have on the lungs?**
    Amiodarone is an iodine-containing antiarrhythmic drug. In some patients, it accumulates in pulmonary macrophages and causes interstitial pneumonia, consolidation, and fibrosis (Fig. 12-7). It also accumulates in the liver and spleen.

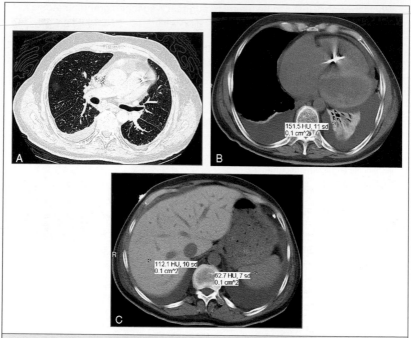

Figure 12-7. Amiodarone toxicity. **A,** High-resolution image through the mid-lung apex shows fine peripheral interstitial lines. **B,** Image through the collapsed lower lobe shows a dense lung secondary to iodine deposition. **C,** Note also the dense liver in this unenhanced CT.

41. **What toxic effect can bleomycin have on the lungs?**
    Bleomycin is an antibiotic and antineoplastic drug. It has lung toxicity in up to 40% of patients. The lung toxicity can be fatal. Although it can have a range of appearances and effects, the most common is chronic interstitial pneumonitis and fibrosis. The CT findings are a predominantly basal mix of ground-glass opacification and fibrotic lines (Fig. 12-8).

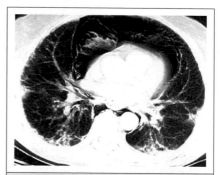

Figure 12-8. Bleomycin toxicity with extensive pulmonary fibrosis. In addition, there is a pneumomediastinum, possibly from mechanical ventilation.

42. **What is Goodpasture syndrome? What does it look like in the lungs?**
    Goodpasture syndrome is a pulmonary-renal syndrome with an anti-basement membrane antibody. It causes repeated episodes of pulmonary alveolar hemorrhage and glomerulonephritis. The pulmonary manifestations usually precede the renal manifestations. After an episode of pulmonary hemorrhage there is an acute alveolar infiltrate, which becomes reticulonodular and then clears in 10–12 days. With multiple episodes, hemosiderin becomes deposited and there is a pattern of chronic interstitial disease and 1- to 3-mm nodules, onto which acute hemorrhagic episodes are superimposed (Fig. 12-9).

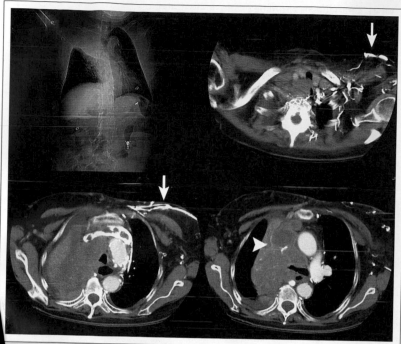

Figure 13-2. Lung cancer in a patient presenting with superior vena cava (SVC) syndrome. Note the chest wall and azygous collateral veins *(arrow)* and complete SVC obstruction *(arrowhead).*

lternative imaging study for staging. Because radiology is not pathology (some things that look e cancer are not, and some normal-sized nodes are sites of metastasis), it is often combined th mediastinoscopy for pathologic staging.

which type of lung cancer is the TNM classification *not* used?

ll cell lung cancer, which is considered metastatic at time of diagnosis. Small cell lung can-
s staged as either limited disease or extensive disease, which determines the role of radia-
herapy.

the TNM classification, what is the T staging?

Carcinoma in situ

alignant cytologic findings with no lesion observed

cm or smaller diameter and surrounded by lung or visceral pleura or endobronchial
distal to the lobar bronchus

meter greater than 3 cm; extension to the visceral pleura, atelectasis, or obstructive
pathy involving less than one lung; lobar endobronchial tumor; or tumor of a main
s more than 2 cm from the carina

al tumor; total atelectasis of one lung; endobronchial tumor of main bronchus within
he carina but not invading it; or tumor of any size with direct extension to the
structures, such as the chest wall mediastinal pleura, diaphragm, parietal peri-
r mediastinal fat of the phrenic nerve

n of the esophagus, trachea, carina, great vessels, recurrent laryngeal nerve,
dy, and/or heart; obstruction of the SVC; malignant pleural or pericardial effusion;
ulmonary nodules within the same lobe as the primary tumor

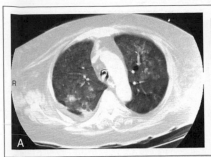
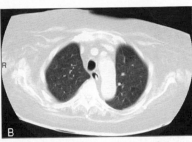

Figure 12-9. Goodpasture syndrome. *A,* Initial image during an acute hemorrhagic episode shows areas of ground-glass infiltrate and consolidation. *B,* On follow-up study 6 weeks later they have cleared.

KEY POINTS: THORACIC INFLAMMATORY CONDITIONS ✓

1. Sarcoidosis causes changes that include adenopathy and pulmonary nodules and interstitial lung disease. The appearance can be characteristic but also can mimic and needs to be differentiated from lung cancer.

2. Scleroderma causes esophageal dysmotility and characteristic basal and posterior fibrosis secondary to aspiration.

3. Wegener's granulomatosis causes pulmonary nodules, some cavitated. It must be differentiated from lung metastases.

BIBLIOGRAPHY

1. Dahnert W: Radiology Review Manual, 3rd ed. Baltimore, Lippincott, Williams & Wilkins, 1996.

2. Kim EA, Lee KS, Johkoh T, et al: Interstitial lung diseases associated with collagen vascular diseases: Radiologic and histopathologic findings. Radiographics 22(Suppl):S151–S165, 2002.

3. Mayberry JP, Primack SL, Muller NL: Thoracic manifestations of systemic autoimmune diseases: Radiographic and high resolution CT findings. Radiographics 20:1623–1635, 2000.

4. McLoud T: Thoracic Radiology Requisites. St. Louis, Mosby, 1998.

5. Muller N, Fraser R, Colman N, Pare P: Radiologic Diagnosis of Diseases of the Chest. Philadelphia, W.B. Saunders, 2001.

6. Stern EJ, Swensen SJ: High-resolution CT of the Chest. Philadelphia, Lippincott-Raven, 1996.

7. Webb WR, Muller N Naidich D: High-Resolution CT of the Lung, 2nd ed. Philadelphia, Lippincott-Raven, 1996.

8. Weissleder R, Rieumont MJ, Writtenburg J: Primer of Diagnostic Imaging, 2nd ed. St. Louis, Mosby, 1997.

CHAPTER 13

NEOPLASMS OF THE LUNG AND AIRWAY

Matthew Cham, MD, and John G. Strang, MD

1. How common is lung cancer?
Lung cancer is the leading cause of cancer mortality in men and women in the United States, surpassing breast cancer as the leading cause of cancer death in women since 1987. It is estimated that 1 in 13 men and 1 in 17 women will die of lung cancer.

2. If your institution provides imaging for a population of 250,000 people, how many new cases of lung cancer would be diagnosed per year?
Given the lung cancer incidence of 174,000 new cases in the U.S. population of 295 million, you would expect to find about 150 new lung cancer cases annually—almost three new cases per week!

3. How many people die of lung cancer per day?
In the United States, there are 160,000 lung cancer deaths each year, compared with 41,000 deaths in automobile accidents, 19,000 homicides, and 17,000 deaths due to acquired immunodeficiency syndrome (AIDS). On average, 420 Americans die from lung cancer each day—that is the equivalent of a Boeing 747 Jumbo Jet crash every 24 hours.
 Worldwide, about 1.25 million people die of lung cancer annually—one person every 30 seconds!

4. What is the survival rate for lung cancer?
The 5-year survival rate is 14% in the United States and 8% in Europe. Finding all lung cancer at stage I by early detection could raise the survival rate to approximately 80%.

5. What is the relationship between lung cancer and tobacco?
Eighty-five to 90% of lung cancer deaths are attributed to cigarette smoking. Twenty-five percent of lung cancer in nonsmokers is attributed to passive or second-hand smoke. The likelihood of lung cancer increases with the number of cigarettes smoked, depth of inhalation, and age at which smoking began.

6. What percentage of smokers will develop lung cancer?
Between 10 and 20% of smokers will develop lung cancer in their lifetime. Of these, about 95% will die within 5 years of diagnosis.

7. How long does it take between starting smoking and developing lung cancer?
Lung cancer is estimated to take about 20 years to develop, depending on age, pack-years smoked, and genetic factors.

8. What are the most common presenting symptoms of lung cancer?
Cough, wheezing, hemoptysis, and postobstructive pneumonia are seen with central tumors. Pain, Pancoast syndrome, and superior vena cava (SVC) syndrome are seen with extrapulmonary invasion. Paraneoplastic syndrome is occasionally seen. Ten percent are asymptomatic.

9. What is Pancoast syndrome?
Pancoast syndrome is characterized by a malignant neoplasm along the superior sulcus of the lung with involvement of the thoracic inlet, brachial plexus, and cervical sympathetic nerves. This presents with characteristic pain in the shoulder region (eighth cervical distribution and second thoracic trunk), hand muscle atrophy, Horner's syndrome (ptosis, miosis, hemianhidrosis, enophthalmos), and SVC syndrome (Fig. 13-1).

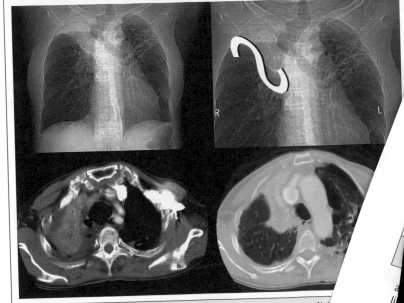

Figure 13-1. Lung carcinoma in a patient presenting with Pancoast syndrome. No[...] "S sign of Golden" formed by the inferior tumor margin on plain radiograph.

10. What is SVC syndrome?
SVC syndrome results from SVC obstruction and is characterized by [...] toms including facial and neck swelling, bilateral upper extremity s[...] and dyspnea (Fig. 13-2).

11. What are some paraneoplastic syndromes?
Paraneoplastic syndromes include cachexia, malaise, fever, cl[...] osteoarthropathy, nonbacterial thrombotic endocarditis, mig[...] ectopic hormone production (adrenocorticotropic hormone [...] [ADH], hypercalcemia).

12. What is the TNM classification for lung cancer
T represents the degree of spread of the primary tumor [...] lymph node involvement; and **M** represents the prese[...]

13. What is the role of CT in lung cancer stagi[...]
CT can confirm the abnormality and differentiate f[...] the size and location of primary tumor, extent of i[...] presence of metastatic disease. Positron emissi[...]

14. Fo[...]
Sm[...]
cer [...]
tion [...]

15. Und[...]
 ▪ **Tiss**[...]
 ▪ **Tx:** [...]
 ▪ **T1:** 3[...]
  tumor[...]
 ▪ **T2:** Di[...]
  pneum[...]
  bronch[...]
 ▪ **T3:** Apic[...]
  2 cm of [...]
  adjacent [...]
  cardium, [...]
 ▪ **T4:** Invasi[...]
  vertebral b[...]
  or satellite [...]

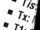
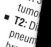

16. **Under the TNM classification, what is the N staging?**
   - **N0:** No lymph nodes involved
   - **N1:** Ipsilateral bronchopulmonary or hilar nodes involved
   - **N2:** Involvement of ipsilateral mediastinal nodes, including upper and lower paratracheal nodes, pretracheal and retrotracheal nodes, aortic and aortic window nodes, para-aortic nodes, para-esophageal nodes, subcarinal nodes, and the pulmonary ligament
   - **N3:** Involvement of contralateral mediastinal or hilar nodes and any scalene or supraclavicular nodes

17. **Under the TNM classification, what is the M staging?**
   - **M0:** No metastases
   - **M1:** Metastases present
   Lung cancer staging and 5-year survival rates are summarized in Table 13-1.

TABLE 13-1. LUNG CANCER STAGING AND 5-YEAR SURVIVAL RATES		
Stage	**TNM Classification**	**5-Year Survival Rate**
Stage IA	T1N0M0	75%
Stage IB	T2N0M0	55%
Stage IIA	T1N1M0	50%
Stage IIB	T2N1M0 or T3N0M0	40%
Stage IIIA	T1–3N2M0 or T3N1M0	10–35%
Stage IIIB	Any T4 or any N3M0	5%
Stage IV	Any M1	1%

18. **Which stages of lung cancer are considered unresectable?**
   Stage IIIB and stage IV. The important divisions that decide resectability are thus between T3 and T4, N2 and N3, and M0 and M1.

19. **When patients present with lung cancer symptoms, what stage of lung cancer do we typically find?**
   Stages III to IV are typically found.

20. **Why has CT made the solitary pulmonary nodule (SPN) problematic for the radiologist?**
   Because small SPNs are easy to detect with CT but hard to characterize. In a high-risk population of heavy smokers older than 50 years of age, about 70% of subjects will have pulmonary nodules (and thinner slices with automated nodule detection software will likely find even more). The majority of nodules <2 cm in diameter are missed on chest x-ray. So CT finds these nodules, most of which are benign, but often too small to biopsy, too small for accurate PET characterization, and too morbid to resect.
   Swensen SJ: CT screening for lung cancer. AJR 179:833–836, 2002.

21. **What is the likelihood ratio (LR) for SPNs?**
   The LR is the likelihood that a particular characteristic of a nodule or of a patient will be associated with malignancy versus benignity. Mathematically, it is defined as:

   $$LR = \frac{\text{Number of malignant nodules with this feature}}{\text{Number of benign nodules with this feature}}$$

LR < 1.0 suggests that the characteristic is more often seen in benign lesions, LR = 1.0 suggests a 50% chance of appearing in a benign lesion, and LR > 1.0 suggests that the characteristic is more often seen in malignant lesions.

22. **What are the LRs for radiologic features of SPNs?**
See Table 13-2.

TABLE 13-2. LIKELIHOOD RATIOS (LR) FOR RADIOLOGIC FEATURES OF SOLITARY PULMONARY NODULES

Radiologic Feature	LR
Spiculated margin	5.54
Malignant growth rate	3.40
Smooth margin	0.30
Age 30–39	0.24
Never smoked	0.19
Age 20–29	0.05
Benign growth rate	0.01

Data from Gurney JW: Determining the likelihood of malignancy in solitary pulmonary nodules with Bayesian analysis. Part I: Theory. Radiology 186:405–413, 1993.

23. **What are the two radiologic criteria that are generally accepted as proof of lung nodule benignity?**
   - Lack of nodule growth over 2 years
   - Nodule calcification in a benign pattern
Interestingly, these two criteria were first described in the late 1940s to early 1950s, long before CT.

   Aufses AH: Differential diagnosis between the early infiltrate or tuberculous and carcinoma of the lung. Tuberculology 210:72–78, 1949.
   Good CA, Hood RT Jr, McDonald JR: Significance of a solitary mass in the lung. AJR 70:543–554, 1953.
   Hood RT Jr, Good CA, Clagett OT, McDonald JR: Solitary circumscribed lesions of the lung. JAMA 152:1185–1191, 1953.
   Lillington GA: Management of solitary pulmonary nodules. Postgrad Med 101:145–150, 1997.

24. **What patterns of calcification are considered benign?**
Diffuse, central, concentric (laminar), and popcorn-like calcifications are considered benign patterns. Eccentric and stippled calcifications are not considered benign.

25. **Why not biopsy all CT-detected SPNs?**
Among all CT-detectable noncalcified lung nodules in a high-risk population, up to 98% are benign. Many small lesions are not amenable to percutaneous biopsy, whereas more invasive diagnostic interventions are associated with higher complication rates that are difficult to justify given the rate of benignity.

26. **So if we cannot biopsy all SPNs, what can we do?**
We can follow their growth rate.

27. **What are the typical volume doubling times of lung cancers?**

Volume doubling times (the time it takes the volume of the tumor to double) are approximately 30 days to 18 months. Some lung cancer cell types tend to be faster (i.e., squamous cell carcinoma) and others slower (bronchoalveolar carcinoma) (Fig. 13-3).

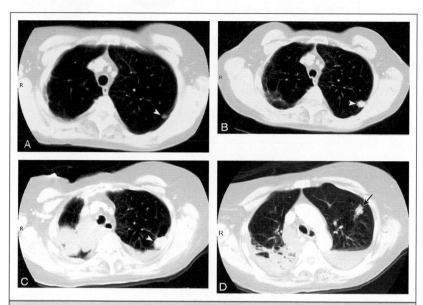

Figure 13-3. **A,** Baseline scan shows growing left upper lobe lung carcinoma *(arrowhead)*. The cancer was not resected because of comorbidities (emphysema). **B,** 16-month follow-up. **C,** 33-month follow-up. **D,** Lung metastases *(arrow)* and bony metastases (not shown) develop on 33-month scan. Volume doubling time is approximately 6 months.

28. **How is interval nodule growth evaluated?**

- Manual measurement from film
- Electronic calipers
- Three-dimensional (3D) segmentation/volume evaluation

More accurate measurements detect smaller changes more reliably and so detect growth sooner.

29. **What is the relationship between volume and diameter?**

Volume of a sphere = $1.33\pi \, (d/2)^3$

where $\pi = 3.14$ and d = diameter of sphere.

30. **If a perfectly spherical nodule doubles in diameter, how much has its volume increased?**

A twofold increase in the diameter of a sphere corresponds to an eightfold increase in volume (Fig. 13-4).

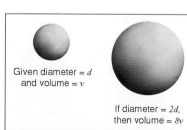

Given diameter = d
and volume = v

If diameter = $2d$,
then volume = $8v$

Figure 13-4. The sphere on the right measures two times the diameter but eight times the volume compared to the sphere on the left.

31. **If a perfectly spherical nodule doubles in volume, how much has its diameter increased?**
A twofold increase in volume corresponds to only a 26% increase in diameter (Fig. 13-5).

32. **If a 4-mm diameter nodule grows to 5 mm, how much has its volume increased?**
The volume has nearly doubled! Can you reliably distinguish 4- and 5-mm nodules by eye or calipers? How about if they are minified by a factor of 2 or more when you view them on your picture archiving and communications system (PACS) (Fig. 13-6)?

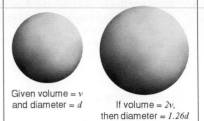

Given volume = v and diameter = d If volume = $2v$, then diameter = $1.26d$

Figure 13-5. The sphere on the right has twice the volume but only 1.25 times the diameter compared to the sphere on the left.

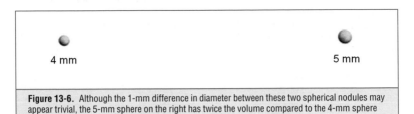

4 mm   5 mm

Figure 13-6. Although the 1-mm difference in diameter between these two spherical nodules may appear trivial, the 5-mm sphere on the right has twice the volume compared to the 4-mm sphere on the left.

33. **How often do pulmonary nodules present as a perfect sphere?**
Never. This is the reason why tumor volume measurements cannot be derived from simple electronic caliper measurements of diameter. Many investigators are developing more accurate volumetric segmentation techniques and computer-aided detection/diagnosis (CAD) algorithms necessary for accurate growth rate measurements.

34. **What technical parameters affect the volumetric evaluation of nodules detected on CT screening?**
Collimation thickness, field of view, and segmentation algorithm all affect the accuracy of volumetric evaluation. Thinner collimation, small field of view, and accurate segmentation algorithms are all required for accurate volumetric nodule analysis. A narrow field of view with thin sections generates a more accurate volumetric approximation of the actual nodule (Fig. 13-7).

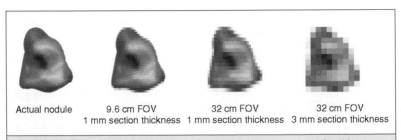

Actual nodule   9.6 cm FOV   32 cm FOV   32 cm FOV
          1 mm section thickness 1 mm section thickness 3 mm section thickness

Figure 13-7. A narrow field of view with thin sections generates a more accurate volumetric approximation of the actual nodule.

35. **What are the limitations of CT volumetric measurement?**
    - Acquisition parameters: nodules < 3 mm
    - Methodologic variations
    - Motion artifacts
    - Segmentation artifacts
    - Temporal and respiratory variation

36. **How can CAD help?**
    - Improve sensitivity (early detection)
    - Evaluate complex imaging features (nodule characterization)
    - Simplify repetitive tasks (automate nodule registration between studies)
    - Minimize interobserver variability (improved standardization)

37. **What are the limitations of CAD?**
    - Variation in patient selection/scan technique
    - Lack of standards in reporting data; number of false positives per scan or per patient group
    - Reliance on expert readers; no histologic standard
    - Absence of interpretive guidelines; no consensus on definition of nodule
    - Limited by CT capability and resolution
    - Limited by nodule density, size, and location

38. **How often should SPNs be followed radiologically?**
    This is a constantly changing field in radiology. Over the course of 30 years, pulmonary nodule evaluation has changed from chest x-ray to conventional CT, helical CT, and 4-, 16-, 40-, 60-, and 256-detector row CT. The current nodule follow-up recommendations are dependent on nodule size:
    - Many noncalcified nodules < 5 mm are benign or inflammatory. nodules that that resolve in 12 months. Repeat CT scan in 12 months.
    - Noncalcified nodules 4- to 7-mm are indeterminate. Order thin-section CT scan in 3 months.
    - Noncalcified nodules 8- to 20-mm are indeterminate. Order thin-section CT scan as soon as possible.
    - Noncalcified nodules larger than 20 mm are indeterminate. Perform biopsy or surgery.

    Henschke CI, Yankelevitz DF, Naidich DP, et al: CT screening for lung cancer: Suspiciousness of nodules according to size on baseline scans. Radiology 231:164–168, 2004.

    Swensen SJ, Jett JR, Sloan JA, et al: Screening for lung cancer with low-dose spiral computed tomography. Am J Respir Crit Care Med 165:508–513, 2002.

39. **What is the role of fluorine-18-fluorodeoxyglucose (FDG)-PET in the diagnosis of a SPN?**
    Lung cancer cells have a higher metabolic rate than normal cells; therefore, glucose uptake is higher. FDG-PET imaging uses the isotope fluorine-18 bound to a glucose analog to make FDG. Increased FDG uptake is seen in most malignant tumors and is the basis of the PET study used to differentiate malignant from benign nodules. Overall FDG-PET sensitivity for malignancy is 67–91% (median of 81%) and specificity is 82–96% (median of 90%) (Fig. 13-8). PET has a role in diagnosing, staging, and restaging lung carcinoma.

    Gould MK, Kuschner WG, Rydzak CE, et al: Test performance of positron emission tomography and computed tomography for mediastinal staging in patients with non–small-cell lung cancer: A meta-analysis. Ann Intern Med 139:879–892, 2003.

40. **Which cancer subtypes are often falsely negative on FDG-PET?**
    Tumors that behave in a more indolent fashion, such as carcinoid tumors and bronchioloalveolar carcinoma, are more commonly falsely negative on FDG-PET. However, up to 44% of lung cancers that have falsely negative PET scans are more indolent non-small cell cancer.

41. **What lesions can be falsely positive on FDG-PET?**
    Granulomatous disease, infection, inflammation, reactive lymph node hyperplasia, and sarcoidosis can all be falsely positive on FDG-PET. Not surprisingly, lymph node volume has been found to be significantly correlated with FDG accumulation.

42. **What is the most common benign neoplasm of the lung?**
    Hamartomas are the most common benign neoplasm of the lung. They contain a mixture of connective tissue, epithelial-lined clefts, and variable amounts of bone, cartilage, fat, vessels, and smooth muscle. Hamartomas may be diagnosed confidently on CT scans when the nodule is less than 2 cm in diameter, appearing spherical with a smooth contour, sharp outline, and containing fat with "popcorn-shaped" calcifications.

    Other common benign lung tumors and tumor-like lesions include papillomas, inflammatory pseudotumors, and granulomas. Collectively, these benign lesions comprise 51% of SPNs seen on chest x-ray (Figs. 13-9 and 13-10).

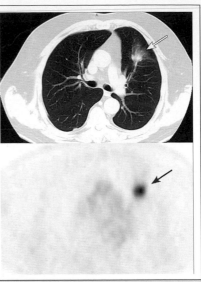

Figure 13-8. A solitary pulmonary nodule found on CT demonstrates increased FDG uptake on PET scan *(arrow),* confirmed on pathology to be lung adenocarcinoma.

43. **What other benign entities can present as pulmonary nodules?**
    - Arteriovenous malformation (Fig. 13-11)
    - Round atelectasis, which is a pseudotumor caused by infolding of pleura and containing pleural effusions (Fig. 13-12)
    - Pulmonary sequestrations, which are congenital and associated with ectopic arteries and draining veins (Fig. 13-13)
    - Pulmonary infarcts (Fig. 13-14)
    - Endobronchial/endotracheal mucus (Fig. 13-15)

44. **What are the requirements for cancer screening?**
    Screening is the testing of asymptomatic people (they are not yet patients!). Requirements for cancer screening include the following:
    - Disease must be treatable and common.
    - Test must be easily performed, inexpensive, and reproducible.
    - Test must be highly sensitive and widely available.

45. **Why is there a demand for CT lung cancer screening?**
    - Early stage lung cancer has a better prognosis.
    - Without screening, only 20% of cancers are diagnosed when resectable.
    - There are a tremendous number of smokers and ex-smokers.

46. **What is I-ELCAP? What is the evidence that CT screening can be effective?**
    The International Early Lung Cancer Action Program (I-ELCAP) has been performing CT screening of smokers and ex-smokers. ELCAP published their initial results in a landmark article in

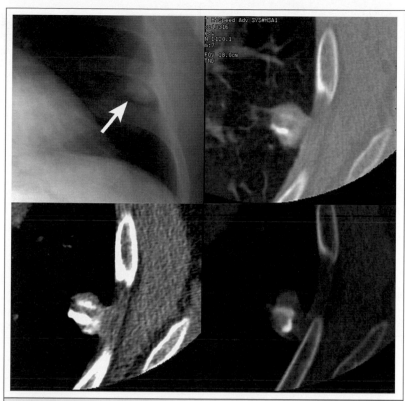

Figure 13-9. Pulmonary hamartomas classically present as a calcified solitary coin lesion on plain chest radiographs *(arrow)*. Pulmonary hamartoma on CT demonstrates typical popcorn calcification.

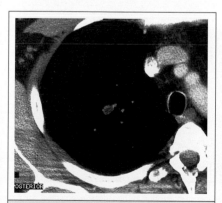

Figure 13-10. Pulmonary hamartoma in a different patient containing lipid (−50 Hounsfield units).

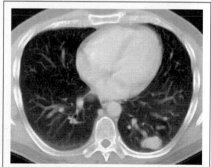

Figure 13-11. Arteriovenous malformation presenting as a mass in a patient with Osler-Weber-Rendu syndrome.

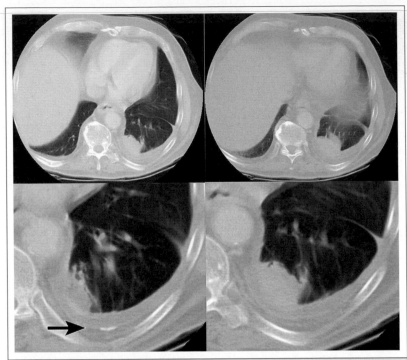

Figure 13-12. Round atelectasis typically presents as a round mass abutting the pleura in the lung periphery. It is usually associated with vessels and bronchi that swirl toward the mass, referred to as the "comet-tail" sign. Note the pleural calcification *(arrow)*.

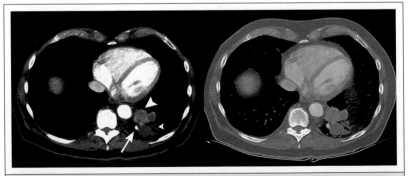

Figure 13-13. Pulmonary sequestration with coincidental lung carcinoma. The sequestration *(small arrowhead)* is more lateral and can present as a mass on radiograph or CT. Note the large adjacent feeding vessel *(arrow)* from the aorta. In this case, there is also a lung carcinoma *(large arrowhead)* medial to the sequestration.

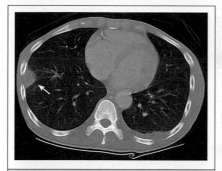

Figure 13-14. A pulmonary infarct *(arrow)* may occur as a sequela of pulmonary embolism. Infarcts are uncommon due to the lungs' dual arterial blood supply arising from the bronchial and pulmonary arteries. They resolve gradually over the course of weeks, melting away like an ice cube.

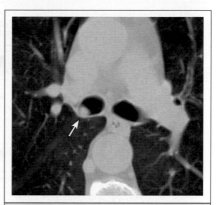

Figure 13-15. A mucus plug *(arrow)* can mimic endobronchial tumors not only by its appearance but also by its tendency to cause obstructive atelectasis. These will sometimes move if you rescan the patient prone, showing that they are mucus. These generally do not move just by having the patient try to cough.

Lancet in 1999, demonstrating that low-dose CT not only detected lung cancer in the screening population but also had a strong stage shift to early stage, potentially curable cancers.

Henschke CI, McCauley D, Yankelevitz DF, et al: Early lung cancer action project: Overall design and findings from baseline screening. Lancet 354:99–105, 1999.

47. **If screening changes staging, and staging changes mortality, then why hasn't CT lung cancer screening become routine?**
Improvement in prognosis is not synonymous with reduction in mortality. Concerns include potential over diagnosis, morbidity from false positive findings, radiation dose, the single arm methodology of ELCAP (all enrolled subjects received CT), and the potential enormous overall cost of national lung cancer screening. The effect of CT screening on lung cancer mortality is currently being evaluated by several large studies including ELCAP (which continues) and the National Cancer Institute sponsored National Lung Screening Trial (NLST) a large randomized controlled trial comparing x-ray to CT for lung cancer.

48. **What is the death rate from diseases *other* than lung cancer in the screened population?**
Data on about 5000 screened patients enrolled in the CT screening for lung cancer program in New York City suggest that the overall 10-year death rate from all causes other than lung cancer to be 7% in those who were 75 years of age or younger at the time of enrollment and 11% for those older 75 years of age.

Consensus Statement of The 11th International Conference on Screening for Lung Cancer, Rome, October 15-17, 2004. Available at http://www.ielcap.org/professionals/m_conf_11_sum.htm

49. **What is the effect of CT screening on smoking cessation?**
Smokers who underwent CT screening had a 14% smoking abstinence rate at 1-year follow-up, higher than the expected 5–7% smoking abstinence rate for spontaneous smoking cessation in the general population. CT screening for lung cancer can serve as a catalyst for smoking cessation in more than half of screened patients, potentially increasing the overall cancer prevention benefit of CT screening.

Cox LS, Clark MM, Jett JR, et al: Change in smoking status after spiral chest computed tomography scan screening. Cancer 98:2495–2501, 2003.

Ostroff JS, Buckshee N, Mancuso CA, et al: Smoking cessation following CT screening for early detection of lung cancer. Prevent Med 33:613–621, 2001.

50. **What are the radiographic features of squamous cell cancer?**
Squamous cell carcinoma is often occult on chest x-ray and may present as atelectasis that does not clear due to obstructing central mass. When seen, it presents as a hilar or perihilar mass with bronchial wall thickening that is often focal (Fig. 13-16). A peripheral nodule or mass is seen in 30%. The mass or nodule may cavitate. Local invasion is rapid, and metastasis occurs later.

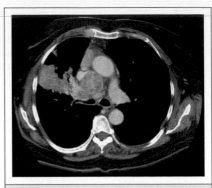

Figure 13-16. Squamous cell lung cancer demonstrating the characteristic perihilar location and central necrosis. Note the large adenopathy.

51. **What are the clinical features of squamous cell cancer?**
    - Pancoast syndrome when apical
    - Hyperparathyroidism (due to secretion of a parathyroid-like substance)
    - Strong association with cigarette smoking

52. **Which type of lung cancer has the strongest association with cigarette smoking and the poorest survival rates?**
Small cell lung cancer is associated with the poorest survival rates. It is considered metastatic at presentation and has the strongest association with cigarette smoking. When untreated, small cell lung cancer median survival is 2–4 months. When treated with chemotherapy and radiation, median survival is 9–18 months. At best, 15–25% survive 24 months.

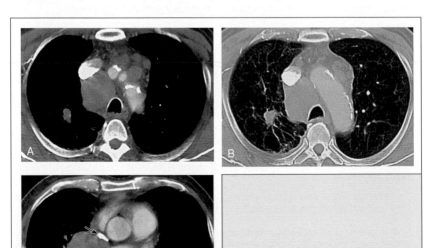

Figure 13-17. Small cell lung cancer. Note the large central mass and adenopathy *(A)* with relatively small right upper lobe tumor *(B, arrow)*. *C*, The adenopathy is compressing the SVC *(arrow)* and right hilar vessels *(arrowheads)*. (Courtesy of Patrick Fultz, MD.)

53. **What are the typical radiographic features of small cell lung cancer?**
    Central hilar or perihilar mass in 90% with mediastinal adenopathy (Fig. 13-17). Bronchial compression is common. Endobronchial lesions are unusual. The primary tumor is relatively small and sometimes undetectable. Although the tumor is usually necrotic on gross pathology, cavitation is rarely seen radiographically. Small cell cancer is considered metastatic at time of diagnosis (Fig. 13-18).

54. **Which type of lung cancer is the most common cause of SVC syndrome?**
    Small cell lung cancer is the most common cause of SVC syndrome. Other syndromes associated with small cell lung cancer include Cushing's syndrome, syndrome of inappropriate antidiuretic hormone (SIADH), and Eaton-Lambert syndrome.

55. **Histologically, which lung cancer type is often a diagnosis of exclusion?**
    Large cell carcinoma is poorly differentiated and often a diagnosis of exclusion histologically. It is characterized by rapid growth and early metastasis. It has a strong association with cigarette smoking.

56. **What are the radiographic features of large cell cancer?**
    They are usually peripheral, with 70% of tumors measuring 3–4 cm or larger at presentation.

57. **What are the neuroendocrine types of lung cancer?**
    Typical bronchial carcinoid, atypical bronchial carcinoid, large cell neuroendocrine carcinoma, and small cell carcinoma. These tumors are almost always malignant. Because they are metabolically active, they can be very small at presentation (Fig. 13-19).

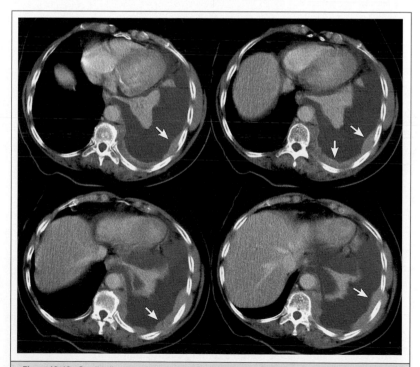

Figure 13-18. Small cell cancer metastatic to pleura at time of presentation.

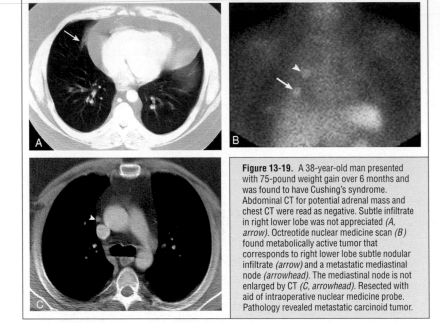

Figure 13-19. A 38-year-old man presented with 75-pound weight gain over 6 months and was found to have Cushing's syndrome. Abdominal CT for potential adrenal mass and chest CT were read as negative. Subtle infiltrate in right lower lobe was not appreciated *(A, arrow)*. Octreotide nuclear medicine scan *(B)* found metabolically active tumor that corresponds to right lower lobe subtle nodular infiltrate *(arrow)* and a metastatic mediastinal node *(arrowhead)*. The mediastinal node is not enlarged by CT *(C, arrowhead)*. Resected with aid of intraoperative nuclear medicine probe. Pathology revealed metastatic carcinoid tumor.

58. What are the clinical features of typical and atypical bronchial carcinoid tumors?
- Wide age range that is generally younger
- No gender predilection
- 20–40% of patients are nonsmokers
- Associated with multiple endocrine neoplasia (MEN) type I, presenting with cough, hemoptysis, and dyspnea

59. What differentiates typical and atypical carcinoid?
Mitotic rates. Typical carcinoid mitotic rate is <2 per 10 high-power field (HPF), whereas atypical carcinoid mitotic rate is <10 per 10 HPF. Typical carcinoids are slow growing with a 95% 5-year survival. Atypical carcinoids are more aggressive, more likely to metastasize, and more likely to be peribronchial.

60. What are the typical CT features of bronchial carcinoid tumors?
Sharply marginated nodule or mass that involves the central bronchi in 80% of patients. They may be endobronchial, partially endobronchial, bronchial, or peribronchial. They sometimes calcify. They can be associated with other nonspecific findings including lymphadenopathy, consolidation, atelectasis, and pleural effusions.

61. Who gets small cell and large cell neuroendocrine carcinoma?
They occur in older smokers.

62. What differentiates small cell and large cell neuroendocrine tumors?
Immunohistochemistry. Both types have marked histologic heterogeneity with >70 mitoses per 10 HPF.

63. What are the radiographic features of lung adenocarcinoma?
Located peripherally in 75%. Usually a solitary lobulated mass or nodule in an upper lobe. It may have ill- or well-defined borders (Fig. 13-20). It can be a central mass, however (Fig. 13-21).

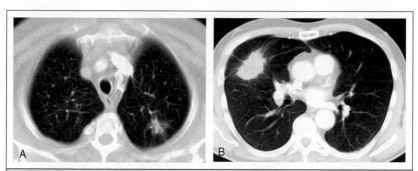

Figure 13-20. *A* and *B,* Lung adenocarcinoma most commonly appears as a peripheral, small or larger spiculated mass.

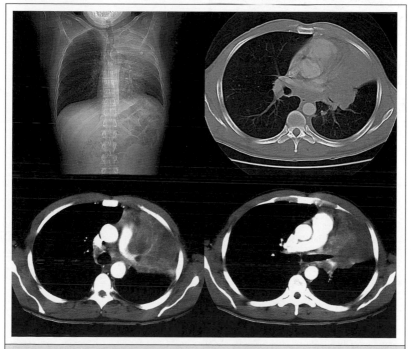

Figure 13-21. Lung adenocarcinoma. Although lung adenocarcinomas most commonly involves the peripheral lung zones, it may also arise along the hilum, as seen in this example.

64. **Why is bronchioloalveolar carcinoma unique among other types of lung adenocarcinoma?**

It often presents as a solitary lesion with slower growth, superior resectability, and excellent prognosis. It may present as a consolidation that does not clear.

65. **What is atypical adenomatous hyperplasia (AAH)?**

A preinvasive lesion often found in lung cancer specimens and thought to be a precursor for bronchioalveolar carcinoma and invasive adenocarcinoma. Lesions are composed of atypical cuboidal epithelium originating from alveolar and bronchiolar lining.

66. **Summarize the important facts about the most common types of lung cancers.**
See Table 13-3.

TABLE 13-3. SUMMARY OF THE MOST IMPORTANT FACTS ABOUT THE COMMON TYPES OF LUNG CANCER

	Relative Frequency	Usual Location in Lung	Association with Smoking	Progression Rate	Metastatic Rate	Surgical Resection	Average 5-Year Survival
Lung adenocarcinoma	35%	Peripheral	Low	Average	Average	Maybe	<10%
Squamous cell carcinoma	30%	Usually hilar	High	Slow	Late	Maybe	>50%
Large cell carcinoma	10%	Central or peripheral	High	Rapid	Early	Maybe	<10%
Small cell carcinoma	20%	Hilar	High	Rapid	Very early	Never	<1%

67. **What are the rare histologic types of lung cancer?**
   - Adenoid cystic carcinoma (cylindroma)
   - Mucoepidermoid carcinoma
   - Carcinosarcoma
   - Pulmonary blastoma

68. **Which nonpulmonary cancers are most likely to present as pulmonary metastases?**
Breast, colon, renal, melanoma, sarcoma, and thyroid cancer (Fig. 13-22). Renal cancer in particular favors an endobronchial metastasis (Fig. 13-23). Thyroid cancer classically gives multiple small—even military—nodules.

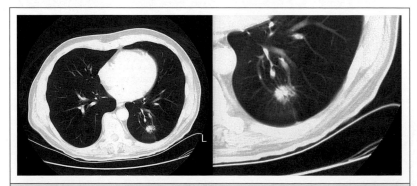

Figure 13-22. Pancreatic cell carcinoma with metastasis to the lung. Most metastases are smooth, but they can be speculated, as in this case.

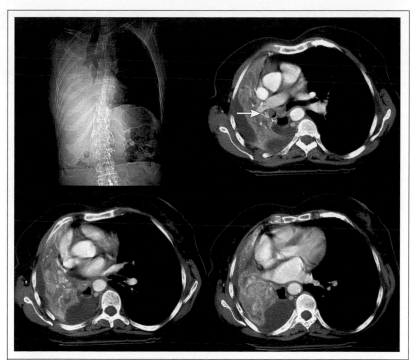

Figure 13-23. Endobronchial metastatic renal cell carcinoma of the right mainstem bronchus *(arrow)* causing right lung atelectasis.

69. **What is the most common primary malignancy of the trachea?**

Squamous cell carcinoma of the trachea, which accounts for 45% of primary tracheal neoplasms. The typical presentation is a male in his 50s or 60s, with multiple respiratory malignancies. There is no predominant location, and recurrence is frequent at the site of resection. Other primary malignancies of the trachea include adenoid cystic, carcinoid, mucoepidermoid carcinoma, and squamous papilloma.

70. **What is the second most common primary tracheal malignancy?**

Adenoid cystic carcinomas, also known as cylindromas, are the second most common primary tracheal neoplasms, comprising 20–35% of all tracheal tumors and 80% of all bronchial gland tumors. The mean presenting age is 40–50 years, has no sex predilection, and often presents with symptoms of tracheobronchial obstruction including wheezing, cough, hemoptysis, and dyspnea. Despite rare extrathoracic metastasis, prognosis is poor due to common local recurrence.

71. **What are the typical CT features of adenoid cystic carcinomas?**

Intraluminal tumor or annular constricting lesion, predominantly along the central trachea and bronchi. It is locally invasive, with 10–15% located in the lung periphery.

72. **What are the clinical features of mucoepidermoid carcinomas?**

Wide age range with slight male predominance. Symptoms are nonspecific. Prognosis is excellent for low-grade tumors.

KEY POINTS: LUNG CANCER

1. Lung cancer is incredibly common, and the radiologist is often the first to know. Always suspect it. Most symptomatic patients at time of diagnosis will die of their disease.

2. Carefully distinguish between "work-up" and "follow-up." Work up more suspicious nodes (i.e., determine the need for resection *now,* through biopsy, PET, etc.). Follow up smaller, less suspicious nodes (i.e., rescan for growth in several months). The size threshold is approximately 1 cm. Don't say follow-up when you mean work-up.

3. Significant growth in small tumors can be difficult to measure with present tools because of the volumetric nature of growth.

4. Lung cancer screening trials are in progress. The ELCAP study showed that CT screening can downstage lung cancer. Randomized trials are evaluating whether long-term morbidity and mortality are also changed.

---

73. **What are the CT features of mucoepidermoid carcinomas?**
Endobronchial, exophytic, or polypoid lesions of the central bronchi, less commonly in the trachea. Smooth margins when low-grade; ragged or ill-defined when high-grade.

74. **What are the clinical features of carcinosarcoma?**
It is rare, comprising 0.3% of all lung cancers, affecting middle-aged and elderly men. Prognosis is poor with rapid local invasion and widespread metastasis.

75. **What are the CT features of carcinosarcoma?**
Peripheral tumors present as a large mass, 6 cm in diameter on average, with associated central necrosis and hemorrhage. There is an upper lobe predominance. Chest wall and mediastinal invasion may occur. Central tumors present as an endobronchial lesion, resembling a mucus plug, with parenchymal invasion.

76. **What are the clinical features of pulmonary blastoma?**
   ■ Biphasic age distribution affecting males in their first and seventh decades
   ■ Thought to be a variant of carcinosarcoma due to histologic, clinical, and radiologic resemblance

77. **What do carcinosarcoma and pulmonary blastoma have in common?**
Both are mixed tumors with malignant epithelial and mesenchymal components.

78. **What is the most common pleural neoplasm?**
Malignant mesothelioma. It occurs in 10% of asbestos-exposed individuals, typically males in their 60s to 80s. Median survival time is 10 months. At best, the 5-year survival rate is 25–30%.

79. **What are the CT features of malignant mesothelioma?**
CT features are mass-like pleural thickening, fissural thickening, pleural effusions, and pleural calcifications (Fig. 13-24).

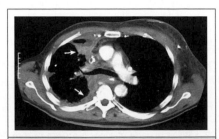

Figure 13-24. Malignant mesothelioma along the medial right pleura *(arrows).*

80. **What is the diagnostic test of choice for malignant mesothelioma?**
Video-assisted thoracoscopic surgery (VATS) has a sensitivity of 98%. Open surgery is an option when adhesions preclude VATS. Fine needle aspiration and cytology are of limited use.

81. **What is the most common cause of malignant pleural effusion?**
Lung cancer (see Fig. 12-18). The second most common cause is breast cancer. Metastases favor the costophrenic angles (Fig. 13-25).

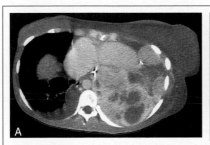
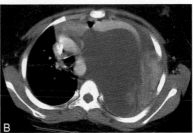

Figure 13-25. *A,* Malignant fibrous histiocytoma with left pleural invasion. *B,* Primitive neuroectodermal tissue (PNET) invading the left lung and pleura.

82. **What is the pathophysiology of malignant pleural effusion?**
The pathophysiology is direct tumor invasion of pleura, lymphatic obstruction, severe hypoproteinemia, and pneumonia/atelectasis.

WEBSITES

1. International Early Lung Cancer Action Program
http://www.ielcap.org/professionals.htm
2. National Lung Screening Trial
http://www.cancer.gov/nlst

BIBLIOGRAPHY

Lung Neoplasms
1. Rosado-de-Christenson ML, Templeton PA, Moran CA: Bronchogenic carcinoma: Radiologic-pathologic correlation. Radiographics 14:429–446, 1994.

Pleural Neoplasms
2. Dynes MC, White EM, Fry WA, Ghahremani GG: Imaging manifestations of pleural tumors. Radiographics 12:1191–1201, 1992.
3. Weyant MJ, Flores RM: Imaging of pleural and chest wall tumors. Thorac Surg Clin 14:15–23, 2004.

Airway Neoplasms
4. McCarthy MJ, Rosado-de-Christenson ML: Tumors of the trachea. J Thorac Imag 10:180–198, 1995.
5. Wilson RW, Frazier AA: Pathological-radiological correlations: Pathological and radiological correlation of endobronchial neoplasms. Part II: Malignant tumors. Ann Diagn Pathol 2:31–34, 1998.
6. Wilson RW, Kirejczyk W: Pathological and radiological correlation of endobronchial neoplasms. Part I: Benign tumors. Ann Diagn Pathol 1:31–46, 1997.

CT Screening for Lung Cancer

7. Aberle DR, Gamsu G, Henschke CI, et al: A consensus statement of the Society of Thoracic Radiology: Screening for lung cancer with helical computed tomography. J Thorac Imag 16:65–68, 2001.

8. Humphrey LL, Teutsch S, Johnson M: U.S. Preventive Services Task Force. Lung cancer screening with sputum cytologic examination, chest radiography, and computed tomography: An update for the U.S. Preventive Services Task Force. Ann Intern Med 140:740–753, 2004.

9. Miettinen OS, Henschke CI: CT screening for lung cancer: Coping with nihilistic recommendations. Radiology 225:920, 2002.

10. Swensen SJ, Jett JR, Midthun DE, Hartman TE: Computed tomographic screening for lung cancer: Home run or foul ball? Mayo Clin Proc 78:1187–1188, 2003.

CAD for Lung Cancer

11. Reeves AP, Kostis WJ: Computer-aided diagnosis for lung cancer. Radiol Clin North Am 38:497–509, 2000.

12. Yankelevitz D, Henschke CI: State-of-the-art screening for lung cancer. Part 2: CT scanning. Thorac Surg Clin 14:53–59, 2004.

PET for Lung Cancer

13. Mavi A, Lakhani P, Zhuang H, et al: Fluorodeoxyglucose-PET in characterizing solitary pulmonary nodules, assessing pleural diseases, and the initial staging, restaging, therapy planning, and monitoring response of lung cancer. Radiol Clin North Am 43:1–21, 2005.

CHAPTER 14

CT CAD

Waqar Shah, MD

1. **What does CAD stand for?**
   Computer-assisted detection. Sometimes it is interpreted as computer-aided diagnosis, but because present systems only help you find lesions, diagnosis really remains in the future.

2. **What is the difference between visualization software and CAD?**
   Visualization software displays the data set for the radiologist. Virtual colonoscopy, maximum intensity projections (MIP), volume rendering—they all manipulate the data for display. CAD analyzes the images in search of patterns to bring to the radiologist's attention.

3. **What applications are there for CAD in CT?**
   CAD in CT has been shown to be helpful in detecting lung nodules, tracking the growth of lung nodules, detecting pulmonary emboli, measuring emphysematous lung, and aiding virtual colonoscopy (polyp detection).

4. **What are the advantages of using CAD?**
   CAD provides a "second pair of eyes." It has the inherent advantages of a computer over a human being (it does not require sleep or food, does not get bored, and is consistent over time in finding patterns). CAD can handle very large data sets created by thin-slice multidetector CT.

5. **Does CAD effectively improve sensitivity or specificity?**
   Sensitivity. CAD (at present) is set up to find possible lesions and so leans toward sensitivity.

6. **Who makes CAD software?**
   Vendors include R2 Technology, iCAD (incorporating CADx systems), Medicsight, TeraRecon, and the major equipment manufacturers.

7. **How was CAD first used in clinical radiology?**
   It was first used in mammography.

8. **When was CAD first introduced in CT? For what application?**
   The world's first CT CAD system was installed in Athens, Greece, by R2 Technology in October of 2003 for detection of lung nodules.

9. **How effective is CAD in plain film or digital mammography for detecting breast cancer?**
   As of early 2005, more than 1200 centers across the United States use CAD, and more than 8 million women have had their mammograms interpreted with its aid. CAD has been shown to increase early detection of breast cancer by up to 23%.
   In the evaluation of 19,596 screening mammograms performed with CAD, Stamatia Destounis, staff radiologist at the Elizabeth Wende Breast Clinic in Rochester, New York, determined that a 7% higher yield is possible when double reading is performed and CAD software is implemented. Without CAD, the sensitivity of double reading was 86%. With the implementation of CAD software, it rose to 93%.

10. **When did the Food and Drug Administration (FDA) approve CAD for CT?**
The ImageChecker CT CAD system from R2 Technology was the first CAD system for the detection of lung nodules on CT exams available in the United States. It was approved by the FDA on July 8, 2004.

11. **What percentage of lung nodules (approximately) is missed by the human eye?**
About 20%. Of course, this estimate is size-dependent.

12. **Why are pulmonary nodules important to detect?**
Lung cancer is the world's most common lethal cancer. It accounts for more than 1.2 million new cases annually. Lung cancer is difficult to detect in its earliest stage, when it is an asymptomatic lung nodule. Early-stage lung cancers are detected incidentally by imaging studies that were performed for an unrelated medical problem. The 5-year survival rate for all stages of lung cancer is 14%. When lung cancer is localized at the time of diagnosis, the 5-year survival rate increases to 42%. Approximately 15% of lung cancers are found in the early stages.

13. **What does the receiver operator curve (ROC) look like for interpretation of a chest CT for pulmonary nodules with and without CAD?**
See Figure 14.1.

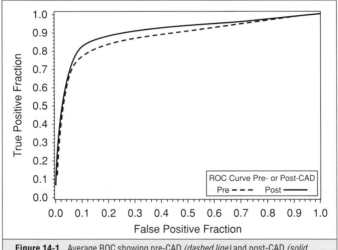

Figure 14-1. Average ROC showing pre-CAD *(dashed line)* and post-CAD *(solid line)* performance for 90-cases study. Thus, the study showed a statistically significant improvement in the area under the ROC with the use of CAD.

14. **How is CAD for pulmonary nodule detection used?**
The CAD software is a detection aid not an interpretative aid. It should be reviewed on completion of a radiologist's initial reading of the scan. Its purpose is to draw attention to areas that may represent nodules. The radiologist decides whether to accept or reject the additional "nodules" found by the CAD program. Its benefit will bring the greatest yield if it is used after the first reading of the images. If there is a potential positive finding that CAD does not mark, the radiologist should not be swayed in making his or her call.

15. **Can the software detect disease other than pulmonary nodules?**
The algorithm looks for solid lung nodules. In general, CAD does not look for non-nodular abnormalities (e.g., scars, atelectasis, bronchiectasis), nodules or other abnormalities outside

the lung parenchyma (e.g., in the mediastinum or in the chest wall), or ground-glass opacities or other nonsolid or part-solid nodules that may represent malignancies.

16. **What limitations are there for nodule detection by CAD?**
CAD software is not designed to detect changes from other CT exams. Therefore, comparisons are not readily made. CAD software is more sensitive for the detection of solid spherical nodules than for nodules that are partly solid or nonsolid or that have very irregular shapes. In addition, CAD software cannot detect ground-glass opacities.

17. **How does CAD differentiate true pulmonary nodules from small vessels that may appear to be nodules on a single CT slice?**
Shape analysis is performed in three dimensions. As a result an object that appears circular in a two-dimensional (2D) axial slice may not be marked, because in three dimensions it is very flat or elongated, such as a vessel. A solitary nodule will be round and compact in every direction.
　　The algorithm can differentiate between nodules and blood vessels based on density, size, texture, and other properties. Nodule volumes can be ascertained. This task can otherwise be very time consuming for a radiologist. Based on each finding's size, shape, density, and other characteristics, the algorithm assigns the finding a likelihood. All findings whose likelihood exceeds a fixed threshold are presented to the user as potential nodules.

18. **What is the next step after a nodule is discovered?**
- Determine if it is a true nodule (radiologist).
- Determine its size (radiologist plus CAD).
- Determine whether it should be biopsied/excised or followed for growth (clinician and radiologist).
- If followed for size, measure it accurately (CAD) and store result awaiting the follow-up scans.

19. **Which is more important—good reproducibly or good calibration?**
Good reproducibility. Our present treatment algorithms depend more on change in size than on absolute size. If we can measure a nodule with high reproducibility (even though there may be a positive or negative bias in size), we can determine if it is growing. The definition of the precise size (should spiculations be included?) is difficult, and calibrating these systems to real human nodules in living breathing patients is impossible.
　　The disadvantage of poor calibration is that it makes difficult comparing nodules measured by different systems with different measurement algorithms for clinical or research purposes.

20. **Is there an acquisition protocol for CT scans acquired for CAD?**
Yes. In general, the protocol is as follows:
- The scan is acquired with minimum four-detector multiple-row detector CT (MDCT) scanner.
- Acquisition protocol is with collimation of 3 mm or less (minimum 0.5 mm), which results in image reconstruction with slice thickness of 3 mm or less.
- Image spacing is less than or equal to slice thickness (image overlap is acceptable, but gaps are not).
- Slices are contiguous (reconstructions where image spacing is larger than the slice thickness are not acceptable).
- Slice thickness is the same throughout the series.
- Slice spacing is the same throughout the series.
- Exposure is no less than 15 mAs (maximum 250 mAs).
- Series containing lung should not have more than 800 images.
- Minimal field of view is 18 cm.
- Scan must be completed in a single breath-hold (to avoid motion artifacts).
- Scan should be acquired with values of pitch and other parameters such that the reconstructed data are of acceptable quality for reading by a radiologist.

KEY POINTS: CT CAD

1. CAD has promising results for the detection of pulmonary nodules and virtual colonoscopy. It improves sensitivity for nodule detection. The number of false-positive nodules detected, however, remains high.

2. Coronary artery calcification measurement is a third application for CAD. CAD is already widely used with mammography. These are the leading causes of neoplastic and nonneoplastic death.

3. CAD is a partial answer to growing image overload. It should let us take advantage of the high-quality thin-slice data sets produced by MDCT.

21. Do patients with staples or other metallic objects in the thorax or mediastinum cause problems for CAD?

These cases are acceptable for review. However, they will need to be preprocessed for CAD to minimize streak artifacts.

22. How is CAD done for virtual colonoscopy?

The first step is the digital extraction of the colon using CT slices and the generation of an isotropic volume rendering through graphic interpolation.

The second step is a shape-based analysis of the data set to discriminate between normal and abnormal colonic structures. Volume rendering is used to identify three shapes that are indicative of colorectal cancer. These shapes include the following:

- The ridge, associated with normal folds in the colon wall
- The cap, associated with polyps
- The cup or recesses in the colon wall

Additional software analysis evaluates the internal features of suspected abnormalities to reduce the false-positive rate. The software recognizes the inhomogeneous, mottled appearance of residual stool. For example, final results are generated after the shape-based and feature-guided analyses are completed. The program automatically calculates its confidence in each finding, which is colorized accordingly.

23. What is the sensitivity of polyp detection by CAD?

For polyp/mass analysis, the CAD scheme is 96% sensitive for detecting suspicious polyps. Abraham H. Dachman at the University of Chicago retrospectively studied 20 CT colonography data sets: 10 sets containing a total of 11 polyps, 5–12 mm in size, and 10 were normal. Readers missed 42% of the polyps without CAD; they later identified 75% of the missed polyps with the help of the CAD system. CAD detected all the polyps missed by the readers, whereas readers correctly dismissed 77% of the computer's false positives.

24. What is the minimum size of a polyp that would be detected by CAD?

The minimum size is 3 mm.

25. What causes false positives in CAD in CT colonography?

The ileocecal valve, haustra (especially in an underdistended colon), rectal tube, extrinsic compression, and stool cause false positives.

26. How does CAD differentiate stool from a polyp in CT colonography?

Stool differentiation is based on differences in the internal density variation between polyps and stool. These density variations are caused by the tendency of stool to contain air bubbles that can be recognized on CT images as an inhomogeneous textural pattern, or mottle pattern.

In contrast, polyps tend to have a homogeneous textural pattern, or solid pattern. In addition, stool tagging (administering an agent to increase stool density) can be used.

27. What will be the impact of CAD on the radiologist?
It should improve the quality of work as well as aid in interpreting the growing quantity of images that need evaluation.

BIBLIOGRAPHY

1. Acar B, Beaulieu CF, Paik DS, et al: Computer-aided detection of colonic polyps in CT colonography using optical flow. Radiology 221(P):331, 2001.

2. Chan HP, Sahiner B, Helvie MA, et al: Improvement of radiologists' characterization of mammographic masses by using computer-aided diagnosis: An ROC study. Radiology 212:817–827, 1999.

3. Destounis SV, DiNitto P, Logan-Young W, et al: Can computer-aided detection with double reading of screening mammograms help decrease the false-negative rate? Initial experience. Radiology 232:578–584, 2004.

4. Dorfmann DD, Berbaum KS, Metz CE: Receiver operating characteristic rating analysis. Invest Radiol 27.723–731, 1992.

5. Johnson CD, Toledano AY, Herman BA, et al: Computerized tomographic colonography: Performance evaluation in a retrospective multicenter setting. Gastroenterology 125:688–695, 2003.

6. Kobayashi T, Xu XW, MacMahon H, et al: Effect of a computer-aided diagnosis scheme on radiologists' performance in detection of lung nodules on radiographs. Radiology 199:843–848, 1996.

7. Nappi J, Yoshida H: Feature-guided analysis for reduction of false positives in CAD of polyps for CT colonography. Med Phys 30:1592–1601, 2003.

8. Nappi J, Yoshida H: Automated detection of polyps with CT colonography: Evaluation of volumetric features for reduction of false-positive findings. Acad Radiol 9:386–397, 2002.

9. Rutter C: Bootstrap estimation of diagnostic accuracy with patient-clustered data. Acad Radiol 7:413–419, 2000.

10. Summers RM, Johnson CD, Pusanik LM, et al: Automated polyp detection at CT colonography: Feasibility assessment in a human population. Radiology 219:51–59, 2001.

11. Yoshida H, Nappi J, MacEneaney P, et al: Computer-aided diagnosis scheme for the detection of polyps in CT colonography. Radiographics 22:963–979, 2002.

WEBSITES

Leading independent CAD manufacturers websites in 2005. Expect turnover in this evolving industry.

www.r2tech.com

www.icadmed.com

www.medicsight.com

www.eddatech.com

www.mediantechnologies.com

www.medical.siemens.com (search for "LungCare")

CHAPTER 15

ANTERIOR MEDIASTINUM

Igor Mikityansky, MD, and Deborah Rubens, MD

1. **What is the mediastinum?**
   Mediastinum means middle or partition. In the chest, it is the tissues and organs between the two pleural sacs, bordered anteriorly by the sternum, posteriorly by the vertebral column, superiorly by the thoracic inlet, and inferiorly by the diaphragm. It contains the heart and pericardium, the bases of the great vessels, the trachea and bronchi, esophagus, thymus, lymph nodes, thoracic duct, and phrenic and vagus nerves.

2. **What are the mediastinal compartments?**
   The mediastinum is divided into anterior, middle, and posterior compartments. Some classifications include an additional superior compartment, which comprises the thoracic inlet and includes portions of the other three compartments. This is best conceptualized by a lateral diagram of the chest (Fig. 15-1).

3. **What are the boundaries of the anterior mediastinum?**
   The anterior mediastinum occupies the space between the sternum anteriorly and the pericardium, aorta, and brachiocephalic vessels posteriorly. It is defined superiorly by the thoracic inlet, inferiorly by the diaphragm, and laterally by the parietal pleura.

4. **What lies within the anterior mediastinum?**
   The major structures are the thymus, lymph nodes, fat, and the internal mammary vessels.

5. **What is the superior mediastinum?**
   This is the superior portion of the anterior mediastinum. It extends from the thoracic inlet to a line drawn from the sternal angle

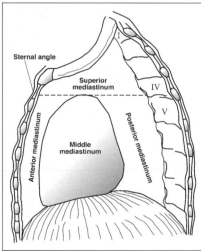

Figure 15-1. The mediastinal compartments are best understood from a sagittal view of the chest.

to the fourth intervertebral disc. It has no unique structures but contains components that continue from the anterior mediastinum or from the neck (intrathoracic continuation of the thyroid).

6. **What are the four "T's"?**
   These are the most important masses of the anterior mediastinum: thyroid, thymoma, teratoma (or any germ cell neoplasm), and terrible lymphoma.

7. **What is the thymus?**
   The thymus is a lymphatic organ located in the superior part of anterior mediastinum. It is responsible for differentiation of lymphocytes.

8. **What is the natural history of the thymus?**

Although weighing only 10–15 gm at birth, the thymus reaches maximum weight at puberty (30–40 gm) with subsequent fatty involution over a 5- to 15-year period. By the age of 35 most of the thymus has been replaced by fat. A residual soft tissue mass in a 30-year-old is unusual, unless the patient has been stressed (*see* thymic rebound).

9. **What is the CT appearance of the thymus?**

From birth to puberty, the thymus fills the anterior mediastinum. It has a soft tissue density similar to muscle. Its shape is triangular or bilobed with convex lateral margins. From puberty to 25 years of age, fat appears in the anterior mediastinum and the thymus is a discrete soft tissue structure, separated from the heart and the great vessels. After 25, more fat appears within and around the thymus, which gradually disappears until the anterior or mediastinal tissue is entirely fatty, at age 40 and beyond. The normal-sized thymus is up to 1.8 cm thick (short axis) up to age 20 and less than 1.3 cm in short axis after that (Fig. 15-2).

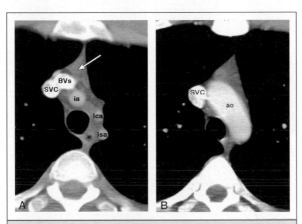

Figure 15-2. *A,* Triangular soft tissue of the normal thymus *(arrows)* extends from the great vessels to the anterior pleural surface in this 20-year-old man. Proximally the lateral margins are slightly concave. *B,* More caudally at the level of the aortic arch, the thymus broadens slightly and may become slightly convex, as shown here. BVs = brachiocephalic veins, ia = innominate artery, lsa = left subclavian artery, lca = left common carotid artery, SVC = superior vena cava, ao = aorta.

10. **What is the most common thymic abnormality that presents as an anterior mediastinal mass?**

Thymoma is most common. It may be either benign or malignant. Age at presentation is between 40 and 60, and men and women are equally affected.

11. **What conditions are associated with thymoma?**

Thymoma is usually an incidental finding in healthy people. However, it may occur in association with myasthenia gravis, red cell aplasia, and hypoglobulinemia.

12. **What association exists between myasthenia gravis and thymoma?**

Fifteen percent of patients with myasthenia gravis have thymoma, whereas 50% of patients with thymoma have myasthenia gravis.

13. **What is the CT appearance of thymoma?**
    This is a well-defined, round, or oval mass, of homogeneous soft tissue density located anterior to the junction of heart and great vessels (Fig. 15-3). However, thymomas can be found at any level from the thoracic inlet to the diaphragm. There is usually an isoattenuating homogeneous bulge or change from concave to convex appearance of the thymic edge. The enhancement of the tumor is similar to the normal thymus. In 20% of cases there is curvilinear calcification. Areas of cystic degeneration with lower CT attenuation can also be found in some cases. Both calcifications and cystic degeneration are equally common in invasive and noninvasive thymomas.

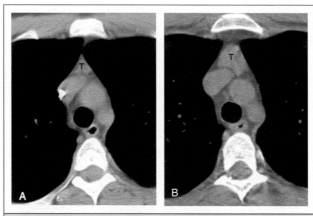

Figure 15-3. Twenty-year-old patient with osteosarcoma after chemotherapy. **A,** Pretreatment image at the level of the great vessels shows normal thymic tissue (T) with convex margins. **B,** Postchemotherapy image at the same level reveals a lobulated soft tissue mass (T) with convex margins.

14. **Can thymomas be symptomatic?**
    Fifty percent of the cases are asymptomatic and are found incidentally. About 25–30% of the patients present with signs of mediastinal compression, such as cough, dyspnea, chest pain, respiratory infection, hoarseness, or dysphagia. Rarely, patients present with superior vena cava obstruction.

15. **What is the distribution of benign versus malignant tumors?**
    Thirty percent of thymomas are invasive with extension through the fibrous capsule, into the chest wall, and contiguous spread along pleural surfaces, usually unilateral. If resected there is a 2% chance of tumor recurrence.

16. **What is the CT appearance of invasive thymoma?**
    An irregular, ill-defined mass, with obliteration of normal fat planes is a good indicator of invasion and is the only characteristic differentiating invasive and noninvasive thymomas. The most commonly invaded organs are the trachea, the great vessels, mediastinal pleura, and the pericardium. Fifteen percent of advanced cases have pleural extension without connection with the primary tumors. There is no histologic difference between benign and invasive thymoma.

17. **How are invasive thymomas classified?**
    Thymomas are classified, according to the Masaoka staging system, as stage I through stage IV. Stage I has an intact capsule, stage II extends into the mediastinal fat or pleura, and stage III

invades neighboring organs (pericardium, great vessels, or lungs). Stage IVa has pleural or pericardial implants and IVb has lymphatic or hematogenous metastases.

18. **What is the treatment and prognosis of invasive thymoma?**
    Treatment includes radical excision of the tumor for all stages with radiation therapy for stage II and beyond and chemotherapy in stages III and IV. The 5-year survival rate is 93% for stage I, 86% for stage II, 70% for stage III, and 25% for stage IV. Thymomas associated with myasthenia gravis tend to be less aggressive.

19. **What is thymic hyperplasia?**
    This is a gland that has increased lymphoid follicles, many with active germinal centers. The gland itself is not necessarily enlarged. Hyperplasia is associated with hyperthyroidism, acromegaly, Addison's disease, myasthenia gravis, systemic lupus erythematosus, scleroderma, and rheumatoid arthritis.

20. **What is "rebound" thymic hyperplasia?**
    This condition follows a systemic stress, such as chemotherapy, burns, or surgery, which cause the thymus to involute. Following elimination of the stress the thymus "rebounds" and enlarges, often to 50% greater than normal size for age. CT shows an enlarged thymus with normal bilobed, "arrowhead" configuration (Fig. 15-4). Unlike lymphoid thymic hyperplasia, the gross architecture and histologic appearance are completely normal.

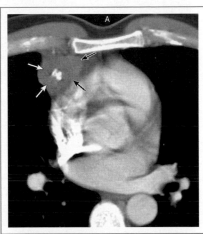

21. **What is thymic carcinoid?**
    This is a tumor arising from thymic cells of neural crest origin. It presents as a mediastinal mass in a patient with endocrine symptoms. It may be associated with Cushing's syndrome, syndrome of inappropriate antidiuretic hormone (SIADH), hyperparathyroidism, and multiple endocrine neoplasia (MEN) I syndrome. These tumors are bulky and lobulated. Up to 50% are invasive.

Figure 15-4. Well-defined mediastinal mass *(arrows)* with central calcification. Despite relatively benign features (smooth margins, no lymphadenopathy or evidence of spread to heart, chest wall or pleura) this mass was malignant on histology.

22. **What are the features of primary thymic carcinoma?**
    This tumor is extremely rare, such that it is diagnosed by excluding metastatic carcinoma. Its CT appearance is nonspecific but typically is a solid mass with poorly defined margins. Thymic carcinoma tends to be large, ranging from 5 to 15 cm in diameter. Its behavior is very aggressive, often locally invasive, and it may metastasize hematogenously to distant organs. Patients are often symptomatic at presentation, complaining of cough, chest pain, fever, weight loss, night sweats, and/or fatigue.

23. **How does lymphoma involve the thymus?**
    Lymphoma frequently occurs in the thymus, especially in Hodgkin's disease, in which more than one third of the patients have thymic tumor. Lymphoblastic lymphoma, a T-cell lymphoma, also commonly affects the thymus.

24. **What is the CT appearance of thymic lymphoma?**

The thymus is replaced by a homogeneous, round, soft tissue mass without calcifications and often with other mediastinal lymph node enlargement. Nodular sclerosing Hodgkin's lymphoma has a tendency to cystic degeneration, particularly post therapy (Fig. 15-5).

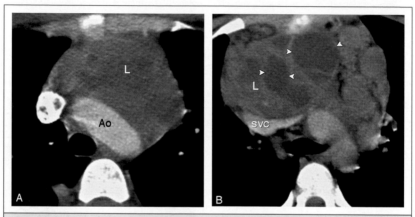

Figure 15-5. **A,** Axial image of nodular sclerosing Hodgkin's lymphoma (L) replaces and enlarges the thymus at the level of the aortic arch. **B,** More caudally there are lower attenuation nodules *(arrowheads),* typical of nodular sclerosing Hodgkin's lymphoma. Even fairly bulky masses may not displace the vessels, but as the mass enlarges, the superior vena cava (SVC) is eventually compressed and the patient may present with SVC syndrome (facial and upper extremity swelling, shortness of breath). Ao = aorta.

25. **What are thymic cysts?**

True thymic cysts are rare, accounting for only 2–3% of anterior mediastinal masses. These may be congenital or acquired and can be seen at any age. Acquired cysts are thought to result from thymic inflammation. Congenital cysts are unilocular. Benign thymic cysts may be difficult to differentiate from cystic degeneration of tumors such as Hodgkin's disease, thymoma, or seminoma.

26. **What is the CT appearance of a thymic cyst?**

This is no different from any other cyst by CT. It is a nonenhancing, well-defined mass with an imperceptible wall. CT Hounsfield unit attenuation is usually that of water (0–10 HU); however, it may be increased if there is hemorrhage or an infection involving the cyst. Rarely, curvilinear calcifications occur in the wall. A thickened wall should raise suspicion of an underlying malignancy.

27. **What is a thymolipoma?**

This is a rare, benign thymic neoplasm composed primarily of fat with rare strands of thymic tissue. It is usually discovered incidentally in young adults. On CT it is a large, fat-containing mass draped around the heart and the other mediastinal structures.

28. **Which tumors other than thymoma and lymphoma occur in the anterior mediastinum?**

Germ cell tumors. These include dermoid cysts, benign and malignant teratomas, seminoma, embryonal cell carcinoma, endodermal sinus tumors, and choriocarcinoma. They occur almost exclusively in young men in their 30s.

29. **What is the typical behavior of germ cell neoplasms?**
Sixty to 70% are benign and are either teratomas or dermoid cysts. The rest are malignant, most commonly teratocarcinoma. Malignant lesions occur nearly exclusively in men, whereas benign lesions occur equally in patients of either sex.

30. **How does a dermoid cyst differ from a teratoma? Can they be differentiated by CT?**
A dermoid cyst contains only the ectodermal layer components, whereas a teratoma has all three germinal layers: endoderm, ectoderm, and mesoderm. On CT they have similar features.

KEY POINTS: ANTERIOR MEDIASTINUM

1. The four Ts of the anterior mediastinum are thyroid tumor, thymoma, teratoma, and terrible lymphoma.

2. The thymus varies in appearance with age but should appear "soft" and arrowhead-shaped.

3. Anterior mediastinal masses of thyroid origin connect to the thyroid.

---

31. **What is the CT appearance of benign germ cell neoplasms?**
These are heterogeneous, predominantly cystic masses with smooth, well-defined margins. They can have a solid component and one third to one half have calcifications. The presence of fat suggests a teratoma and identification of a tooth, although rare, is diagnostic. The combination of fat, fluid, and soft tissue elements differentiates teratomas from thymoma or lymphoma (Fig. 15-6).

32. **What is the CT appearance of malignant germ cell neoplasms?**
These are heterogeneous, solid masses with irregular margins. Calcifications are common in transformed teratomas, less so in seminomas, endodermal sinus tumors, or choriocarcinomas. Aggressive lesions are similar in appearance to invasive thymoma, with low density necrotic areas, cystic degeneration, and intratumoral calcifications.

33. **What is prognosis of patients with malignant germ cell neoplasms?**
Overall, it is very poor, with the exception of seminoma, which is radiosensitive and has a 75% long-term survival rate.

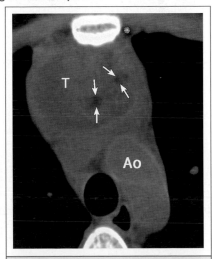

Figure 15-6. Noncontrast CT image of a well-defined anterior mediastinal mass (T), which abuts the aorta (Ao). Centrally the mass is heterogeneous with areas of fat *(arrows)* similar in attenuation to the parasternal and subcutaneous fat *(asterisks)*. Identification of fat separates teratomas from thymoma, lymph nodes, or thyroid masses.

34. **What accounts for majority of the thoracic inlet masses in adults?**
Thyroid masses are, by far, the most common and are found after age 30, more commonly in women (females are affected three to four times as often as males). Nearly 100% are the result

of thyroid overgrowth (thyroid goiter). Malignant thyroid neoplasms infrequently extend into the mediastinum.

35. **How do I know it is thyroid tissue in the mediastinum?**
    - **Location:** This mass is continuous with the cervical thyroid gland, usually in a paratracheal location, with deviation and compression of the trachea (Figs. 15-7 and 15-8). The mass almost always extends posterior to the great vessels. Anterior mediastinal masses located anterior to the great vessels are unlikely to be of thyroid origin. Approximately 25% arise from the posterior aspect of either lobe and extend into the posterior mediastinum (*see* Fig. 15-8).
    - **Appearance:** It is very high attenuation precontrast and enhances intensely post contrast. Commonly there are cystic areas and foci of calcification.

36. **What features of a thyroid mass suggest the possibility of carcinoma?**
    A solid lesion with rapid growth, an irregular ill-defined border, and presence of hemorrhage or central necrosis, especially in a patient with history of neck irradiation,

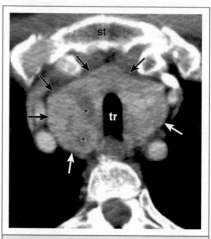

Figure 15-7. Easily identifiable enlarged thyroid *(arrows)* extends beneath the sternum (st) as an anterior mediastinal mass and narrows the trachea (tr) symmetrically. The enlarged thyroid is frequently heterogeneous with decreased attenuation adenomatous nodules *(asterisks)*.

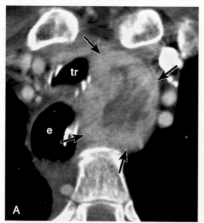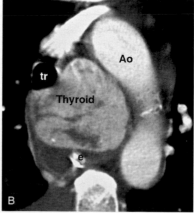

Figure 15-8. *A,* Image at the thoracic inlet shows a large enhancing heterogeneous mass with central necrosis *(arrows)* deviating the trachea (tr) and esophagus (e) to the right and the arch vessels to the left. *B,* More caudally at the level of the aortic arch (Ao) the thyroid is identified as an avidly enhancing slightly heterogeneous mass, displacing the trachea anterolaterally and the esophagus posteriorly.

is highly suspicious for a thyroid carcinoma. Adjacent enlarged lymph nodes in the presence of such a mass also suggest malignancy.

37. **What secondary malignancies occur in the anterior mediastinum?**
Any tumor may metastasize to the mediastinum, the most common are lung cancer (*see* Fig. 15-9) or breast cancer. Typical metastatic lymphadenopathy involving the anterior mediastinum will affect the aortopulmonary (AP) window nodes (Fig. 15-10). (*See* also chapters on middle mediastinum and on lung cancer.)

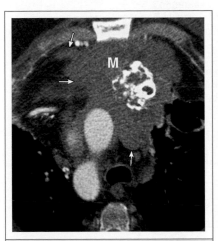

Figure 15-9. Although usually presenting as a parenchymal mass with mediastinal lymphadenopathy (*see* chapters on middle mediastinum and lung cancer), occasionally lung carcinoma presents as an anterior mediastinal mass. Characteristics are nonspecific, as in this large lobulated anterior mediastinal mass (M) with coarse central calcifications. Malignant features include linear extension (*arrow*) into the fat anteriorly. At pathology this was a squamous cell carcinoma.

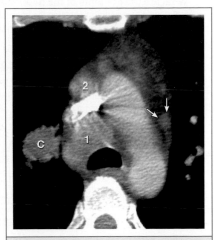

Figure 15-10. Right hilar lung carcinoma (C) with right upper paratracheal lymph node (1), precaval lymph node (2), and smaller nodes in the aortopulmonary window (*arrows*).

BIBLIOGRAPHY

1. Diseases of the mediastinum. In Fraser RS, Pare Peter JA, Fraser RG, Pare PD (eds): Synopsis of Diseases of the Chest, 2nd ed. Philadelphia, W.B. Saunders, 1994, pp 896–942.
2. Mediastinum. In Naidich DP, Zerhouni EA, Siegelman SS (eds): Computed Tomography of the Thorax. New York, Raven Press, 1984, pp 43–81.
3. Miller Q, Kline Letch A, et al: Thymoma. Available at www.emedicine.com/MED/topic2752.htm
4. National Cancer Institute: Malignant thymoma. CancerWeb page. Available at cancerweb.ncl.ac.uk/cancernet/101248.html
5. Thomas CR, Wright CD, Loehrer PJ: Thymoma: State of the art. J Clin Oncol 17:2280, 1999.
6. www.med.wayne.edu/diagRadiology/Anatomy_Modul (This is an overview of mediastinal anatomy online).

CHAPTER 16

MIDDLE MEDIASTINUM

Igor Mikityansky, MD, Nami Azar, MD, John G. Strang, MD, and Deborah Rubens, MD

1. **What are the contents of the middle mediastinum?**
   The middle mediastinum contains the heart and all its entering and exiting vessels, the pericardium, the trachea and main bronchi, paratracheal and tracheobronchial lymph nodes, and the phrenic and vagus nerves.

2. **What are the boundaries of the middle mediastinum?**
   The anterior border is the pericardium, and the posterior boundary is the spine and esophagus. The middle mediastinum is bounded laterally by the pleura, superiorly by the thoracic inlet, and inferiorly by the diaphragm (Fig. 16-1).

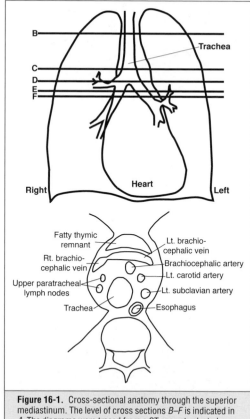

Figure 16-1. Cross-sectional anatomy through the superior mediastinum. The level of cross sections *B–F* is indicated in *A*. The diagrams were traced from a CT scan at selected levels in the superior mediastinum.

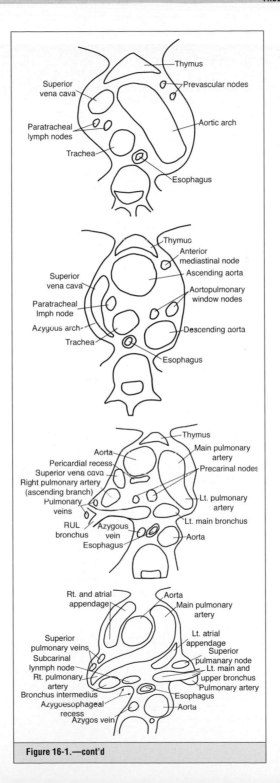

Figure 16-1.—cont'd

3. **What is the most common middle mediastinal mass?**
   Lymph node enlargement is most common, followed by vascular abnormalities (usually aneurysms) and, less commonly, cysts.

4. **What are the locations of mediastinal lymph nodes?**
   - **Anterior:** Internal mammary, paracardiac, prevascular, aorticopulmonary
   - **Middle:** Pretracheal or paratracheal, subcarinal, tracheobronchial, diaphragmatic
   - **Posterior:** Paraesophageal, inferior pulmonary ligament nodes, paravertebral nodes

   The Rouviere classification of the mediastinal lymph nodes is summarized in Table 16-1.

5. **What is the differential diagnosis of mediastinal lymphadenopathy?**
   The causes of mediastinal lymphadenopathy include neoplasms (metastases, especially from bronchogenic carcinoma or extrathoracic primary, lymphoma, leukemia), infections (tuberculosis, fungal, especially histoplasmosis, viral, such as measles and infectious mononucleosis, and bacterial), drug reaction (Dilantin), and inflammatory processes (sarcoidosis, Castleman's disease, and angioimmunoblastic lymphadenopathy) (Fig. 16-2).

6. **Which extrapulmonary primary neoplasms most often metastasize to the mediastinal lymph nodes?**
   Renal tumors, head and neck carcinomas, thyroid carcinoma, melanoma, and breast carcinoma are the most common.

TABLE 16-1. ROUVIERE CLASSIFICATION OF MEDIASTINAL LYMPH NODES

Anterior Mediastinal Nodes
- Internal mammary nodes. These lie parallel to the internal mammary arteries. They are parietal and drain the anterior chest wall, anterior diaphragm, and the medial portion of the breasts.
- Visceral nodes. These lie in the fatty tissues anterior to the large vessels and include the "ductus" node(s) or "aortopulmonary window" node(s), which drain(s) the left upper lobe.
- Cardiophrenic angle nodes.

Middle Mediastinal Nodes (Largest Visceral Group)
- The tracheobronchial nodes or hilar nodes are subdivided into upper and lower groups according to their location relative to the hila.
- The paratracheal nodes, which are subdivided into right, left, and anterior chains; they drain the upper hilar nodes. The lowest node(s) on the right is the azygous node(s).
- The bifurcation or subcarinal nodes, which are located beneath the carina; they drain the lower groups of hilar nodes and preferentially drain into the right paratracheal chain.

Posterior Mediastinal Nodes
- Paravertebral chains. These parietal nodes lie in the proximal intercostal space adjacent to the vertebrae and drain the posterior chest wall, parietal pleura, and vertebrae.
- Periesophageal nodes. Located anteriorly around the esophagus and lower aorta, they drain the posterior diaphragm and pericardium, esophagus, and medial aspect of the lower lobes. They communicate with the thoracic duct, subcarinal, intra-abdominal, para-aortic, and celiac axis nodes.

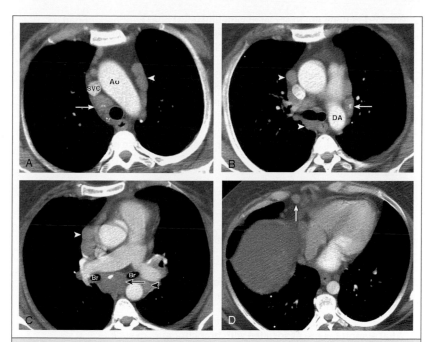

Figure 16-2. Benign mediastinal lymphadenopathy. *A,* Large, irregular pretracheal lymph node *(arrow)* with small irregular calcifications between the trachea (tr) and superior vena cava (SVC). Additional large prevascular lymph nodes *(arrowhead)* are to the left of the aortic arch (Ao). Smaller anterior mediastinal and prevascular lymph nodes are seen on the left. *B,* Large aortopulmonary window lymph node *(arrow)* with dense central calcifications is anterior to the descending aorta (DA). Additional lymph nodes *(arrowheads)* are seen in the tracheoesophageal space and prevascular space on the left. *C,* Large subcarinal lymph node *(arrow)* with small calcification is seen between the two main bronchi (Br). Enlarged para-aortic and right prevascular nodes are also visualized *(arrowhead)*. *D,* Cardiophrenic lymphadenopathy *(arrow)*.

7. **What conditions are associated with low attenuation lymph nodes?**
   These include infections (tuberculosis, *Mycobacterium avium-intracellulare* [MAI], and fungal) and aggressive neoplasms (metastases from seminoma, lung cancer, and lymphoma).

8. **What conditions are associated with calcified lymph nodes?**
   These include infections (fungal, especially histoplasmosis, and tuberculosis), neoplasms (Hodgkin's lymphoma postradiation therapy and metastases, especially mucinous adenocarcinoma), inflammatory processes (sarcoidosis), and inhalational processes (silicosis, which often demonstrates eggshell-type calcifications).

9. **What conditions are associated with prominently enhancing lymph nodes?**
   These include neoplasms (metastases, especially renal cell carcinoma, thyroid carcinoma, and small cell lung cancer) and Castleman's disease, a benign lymph node hyperplasia. Sarcoidosis nodes enhance poorly.

10. **What conditions are associated with "eggshell calcifications" of lymph nodes?**
    Most commonly silicosis or coal worker's pneumoconiosis, but they also may be seen in unusual manifestation of sarcoidosis, granulomatous infection, treated lymphoma, scleroderma, and amyloidosis.

11. **What conditions are associated with unilateral hilar lymphadenopathy?**
    These include metastases (especially from bronchogenic carcinoma or an extrathoracic primary, and lymphoma) and infections (tuberculosis, fungal, and viral).

12. **What conditions are associated with bilateral but asymmetric hilar lymphadenopathy?**
    In addition to the diseases mentioned previously, leukemia frequently involves the hilar nodes in an asymmetric fashion.

13. **What conditions are associated with bilateral symmetric hilar lymphadenopathy?**
    - Castleman's disease
    - Sarcoidosis

14. **What is a bronchogenic cyst?**
    This is a fluid-containing mass that develops due to abnormal foregut development. It is lined by respiratory epithelium and the walls contain cartilage, smooth muscle, and/or mucus glands.

15. **In which mediastinal compartment are bronchogenic cysts are found?**
    The middle mediastinum is the most common site; however, they can occur in all three compartments.

16. **What symptoms are associated with bronchogenic cysts?**
    Bronchogenic cysts are most commonly incidental findings in asymptomatic patients; however, occasionally they cause symptoms secondary to compression of adjacent structures. Rarely bronchogenic cysts become infected.

17. **What are the most common locations of bronchogenic cysts?**
    The most common location is subcarinal. The right paratracheal region is the second most common.

18. **What is the CT appearance of a bronchogenic cyst?**
    This is a well-defined, round, or oval homogeneous mass with water or soft tissue attenuation and thin, often imperceptible wall in characteristic location. Air within the cyst is uncommon and suggests infection. Calcification is uncommon as well but may occur in the wall or within cyst contents.

19. **What causes soft tissue attenuation measurements within bronchogenic cysts?**
    The protein content of these cysts may result in Hounsfield units (HU) from 10–30 HU mimicking a soft tissue mass. However, bronchogenic cysts will not enhance.

20. **What is the differential diagnosis of a cardiophrenic angle mass?**
    The differential diagnosis is pericardial cyst, lipoma, pericardial fat pad, foramen of Morgagni hernia, fibrous tumor of the pleura, and enlarged epicardial lymph nodes secondary to lymphoma or metastasis.

21. **What is a pericardial cyst?**
    This is a cystic structure attached to the parietal pericardium, lined by mesothelial cells and usually containing clear fluid (Fig. 16-3). They usually do not communicate with the pericardial space.

22. **What is the presentation of patients with pericardial cysts?**
    Pericardial cysts are usually incidental findings in asymptomatic patients.

23. What are the common locations of pericardial cysts?
The most common location is in the anterior right cardiophrenic angle. The left cardiophrenic angle and other locations, such as the lower pericardium, are seen in a third of cases. These cysts may insinuate into the major fissure and develop a teardrop configuration.

24. What is CT appearance of pericardial cysts?
These are smooth, thin-walled rounded or oval masses measuring 0–10 HU in a characteristic location. Occasionally they demonstrate soft tissue attenuation (30–40 HU), due to protein or hemorrhage within the cyst.

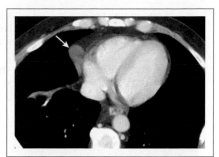

Figure 16-3. Pericardial cyst. Smooth, thin-walled, oval cystic mass *(arrow)* located in the right anterior cardiophrenic angle is a characteristic appearance for a pericardial cyst. The attenuation of the fluid inside the cyst may vary from 0 to 40 Hounsfield units, depending on protein content.

25. What is the appearance of a pericardial fat pad?
A fat-attenuation mass adjacent to the pericardium, usually in the anterior cardiophrenic angle, just lateral to the heart. They are bilateral but may be asymmetric, the right often larger then the left. They may increase over time due to obesity, Cushing's syndrome, and exogenous steroid therapy.

26. What is a foramen of Morgagni hernia? What does it contain?
This is a defect in the anteromedial diaphragm and presents radiographically as a cardiophrenic angle mass, most often on the right. It may contain omentum, liver, small bowel, or colon.

A hernia containing only omentum may appear very similar to a lipoma, except for fine linear densities representing omental vasculature. Both liver and bowel are easily identified on CT and the characteristic location suggests the diagnosis. Most foramen of Morgagni hernias are asymptomatic unless they contain bowel.

27. What is a foramen of Bochdalek hernia? What is its significance?
Unlike the foramina of Morgagni, which are clefts between the diaphragmatic muscle slips, the foramen of Bochdalek is a true gap in the diaphragm posteriorly, with no pleural or peritoneal covering. Hernias occur predominantly on the left as a right-sided defect covered by the liver. Large defects are found in infants, and much of the abdominal contents may present in the chest. In adults, Bochdalek hernias are usually asymptomatic and are discovered incidentally during chest x-ray or CT. The defect is often small, containing intra-abdominal fat or rarely a portion of spleen or kidney (Fig. 16-4).

28. What is Mounier-Kuhn syndrome?
This is a rare condition with sharply demarcated abrupt transition between normal peripheral airways and diffusely dilated trachea and main bronchi likely secondary to a defect in elastic tissues. It occurs primarily in males in their third and fourth decade and may be associated with cutis laxa or Ehlers-Danlos syndrome.

29. What is the presentation of Mounier-Kuhn syndrome?
Patients present in early childhood with recurrent respiratory infections secondary to flaccidity and collapse of the airways.

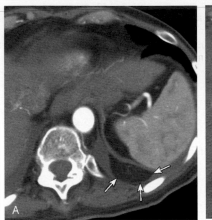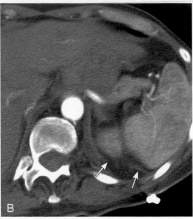

Figure 16-4. Bochdalek hernia. *A,* Image through the caudal chest shows a fat density mass *(arrows)* posterior to the left hemidiaphragm. *B,* Image 2 cm caudal reveals a gap in the diaphragm *(arrows)* through which omental fat has herniated.

30. **What is the CT appearance of Mounier-Kuhn syndrome?**
    This is characterized by tracheobronchomegaly with a corrugated appearance of the trachea and main bronchi secondary to protrusion of the mucosa between the cartilaginous rings and through the trachealis muscle. Bronchiectasis is frequently present.

31. **What are demographics of the primary tracheal tumors?**
    Extremely rare, these tumors equally affect both genders between the ages 30 and 50.
    Ninety percent of tracheal tumors in children are benign, whereas malignant tumors predominate in adults.

32. **What are the most common benign tracheal tumors?**
    These include hemangioma, papilloma, and hamartoma.

33. **What are the most common malignant tracheal tumors?**
    The most common primary malignant tracheal tumors are squamous cell carcinoma and adenoid cystic carcinoma. The most common secondary malignant tracheal tumors are esophageal carcinoma and thyroid carcinoma.

34. **What are characteristics of the squamous-cell carcinoma of the trachea?**
    It accounts for approximately one half of all primary tracheal malignancies, predominately in male smokers older than the age of 40. It tends to be slow growing, is exophytic, and frequently ulcerates. It tends to invade mediastinum. Synchronous or metachronous squamous cell carcinomas of the larynx, lungs, and esophagus are not uncommon.

35. **What is the CT appearance of squamous cell carcinoma of the trachea?**
    The tracheal wall is focally or circumferentially thickened and irregular. There is secondary narrowing of the lumen by a nodular tumor. Extension into adjacent mediastinal fat can be demonstrated in some cases as an irregular soft tissue opacity within mediastinal fat or surrounding adjacent mediastinal vessels, bronchi, or esophagus.

36. **What are characteristics of adenoid cystic carcinoma of the trachea?**
    This accounts for approximately one third of all primary tracheal malignant neoplasms. It is not related to smoking and affects both genders equally in the fifth decade. It grows slowly with endophytic spread extending in the submucosal plane of the trachea and bronchi. It may spread into the surrounding tissues of the neck and mediastinum.

37. **What is the CT appearance of adenoid cystic carcinoma of the trachea?**
    The trachea is thickened with a smooth or nodular appearance. A soft tissue attenuation mass extending into mediastinal fat may be visible. Cervical and mediastinal lymph nodes are the first sites of metastases. Hematogenous metastasis to lungs, liver, and bone can also occur.

38. **What is the treatment and outcome of adenoid cystic carcinoma of the trachea?**
    Resection and reconstruction are curative. Unresectable tumors are irradiated, typically with recurrence several years later.

39. **What is the CT appearance of a benign tracheal tumor?**
    This is a focal, well-defined, smooth or lobulated mass without evidence of tracheal or mediastinal invasion. Hamartomas and chondromas can demonstrate calcifications within chondroid elements.

40. **Which nonneoplastic conditions present as diffuse mediastinal widening (mediastinum >50% of intrathoracic diameter) on a chest radiograph?**
    These include mediastinal lipomatosis, mediastinitis (chronic or acute), diffuse mediastinal lymphadenopathy, and mediastinal hemorrhage.

41. **What is mediastinal lipomatosis?**
    This is an excessive accumulation of unencapsulated fat throughout the mediastinum, most prominently in the anterior and superior mediastinum, where it surrounds the great vessels and displaces the pleural reflections. It also can be detected in the costophrenic angles and the paravertebral, retrocrural, and subcostal regions.

42. **What causes mediastinal lipomatosis?**
    Exogenous obesity may result in mediastinal lipomatosis, but most often it is seen in conditions which results in hypercortisolism, such as Cushing's syndrome, ectopic adrenocorticotropic hormone (ACTH) production, and exogenous steroid therapy.

43. **What is the CT appearance of mediastinal lipomatosis?**
    The corticosteroids mobilize and redistribute body fat with greatest deposition in the upper mediastinum and the pleuropericardial regions. The tissue measures -70 to -30 HU, indicative of fat. The fat does not compress the esophagus or trachea.

44. **What are the etiologies of acute mediastinitis?**
    These include esophageal perforation, extension of infection from adjacent spaces or thoracic structures, postoperative complications following cardiac surgery, or traumatic rupture of the airway (Fig. 16-5).

45. **Which adjacent infectious processes extend into the mediastinum?**
    These include retropharyngeal or nasopharyngeal abscesses, infected pancreatic pseudocysts, subphrenic abscesses, infections of lungs, lymph nodes, pleura (empyema), and pericardium.

46. **What information can CT provide in acute mediastinitis?**
    CT describes the presence and amount of fluid and gas in mediastinum, describes the relationship of mediastinal fluid to adjacent structures, and provides guidance for abscess drainage.

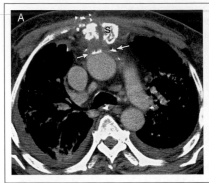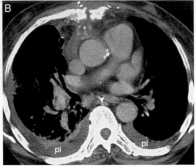

Figure 16-5. Mediastinitis. Patient after cardiac valve replacement 1 month prior with subsequent sternal wound infection and mediastinitis. **A,** Image at the carina shows destruction of the sternum (S) with fragmentary high attenuation sternal wires remaining and an enhancing soft tissue mass anterior to the aorta. **B,** More caudally the soft tissue component is much larger with some liquid centrally. Note also the bilateral pleural effusions (pl).

KEY POINTS: MIDDLE MEDIASTINUM ✓

1. Middle mediastinal masses are most commonly lymphadenopathy. Their distribution and appearance (eggshell calcification, low density) can be a clue to their etiology.

2. The differential diagnosis of middle mediastinal masses also includes vascular masses/aneurysms and bronchogenic or pericardial cysts.

47. **What is chronic mediastinitis?**
    This is the sequela of acute mediastinitis with diffuse fibrosis, sometimes compressing mediastinal structures such as the superior vena cava. Most patients are asymptomatic, however.

48. **What are the causes of chronic mediastinitis?**
    These include infections, such as histoplasmosis, coccidioidomycosis, and tuberculosis; inflammatory processes (sarcoidosis); immunologic processes (systemic lupus erythematosus, rheumatoid arthritis, and Raynaud's phenomenon); side effects of drugs (methysergide); trauma (mediastinal hemorrhage); and idiopathic processes (sclerosing mediastinitis). Histoplasmosis is the most common cause of chronic mediastinitis, especially in the Mississippi and St. Lawrence River valleys where *Histoplasma capsulatum* is endemic.

49. **What is the CT appearance of chronic mediastinitis/mediastinal fibrosis?**
    Mediastinal fibrosis can present as a diffuse process or as a mass, most commonly in the right paratracheal region. If a granulomatous infection is the cause, calcifications may be seen within enlarged mediastinal or hilar lymph nodes. Compression of mediastinal structures can be seen as well.

50. **What is the differential diagnosis for mediastinal fibrosis without calcifications?**
    This includes diffuse mediastinal involvement by either lymphoma or metastatic carcinoma.

51. How common are lymphangiomas in the mediastinum?

Lymphangiomas are more common in the neck and axilla. However, 10% of cases extend into the mediastinum. Isolated mediastinal lymphangiomas represent <1% of lymphangiomas and are more likely to be found in adults.

52. Describe the CT findings of mediastinal lymphangiomas.

- Usually in the superior or anterior mediastinum
- Smoothly marginated cystic mass of water attenuation
- One third have visible septations
- May have areas of high attenuation (hemorrhage) or calcifications
- May displace or insinuate around adjacent mediastinal vessels
- Associated with venous aneurysms

BIBLIOGRAPHY

1. Diseases of the mediastinum. In Fraser RS, Pare Peter JA, Fraser RG, Pare PD (eds): Synopsis of Diseases of the Chest, 2nd ed. Philadelphia, W.B. Saunders, 1994, pp 896–942.

2. Mediastinum. In Naidich DP, Zerhouni EA, Siegelman SS (eds): Computed Tomography of the Thorax. New York, Raven Press, 1984, pp 43–81.

3. www.med.wayne.edu/diagRadiology/Anatomy_Modul (This is a good overview of mediastinal anatomy online.)

CHAPTER 17

POSTERIOR MEDIASTINUM

Igor Mikityansky, MD, Nami Azar, MD, John G. Strang, MD, and Deborah Rubens, MD

1. **What are the common and/or important posterior mediastinal masses?**
   - Hiatal hernia
   - Esophageal carcinoma
   - Megaesophagus
   - Extramedullary hematopoiesis
   - Lymphadenopathy (lymphoma)
   - Neurogenic tumors
   - Bochdalek hernia
   - Musculoskeletal tumors (benign, malignant, metastases)
   - Meningocele/meningomyelocele (consider before biopsy)
   - Esophageal varices

2. **How common is esophageal cancer?**
   The American Cancer Society estimates for 2005 are 14,250 new cases and 13,570 deaths. The extremely high mortality rate is due to diagnosis in late stage and the ease of the tumor spreading locally and to lymph nodes. There are no boundaries to regional spread and adenopathy (Fig. 17-1).

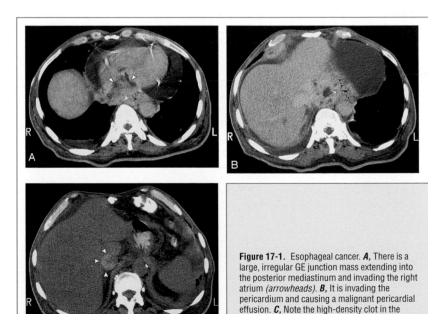

Figure 17-1. Esophageal cancer. **A,** There is a large, irregular GE junction mass extending into the posterior mediastinum and invading the right atrium *(arrowheads).* **B,** It is invading the pericardium and causing a malignant pericardial effusion. **C,** Note the high-density clot in the inferior vena cava seen on the precontrast images *(arrowheads).*

3. **What is the CT appearance of esophageal cancer?**
A thick-walled esophagus with proximal dilation if the mass is obstructive. Lymphadenopathy is common, particularly in the paraesophageal region and along the lesser curvature of the stomach (for low-lying tumors). Detecting esophageal cancer incidentally by CT is unusual, however, due to the normal areas of collapse and dilation of the esophagus in a patient lying supine. The gastroesophageal (GE) junction is particularly difficult when the esophagus runs obliquely, and there may be a small hiatal hernia. Therefore, most CT is done for staging after the diagnosis is known. Lymphadenopathy is the main finding by staging as well as clear extramural extension of tumor in some cases. Transesophageal ultrasound can be useful for determining depth of invasion and detecting adenopathy. Positron emission tomography (PET)/CT is also effective in staging esophageal cancer (Fig. 17-2).

4. **What are GERD and Barrett esophagus? What is their relationship to esophageal cancer?**
GERD is gastrointestinal reflux disease. Barrett esophagus is metaplasia of the distal esophageal mucosa from normal squamous epithelium to columnar epithelium. It is largely caused by irritation from chronic reflux. It may be asymptomatic but raises the risk for adenocarcinoma of the esophagus. However, adenocarcinoma is rare, whereas GERD is extremely common (50% of U.S. adults monthly). Few patients with GERD will get esophageal adenocarcinoma.

5. **What is the difference between squamous cell and adenocarcinoma of the esophagus?**
Squamous cell occurs primarily in the proximal one half to two thirds of the esophagus. Adenocarcinoma arises primarily in the distal third, likely after metaplasia to Barrett esophagus. Adenocarcinoma was uncommon but now accounts for approximately 50% of esophageal cancers.

6. **Describe the staging of esophageal cancer.**
Esophageal cancer is staged using the TNM system (American Joint Committee on Cancer). The key break points are between stage II and stage III (regional nodal metastases with a tumor reaching the adventitia and/or tumor invading adjacent structures) and between stage III and stage IV (development of metastases).

7. **How is esophageal cancer treated?**
Surgical excision is the curative therapy attempted for early-stage esophageal carcinoma. There are various methods for performing esophagectomy. Nonresectable cancer is treated with chemotherapy, irradiation, and chemoradiation with palliative surgery or endoscopic procedures, such as stenting for obstruction.

8. **What are the causes of megaesophagus?**
Achalasia and scleroderma (progressive systemic sclerosis) are the most common causes. Chronic stricture from reflux or mediastinitis may also cause megaesophagus. Chagas disease is the classic disease that is a specific cause of achalasia.

9. **What does *achalasia* mean?**
Achalasia literally means failure of relaxation. The distal esophageal sphincter does not relax, resulting in eventual massive dilation of the esophagus. Loss of the myenteric nervous plexus is sometimes seen. Chagas disease is one specific cause, but in the United States achalasia is predominantly idiopathic.

10. **What is Chagas disease?**
Chagas disease is endemic in South America and is spread from various mammal hosts to humans by the bites of *Trypanosoma cruzi*. Over many years, it causes deterioration of the

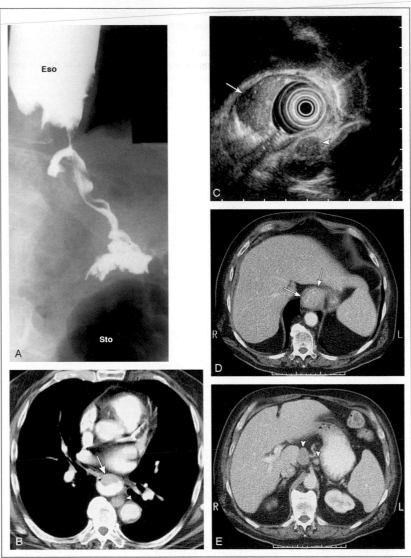

Figure 17-2. Esophageal cancer at the GE junction. This patient presented with dysphagia. **A,** Barium swallow shows a segmental annular constricting mass with abrupt shoulders, typical for esophageal carcinoma. Eso = esophagus; Sto = stomach. **B,** Note the equivalent abrupt overhanging shoulders of the tumor *(arrow)* on the CT at the proximal margin of the tumor. There is also a dilated esophagus and adjacent posterior mediastinal adenopathy *(arrowhead)*. **C,** Note that the adenopathy *(arrowhead)* is also visible on endoscopic ultrasound, which has been used to judge depth of tumor invasion *(arrow)*. **D,** Although the tumor is easily seen at its proximal border, differentiating the distal margin of the mass *(arrows)* from collapsed stomach in a small hiatal hernia can be difficult. **E,** There is also gastrohepatic ligament lymphadenopathy *(arrowheads)*, a common site of regional metastasis for a GE junction tumor.

myenteric nervous plexus of the esophagus and leads to megaesophagus and malnutrition. It also causes cardiomyopathy and megacolon. There are an estimated 24 million infected people in South America and 60,000 annual deaths due to Chagas disease. It is present in the United States due to immigration.

11. **Why is the reduviid bug also known as the "kissing beetle"?**
    It is known by this name because it bites around the lips.

12. **What is extramedullary hematopoiesis?**
    Extramedullary hematopoiesis is compensatory hematopoiesis in patients with chronic ane-
    mias. Erythrocyte-producing cells can cluster in multiple sites: liver, spleen, and paraspinal
    sites. The classic appearance is illustrated in Fig. 17-3. History is usually key; look for tha-
    lassemia, spherocytosis, or other chronic severe anemia.

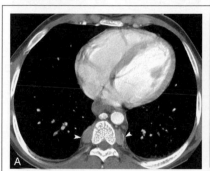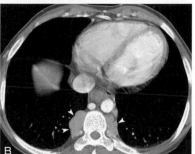

Figure 17-3. Classic appearance of extramedullary hematopoiesis. *A,* Lobulated bilateral homogenous
paraspinal masses in the lower chest *(arrowheads).* The masses can erode adjacent bone. *B,* Note the
expanded medullary space in the adjacent vertebral body causing the lacy appearance to the bone.

13. **What should I know about the neurogenic tumors of the posterior
    mediastinum?**
    - They can arise from a peripheral nerve (intercostal nerves) or the sympathetic ganglia (verti-
      cally oriented).
    - Often they are incidentally discovered by chest x-ray.
    - Neurogenic tumors usually are sharply circumscribed, although plexiform neurofibroma can
      be irregular and invasive.
    - Calcification occasionally occurs but is not a discriminating feature.
    - Some are malignant.
    - Both benign and malignant tumors can erode adjacent ribs, vertebral bodies, or neuroforamina
      (*see* Fig. 17-4).

14. **What is a Bochdalek hernia?**
    A Bochdalek hernia is a posterolateral defect in the development of the diaphragm. It has two
    common presentations:
    - In **infants** they are relatively common (1:2200), may be large, occur overwhelmingly on the
      left, and may cause lung hypoplasia. They carry significant mortality rates.
    - In **adults**, they are small and asymptomatic, usually contain intra-abdominal fat, and become
      very common (>35% older than age 70) with advanced age and chronic obstructive pul-
      monary disease (COPD).
    Bochdalek hernias are usually discovered incidentally by the radiologist. The role of CT is usually
    to show that a paradiaphragmatic mass seen on chest roentgenogram is only a Bochdalek hernia.

15. **What is the role of CT for hiatal hernias?**
    Because hiatal hernias are common and generally benign, CT has little role. CT does, however,
    identify their benign nature when they present as a mediastinal mass on chest x-ray. CT can also
    diagnose complications such as gastric volvulus of the herniated stomach (which presents as
    pain and obstruction) (*see* Fig. 17-5).

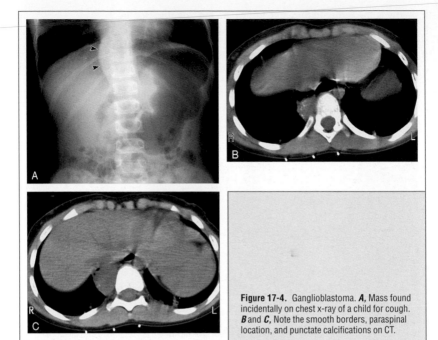

Figure 17-4. Ganglioblastoma. **A,** Mass found incidentally on chest x-ray of a child for cough. **B** and **C,** Note the smooth borders, paraspinal location, and punctate calcifications on CT.

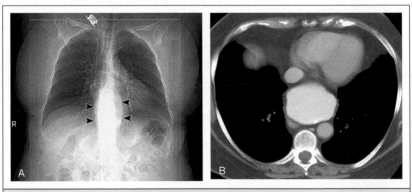

Figure 17-5. A, Fusiform retrocardiac mass on frontal projection in the lower chest *(arrowheads).* **B,** Contrast-filled stomach in hiatal hernia. Differentiate from a dilated esophagus by the presence of rugae and/or an esophageal mass or stricture more distally.

16. **What are some emergent conditions to watch for in the posterior mediastinum?**
    - Esophageal rupture (Boerhaave's syndrome): From forceful repetitive vomiting (Fig. 17-6)
    - Aortic rupture/dissection (*see* aortic pathology)
    - Gastric volvulus in a hiatal hernia
    - Paraspinal abscess
    - Esophageal traumatic perforation (penetrating injuries or iatrogenic from esophagoscopy or dilation of strictures)
    - Paraesophageal abscesses, usually from breakdown of a surgical anastomosis (Fig. 17-7)

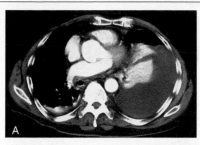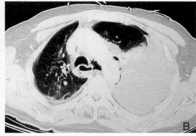

Figure 17-6. Boerhaave's syndrome: esophageal perforation after protracted vomiting. There is a left-sided hydropneumothorax *(A)* as well as pneumomediastinum and esophageal thickening *(B)*.

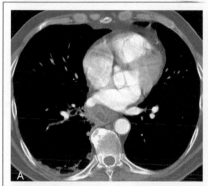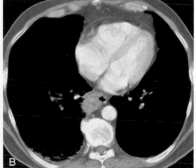

Figure 17-7. A 64-year-old man with history of chronic reflux develops severe chest pain for several days. *A,* CT at time of presentation shows a small paraesophageal abscess, presumably from reflux and perforation. *B,* This resolves with antibiotics.

17. What is the clinical picture of patients with esophageal perforation?

They present with fever, leukocytosis, dysphagia, and retrosternal chest pain radiating to the back. Associated pleural abnormalities (pneumothorax and empyema) are usually left-sided.

18. What causes esophageal perforation?

This may be iatrogenic (esophageal endoscopy or esophageal dilatation) or from impacted foreign body, an obstructing esophageal neoplasm, or repeated episodes of vomiting (Boerhaave's syndrome).

19. What are the complications of esophageal perforation?

The complications include mediastinal abscess and esophagobronchial and esophagopleural fistulas.

20. Why is it important to recognize esophageal perforation?

Morbidity and mortality rates are very high if there is a delay in diagnosis beyond 24 hours.

21. What is the classic cause of a paraspinal abscess?

Tuberculosis of the spine is the classic cause.

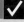
1. Neurogenic tumors often present as smoothly marginated posterior mediastinal masses.

2. Esophageal carcinoma has high morbidity and mortality rates.

3. CT is usually for done staging rather than diagnosis and for detection of local spread, metastases, and lymphadenopathy.

4. PET/CT is an alternative staging modality.

22. **Can esophageal varices from portal hypertension present as a posterior mediastinal mass?**
    Yes, when they are very large (Fig. 17-8).

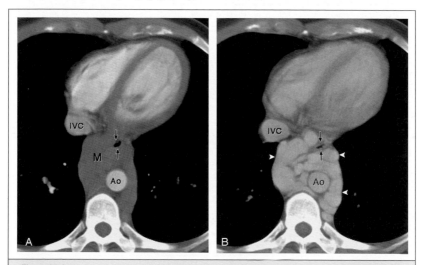

Figure 17-8. Large varices. **A,** Arterial phase image shows the highly contrasted aorta (Ao) and the less contrasted inferior vena cava (IVC). The aorta is surrounded by a relatively nonenhancing homogenous mass (M). The esophagus *(arrows)* is in the anterior portion of the mass. **B,** On delayed (portal venous phase) image, multiple contrast-filled venous varices *(arrowheads)* surround the aorta (Ao). Be wary of biopsying based on a noncontrast study alone!

BIBLIOGRAPHY

1. American Cancer Society: www.cancer.org/docroot/CRI/CRI_2_1x.asp?rnav=criov&dt=12 (Overview of esophageal cancer (and many other cancers).

2. Boiselle P: Mediastinal masses. In McCloud T (ed): Thoracic Radiology: The Requisites. St. Louis, Mosby, 1998, pp 431–462.

3. Kreas B: Michigan Statue University Course on Parasitology: www.msu.edu/course/zol/316/tcru.htm

4. Martínez S, Restrepo CS, Carrillo JA, et al: Thoracic manifestations of tropical parasitic infections: A pictorial review. Radiographics 25:135–155, 2005.

5. Muller N, Fraser R, Colman N, Pare N: Mediastinal masses. In Muller N, Fraser R, Colman N, Pare N (eds): Radiologic Diagnosis of Diseases of the Chest. Philadelphia, W.B. Saunders, 2001, pp 682–747, 753–754.

6. Robbins SL, Cotran RS, Kumar V: Pathologic Basis of Disease 3rd ed. Philadelphia, W.B. Saunders, 1984, pp 798–802.

7. Shaheen N, Ransohoff DF: Gastroesophageal reflux, Barrett esophagus, and esophageal cancer: Scientific review. JAMA 287:1972–1981, 2002.

8. University of Bonn: www.meb.uni-bonn.de/cancer.gov/CDR0000062741.html#REF_53 (Review of esophageal cancer).

CHAPTER 18

VASCULAR ANATOMY OF THE CHEST: NORMAL AND CONGENITAL VARIANTS

Susan Voci, MD, Nael E. A. Saad, MBBCh, and Igor Mikityansky, MD

1. **What are the parts of the thoracic aorta?**
   The thoracic aorta consists of the ascending aorta, aortic arch, and descending thoracic aorta.

2. **What is the anatomy of the ascending aortic arch?**
   The aortic arch extends obliquely posteriorly and to the left. Proximally, the arch is anterior to the trachea and to the left of the superior vena cava (SVC). More distally, the aorta is to the left of the trachea.

3. **What are the branches of the aortic arch?**
   The proximal part of the aortic arch gives rise to the brachiocephalic (innominate), left carotid, and the left subclavian arteries. Variations in the branching pattern of these vessels are common. The left vertebral artery may arise directly from the arch.

4. **What is the difference between the innominate artery and the brachiocephalic artery?**
   There is none. Innominate means without a name; it would seem that the largest branch of the aorta deserves a name! The brachiocephalic artery (or trunk) is a better name, especially because the innominate artery has nothing to do with the innominate bone—another name for the coccyx.

5. **Why isn't it called the "right" brachiocephalic artery?**
   Because there is no left brachiocephalic artery. The left common carotid and the left subclavian artery have separate origins on the aorta.

6. **What are the branches of the descending thoracic aorta?**
   The descending thoracic aorta has four visceral branches: the pericardial, bronchial, esophageal, and mediastinal arteries. It also has three sets of parietal branches: the intercostal, subcostal, and superior phrenic arteries. The largest branches are the intercostal and bronchial arteries.

7. **What does the aortic root consist of?**
   The aortic root is the proximal portion of the ascending aorta and consists of the aortic valve, annulus, and the three sinuses of Valsalva.

8. **Where do the right and left coronary arteries arise?**
   The right and left coronary arteries arise from the right and left sinuses of Valsalva.

9. **Why is the posterior sinus referred to as the noncoronary sinus?**
   The posterior sinus does not give off a coronary artery.

10. **Why does coronary sinus anatomy matter? I will never do coronary angiography.**
    Never say never. Multislice CTA (16 slice or more) can determine if there is a coronary artery anomaly. Even if you are not asked to look for them, coronary artery anomalies occur

incidentally in approximately 0.3% of the population. Look for both the right and left main arteries arising from one sinus and the ectopic artery passing between the aortic root and the pulmonary trunk. There are both benign and potentially malignant coronary artery anomalies. Malignant coronary artery anomalies can present with sudden death, most famously in the case of Pete Maravich, basketball star, who had an absent left coronary artery and died of a myocardial infarction at age 40 during exercise.

11. **What is the aortic isthmus?**
The aortic isthmus is the distal portion of the aortic arch between the origin of the left subclavian artery and the ligamentum arteriosum.

12. **Above the level of the aortic arch, in the superior mediastinum, which five vessels can be identified?**
Three arteries
- Brachiocephalic artery
- Left common carotid artery
- Left subclavian artery
Two veins
- Right brachiocephalic vein
- Left brachiocephalic vein

The right brachiocephalic, the left common carotid, and left subclavian arteries arise from the aortic arch (Fig. 18-1). Variations to this branching portion are common. The most common variation is a bovine arch: a conjoint origin of the brachiocephalic and left common carotid arteries (22–36% cases) (Fig. 18-2).

13. **What is the anatomy of the SVC?**
The SVC is formed by the union of the left and right brachiocephalic veins. It terminates in the right atrium. The SVC is the venous return pathway of the head, neck, upper extremities, and the posterolateral thoracic and abdominal wall.

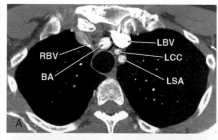
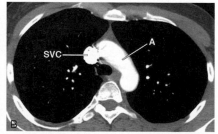
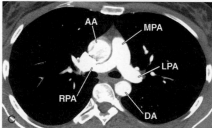

Figure 18-1. *A,* Section through the superior mediastinum showing the usual five vessels: brachiocephalic artery (BA), right brachiocephalic vein (RBV), left brachiocephalic vein (LBV), left common carotid artery (LCC), and left subclavian artery (LSA). *B,* Axial section at the level of the aortic arch. A = aortic arch, SVC = superior vena cava. *C,* Axial section at the level of the pulmonary arteries. AA = ascending aorta, DA = descending aorta, LPA = left pulmonary artery, MPA = main pulmonary artery, RPA = right pulmonary artery.

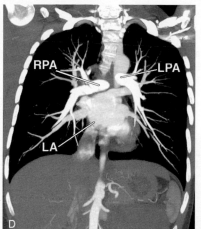

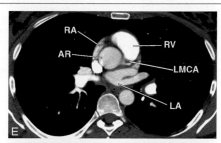

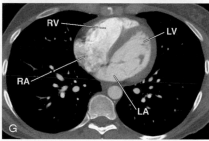

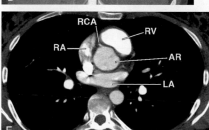

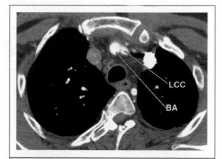

Figure 18-1.—cont'd *D,* Coronal reformat at the level of the pulmonary arteries. LA = left atrium, LPA = left pulmonary artery, RPA = right pulmonary artery. *E,* Axial section at the level of the aortic root (AR). Proximal portion of the left main coronary artery (LMCA) can be seen. LA = left atrium, RA = right atrium, RV = right ventricular outflow tract. *F,* Axial section at the level of the aortic root. Proximal portion of the right coronary artery (RCA) can be seen. AR = aortic root, LA = left atrium, RA = right atrium, RV = right ventricular outflow tract. *G,* Axial section at the level of the heart demonstration the four chambers. LA = left atrium, LV = left ventricle, RA = right atrium, RV = right ventricle.

14. **What is the anatomy of the inferior vena cava (IVC)?**
    The IVC is formed by the union of the common iliac veins. It drains into the right atrium via the inferior vena caval orifice.

15. **Where is the azygous arch located in the chest?**
    The arch of the azygous is typically located at the level of the T5-T6 vertebral bodies.

16. **What is the normal size of the azygous arch?**
    The arch of the azygous is variable in size, measuring up to 15 mm.

Figure 18-2. Axial section just superior to the arch in a patient with a bovine arch, a normal variant. The left common carotid artery (LCC) and the brachiocephalic artery (DA) have a common origin and are just beginning to separate in this image.

17. **What is the anatomy of the azygous arch?**
The arch of the azygous crosses over the right mainstem bronchus. It extends anteriorly along the right side of the distal trachea to join the SVC.

18. **Describe the location and course of the left superior intercostal vein.**
At the level of the aortic arch, the left superior intercostal vein joins the accessory hemiazygous vein. The left superior intercostal vein courses anteriorly around the aortic arch to join the left brachiocephalic vein (Fig. 18-3).

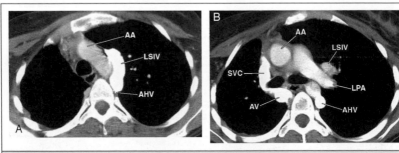

Figure 18-3. **A,** Enlarged left superior intercostal vein (LSIV). AA = aortic arch AHV = accessory hemiazygous vein. **B,** Section at level of azygous arch. Enlarged left superior intercostal vein could be mistaken for lymphadenopathy. AA = ascending aorta, AHV = accessory hemiazygous vein, AV = azygous vein, LPA = left pulmonary artery, LSIV = left superior intercostal vein, SVC = superior vena cava.

19. **Why is recognition of this venous anatomy important?**
The left superior intercostal vein can be mistaken for preaortic lymphadenopathy.

20. **How many pulmonary veins are there?**
There are four pulmonary veins, two from each lung, carrying oxygenated blood from the lungs to the posterosuperior aspect of the left atrium. They have no valves. The pulmonary vein draining the right middle lobe usually drains into the right upper pulmonary vein; however, occasionally it may drain separately into the left atrium. Sometimes the left upper and lower pulmonary veins drain into the left atrium via a common trunk (Fig. 18-4).

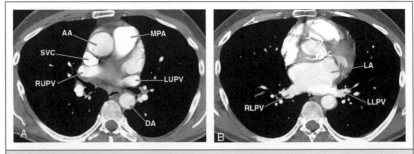

Figure 18-4. **A,** Section through the upper pulmonary veins. AA = ascending aorta, DA = descending aorta, LUPV = left upper pulmonary vein, MPA = main pulmonary artery MPA, SVC = superior vena cava, RUPV = right upper pulmonary vein. **B,** Section through the left atrium (LA). LLPV = left lower pulmonary vein, RLPV = right lower pulmonary vein.

21. **What is the anatomy of the pulmonary arteries?**
    The main pulmonary trunk arises from the right ventricle and divides into the right and left pulmonary arteries.

22. **What is the normal size ratio between the main pulmonary artery and the ascending aorta?**
    The normal pulmonary artery is approximately two-thirds the diameter of the aorta. If the main pulmonary artery is equal in size to the aorta at the same level, then the main pulmonary aorta is enlarged.

23. **Describe the normal bronchial artery anatomy.**
    - The normal anatomy of bronchial arteries shows considerable variability ranging from two to four bronchial arteries. Most commonly there is one right bronchial artery and two left bronchial arteries.
    - The normal bronchial artery diameter is less than 2 mm.
    - The left bronchial arteries arise directly from the aorta.
    - The right bronchial artery arises from the third intercostal artery in about 70% of cases.
    - The bronchial arteries lie along the main bronchi and branch with the airways.
    - The bronchial arteries are present to the level of the terminal bronchioles.

24. **List the common mediastinal sites where the bronchial arteries course.**
    - Retroesophageal space
    - Retrotracheal space
    - Retrobronchial
    - Aortopulmonary window

25. **What is the number and origin of the intercostal arteries?**
    There are 11 in all. The upper two intercostal spaces are supplied by the first intercostal artery, which arises from the costocervical trunk of the subclavian artery. There are nine pairs of intercostal arteries arising from the posterior surface of the aorta and they course along the lower nine intercostal spaces.

26. **What is the relationship of the subclavian artery and vein in the axilla?**
    The subclavian artery lies posterior to the vein in the axilla, allowing blind central venous access.

27. **What are normal sizes of the thoracic aorta and pulmonary artery?**
    - **Ascending aorta:** 4.5 cm at the level of the aortic root, 3.5 cm at the level of the right pulmonary artery
    - **Descending aorta:** 2.0–3.0 cm
    - **Ratio of ascending to descending aorta at aortic root:** ≤1.7 cm
    - **Main pulmonary artery:** 2.8 ± 0.3 cm
    - **Right pulmonary artery:** 2.0 ± 0.4 cm
    - **Left pulmonary artery:** 2.0 ± 0.2 cm

CONGENITAL VASCULAR VARIANTS OF THE CHEST

28. **What is the most common congenital anomaly of the aorta?**
    The most common congenital anomaly of the aorta is an aberrant right subclavian artery that originates from a normal left-sided arch.

29. **What is the prevalence of an aberrant right subclavian artery?**
    This occurs in 0.5–1% of the population.

30. **What is the CT appearance of an aberrant right subclavian artery?**
    A vascular structure arising from the posterior portion of a left-sided arch, coursing from left to right posterior to the trachea and the esophagus (Fig. 18-5).

31. **What is the diverticulum of Kommerell?**
    For a left-sided arch, the distal portion of the embryologic right arch persists, dilates, and gives rise to the aberrant right subclavian artery. This is incorporated into the posterior portion of the left arch (Fig. 18-6).

32. **How many right-sided aortic arch anomalies can potentially occur?**
    Five potential anomalies can occur.

33. **What is the most common right aortic arch anomaly?**
    The most common right aortic arch anomaly is a right aortic arch with an aberrant left subclavian artery (Fig. 18-7).

34. **Is a right aortic arch with an aberrant left subclavian artery associated with congenital heart disease?**
    It is rarely associated.

35. **What is the second most common type of right arch anomaly?**
    A right aortic arch with mirror image branching is the second most common.

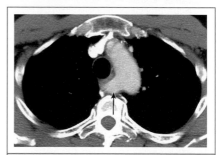

Figure 18-5. Aberrant right subclavian artery (ARSA) with left-sided arch. The right subclavian artery can be seen coursing from left to right posterior to the esophagus (ESO).

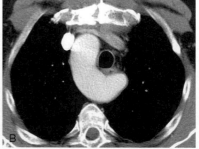

Figure 18-6. Diverticulum of Kommerell *(arrow)* with left-sided aortic arch and aberrant right subclavian artery.

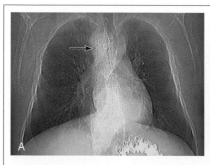

Figure 18-7. Right-sided aortic arch. *A,* Frontal projection shows a right paratracheal bulge *(arrow)* and absence of the normal left sided aortic contour. *B,* Axial image shows the right-sided arch with an aberrant left subclavian artery.

36. **What is the significance of the right aortic arch with mirror image branching?**
This anomaly is significant because congenital heart disease is present in nearly 100% of cases.

37. **What is the most common congenital heart disease associated with a right arch with mirror image branching?**
Tetralogy of Fallot is the most common.

38. **What are the types of double aortic arches?**
There are two types of double aortic arches. The most common form is the functional double aortic arch. In this case, both arches are patent. Both arches join posteriorly to form one descending aorta, which may be midline or left sided. In this anomaly, the right arch is usually larger. The trachea and esophagus are surrounded by the ring formed by the aortic root, the two arches, and the descending thoracic aorta. Less commonly, a double arch is present with atresia of some portion of the left arch.

39. **What is the major difference between double aortic arch with atresia and right aortic arch anomalies?**
With double aortic arch with atresia some portion of the left arch persists; therefore, a vascular ring around the esophagus and trachea is present. With right arch anomalies the left aortic arch is interrupted, and there is seldom a vascular ring.

40. **What are the symptomatic arch anomalies?**
These include double aortic arch, right aortic arch with aberrant left subclavian artery and persistent left ligamentum arteriosum, and cervical arch. All of these can result in tracheal and esophageal compression. Double aortic arch and right arch with aberrant left subclavian artery present in infancy with respiratory and feeding problems.

41. **What is coarctation of the aorta?**
Coarctation of the aorta is a focal narrowing in the proximal descending thoracic aorta, typically in the region of the ductus arteriosus.

42. **What are typical presentations in patients with coarctation of the aorta?**
Infants may present with congestive heart failure when the ductus arteriosus closes. Adults usually present with hypertension and discrepant blood pressure measurements in the arms and legs.

43. **What is the most common cardiac anomaly associated with coarctation of the aorta?**
Bicuspid aortic valve occurs in 75–85% of patients who have coarctations.

44. **What are other cardiovascular anomalies associated with coarctation of the aorta?**
   - Ventricular septal defect
   - Aneurysms of the ascending aorta, ductus, intercostal arteries, and circle of Willis
   - Stenosis of the left subclavian artery
   - Aberrant right subclavian artery
   - Tubular hypoplasia of the transverse arch (50% of patients)

45. **What is pseudocoarctation of the aorta?**
Pseudocoarctation of the aorta is a congenital elongation of the aortic arch resulting in redundancy and kinking. There is no obstruction to blood flow and, therefore, no pressure gradient and no collateral circulation.

46. **What are common collateral pathways resulting from coarctation of the aorta?**
    - Subclavian artery >> internal mammary artery >> intercostal arteries >> descending thoracic aorta
    - Subclavian artery >> thyrocervical and costocervical trunks >> thoracoacromial and descending scapular arteries >> descending thoracic aorta
    - Subclavian artery > > vertebral artery >> anterior spinal artery >> intercostal arteries >> descending thoracic aorta

47. **What are some anomalies of the pulmonary arteries?**
    - Absence of the main pulmonary artery
    - Interruption (absence) of the right or left pulmonary artery
    - Anomalous origin of the left pulmonary artery from the right
    - Pulmonary artery stenosis or coarctation
    - Congenital aneurysms of the pulmonary arteries
    - Direct communication of the right pulmonary artery with the left atrium

48. **What are the CT features of absence or agenesis of a pulmonary artery?**
    Small hemithorax, ipsilateral displacement of the mediastinum, absent main and interlobar arteries, and enlarged contralateral pulmonary arteries and veins are CT features.

49. **Is agenesis of a pulmonary artery an isolated event?**
    Agenesis of a pulmonary artery can be an isolated event or can be associated with congenital heart disease, most commonly tetralogy of Fallot.

50. **What is the scimitar syndrome?**
    Scimitar syndrome is an anomaly of the right pulmonary artery associated with hypoplasia of the right lung with partial anomalous pulmonary venous return to the IVC.

51. **What is the pulmonary artery sling?**
    This is an anomalous left pulmonary artery arising from the right pulmonary artery. This vessel passes posteriorly and to the right side of the distal trachea or right main bronchus, then courses to the left and passes between the esophagus and trachea as it courses to the left hilum. This can result in compression of the right main bronchus and or the trachea.

52. **What is a pulmonary sequestration?**
    A pulmonary sequestration is nonfunctioning lung tissue that derives its blood supply from systemic vessels and is not associated with the bronchi.

53. **What are the two types of sequestrations? How do they differ?**
    Intralobar and extralobar. **Intralobar sequestrations** are contiguous with normal lung and enclosed by pleura. The feeding artery arises from the thoracic aorta most commonly, from the abdominal aortal or celiac artery, and least commonly an intercostal artery. They usually drain to normal pulmonary veins. Intralobar sequestrations are not usually associated with other anomalies and usually discovered incidentally in adulthood.

    Extralobar sequestrations are external to the pleura. They usually derive arterial blood from multiple small vessels. Venous drainage is to systemic veins such as the azygous, hemiazygous, IVC, and the portal vein. They are often associated with other congenital anomalies and therefore identified in the neonatal period or early childhood.

54. **What is the developmental anomaly responsible for persistent left SVC?**
    The anomaly is failure of embryologic regression of a portion of the left common and anterior cardinal veins.

55. What is the prevalence of a persistent left SVC?
It occurs in less than 0.5% of the population.

56. What is the CT appearance of a persistent left SVC?
The left SVC is a vascular structure located lateral to the left common carotid artery and anterior to the left hilum as it courses caudally to drain into the right atrium via a dilated coronary sinus. The right SVC may or may not be present (Figs. 18-8 and 18-9).

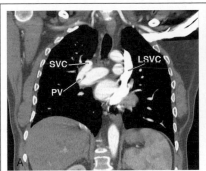
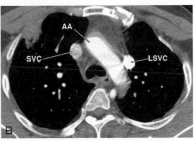

Figure 18-8. *A,* Coronal reformat demonstrating persistent left superior vena cava (LSVC). Note also partial anomalous pulmonary venous return with right pulmonary vein (PV) draining to superior vena cava (SVC) on the right. *B,* Axial section at level of aortic arch (AA). Note that the left SVC does not go to the accessory hemiazygous vein.

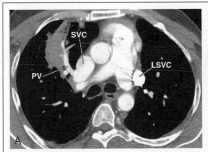
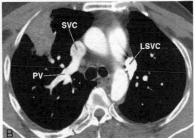

Figure 18-9. *A,* Partial anomalous pulmonary veins drainage. Right upper pulmonary vein (PV), drains to the superior vena cava (SVC). Note persistent left superior vena cava (LSVC). *B,* Right lower PV drains to SVC.

57. What is the clinical significance of a persistent left SVC?
The clinical significance is minor, unless there is an associated atrial septal defect with a left to right shunt. It is significant for surgical planning in heart transplant recipients.

KEY POINTS: FOUR MAJOR COLLATERAL PATHWAYS BETWEEN THE SUPERIOR AND INFERIOR VENA CAVA

1. Via the azygous and hemiazygous veins
2. Via the vertebral venous plexus
3. Via the internal mammary veins/superior epigastric
4. Via the lateral thoracic veins

58. **What is azygous continuation of the IVC?**
    With developmental failure of the hepatic or infrahepatic portion of the IVC, blood returns to the heart via the azygous and hemiazygous veins.

59. **What are the CT findings in azygous continuation?**
    Enlargement of the arch of the azygous, enlargement of the paraspinal portions of the azygous and hemiazygous veins, enlargement of the retrocrural portions of these veins, and absence of the IVC.

60. **With what is azygous continuation associated?**
    It is associated with asplenia and polysplenia syndromes.

61. **What are the four groups of drainage in anomalous pulmonary venous drainage?**
    - Supracardiac, usually to persistent left SVC, 55% of cases
    - Cardiac, direct connection with right atrium or coronary sinus, 30% of cases
    - infradiaphragmatic, common vein that extends below the diaphragm to the portal vein or one of its branches, 15% of cases
    - Mixed, 5% of cases (*see* Figs. 18-4A and 18-5)

KEY POINTS: VASCULAR VARIANTS THAT CAN PRESENT AS MEDIASTINAL MASSES

1. Aberrant right subclavian artery
2. Persistent left SVC
3. Right-sided aortic arch
4. Double aortic arch
5. Azygous continuation

62. **Why is a vascular structure an important aspect of the differential diagnosis of a mediastinal mass?**
    A vascular structure needs to be excluded prior to biopsy.

BIBLIOGRAPHY

1. Dahnert W: Chest. In Dahnert W (ed): Radiology Review Manual. Baltimore, Lippincott, Williams & Wilkins, 1991, pp 191–256.

2. Fraser RS, Pare, Peter JA: Pulmonary abnormalities of developmental origin. In Fraser RS, Pare Peter JA, Fraser RG, Pared PD (eds): Synopsis of Diseases of the Chest, 2nd ed. Philadelphia, W.B. Saunders, 1994, pp 256–283.

3. Gamsu G: The mediastinum. In Moss AA, Gamsu G, Gerart HK (eds): Computed Tomography of the Body with Magnetic Resonance Imaging. 2nd ed. Philadelphia, W.B. Saunders, 1992, pp 43–118.

4. Gutierrez FR, Woodard PK, Fleishman MJ, et al: Thorax: Techniques and normal anatomy. In Lee JKT, Sagel SS, Stanley RJ (eds): Computed Body Tomography with MRI Correlation, 3rd ed. Philadelphia, Lippincott-Raven, 1998, pp 183–259.

5. Hague C, Andrews, G. Forster B: MDCT of a malignant right coronary artery. AJR 182:617–618, 2004.

6. Naidich DP, Webb WR, Muller NL, et al: Aorta, arch vessels, and great veins. In Naidich DP, Webb WR, Muller NL, et al (eds): Computed Tomography and Magnetic Resonance of the Thorax, 3rd ed. Philadelphia, Lippincott-Raven, 1998, pp 505–602.

7. Webb WR, Bran WE, Helms CA: Techniques of thoracic CT. In Webb WR, Bran WE, Helms CA (eds): Fundamentals of Body CT. Philadelphia, W.B. Saunders, 1991, pp 1–4.

8. Webb WR, Bran WE, Helms CA: Mediastinum—vascular abnormalities. In Webb WR, Bran WE, Helms CA (eds): Fundamentals of Body CT. Philadelphia, W.B. Saunders, 1991, pp 5–16.

9. www.emedicine.com/med/topic445.htm (Quick general review of coronary artery anomalies).

CHAPTER 19

VENOUS CT OF THE CHEST

Nael E. A. Saad, MBBCh, Wael E. A. Saad, MBBCh, and Deborah Rubens, MD

1. What are the CT findings in venous thrombosis?

Partial thrombi are identified as nonenhancing blood clots (Fig. 19-1) within a contrast-filled lumen. They may be central or marginal and are often elongated along the path of the vessel. They are usually smoothly marginated (Fig. 19-2). Obstructing thrombi have a varied appearance, depending on age. In the acute phase, the vein is enlarged, sometimes with visible peripheral enhancement. In the chronic phase, the vein loses its peripheral enhancement, becomes smaller, and may eventually calcify.

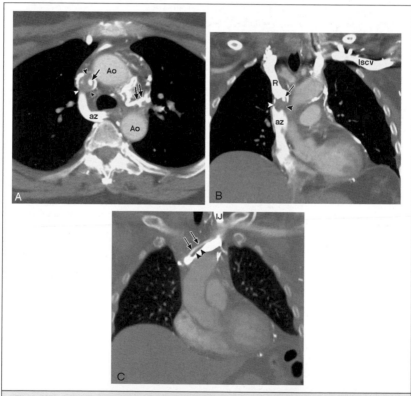

Figure 19-1. A, Axial image at the level of the aortic arch (Ao) shows a smoothly marginated thrombus *(arrowheads)* surrounding a central catheter *(arrow)* in the SVC. The azygous (az) is densely opacified, so this is not a mixing artifact. Collaterals *(paired arrows)* beneath the aortic arch are diverting blood into the azygous system. **B,** Coronal reformat shows the brightly enhanced right brachiocephalic vein (R) and azygous (az) filled by collaterals due to obstruction of the left subclavian vein (lscv) injection. The catheter *(arrow)* is the cause of the clot *(arrowheads)*. **C,** More anterior coronal reconstruction shows an additional thrombus *(arrowheads)*, which has formed on the indwelling catheter *(arrows)*. This is extremely difficult to discern on axial images, as it is parallel to the image plane. Note the abnormal retrograde flow in the left internal jugular vein (IJ).

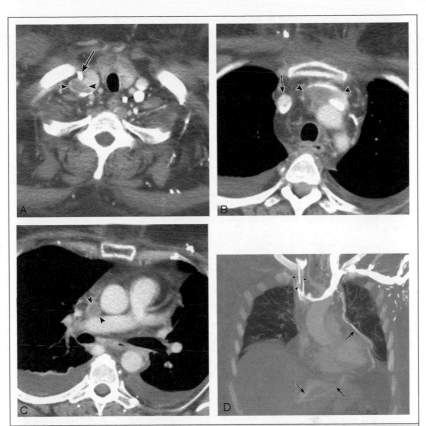

Figure 19-2. *A,* Axial image where catheter *(arrow)* enters the right jugular vein. Directly posterior to the catheter is a large, nonobstructing thrombus *(arrowheads)*. ***B,*** At the level of the great vessels there is an additional nonobstructing thrombus *(arrowheads)* in the left brachiocephalic vein. This thrombus can be differentiated from a mixing artifact because the right brachiocephalic vein *(arrow)* is already opacified. Note the contrast around the clot is brighter than in the right brachiocephalic vein or the aorta. The patient was injected from the left arm and the contrast transit is delayed due to additional thrombi distally. ***C,*** Below the carina the thrombus *(arrowheads)* occludes the SVC while the SVC wall is enhanced. ***D,*** Coronal reformat illustrates the thrombus *(arrowheads)* surrounding the catheter and the collaterals along the heart and below the diaphragm *(arrows)*, which divert blood through the IVC to the heart.

2. **What are the causes of venous thrombosis?**
   The most common cause of upper extremity and thoracic venous thrombosis today is from clots forming on indwelling venous catheters or pacemaker wires *(see* Fig. 19-2). Other causes include hypercoagulable states, such as protein S or protein C deficiency, malignancy, trauma, and venous irritants, such as chemotherapy or intravenous (IV) drug abuse. Primary or effort-induced upper extremity thrombosis (Paget-Schroetter syndrome) is rare.

3. **What is the pathogenesis of the peripheral enhancement in acute venous thrombosis?**
   It is not clearly understood. The peripheral enhancement may represent the vasa vasorum in the wall of the vein and reflect the "itis" part of thrombophlebitis *(see* Fig. 19-1C).

4. **What is a common pitfall in the diagnosis of thrombosis?**
   A mixing artifact frequently causes a low-attenuation area in the superior vena cava (SVC), which mimics thrombosis. This is due to unenhanced blood from the contralateral brachiocephalic vein mixing with enhanced blood from the side of the injection. Unenhanced blood from the azygous as it enters the SVC also is a common site of "pseudothrombosis" (Fig. 19-3).

5. **How can you differentiate between flow artifacts and true thrombus?**
   Viewing multiple contiguous images usually determines artifacts because the shape of the nonopacified area successively tapers. Knowing the sites of venous confluence and direction of blood flow permits one to predict the common sites of incomplete mixing and where distal resolution should occur.

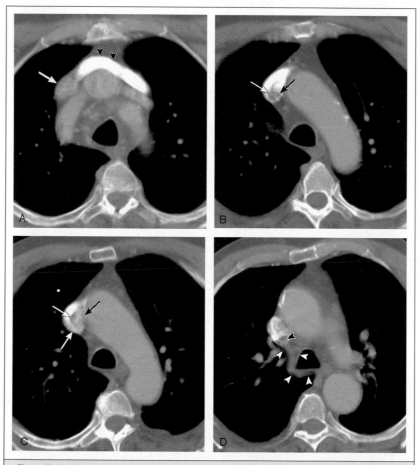

Figure 19-3. **A,** Unopacified blood *(arrow)* from the right brachiocephalic vein joins the opacified blood from the left brachiocephalic vein *(arrowheads)* to form the SVC. **B,** Ten millimeters caudally at the level of the aortic arch, the blood from the right forms a pseudoclot *(arrows)* in the SVC. **C,** As the blood mixes, the pseudoclot *(arrows)* enlarges and becomes more heterogeneous. **D,** At the level of the azygous more unopacified blood *(arrowheads)* joins the SVC.

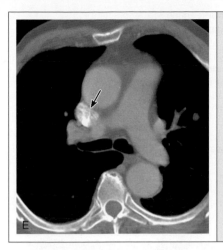

Figure 19-3.—cont'd *E*, Just above the right atrium the unopacified blood has dispersed and is more uniformly mixed throughout the SVC lumen *(arrow)*.

6. **What is the SVC syndrome?**
   This is obstruction of the SVC or both brachiocephalic veins with engorgement of proximal neck veins. Extrinsic obstruction is caused by tumors or other masses. Intrinsic obstruction is due to thrombosis.

7. **What are the causes of SVC syndrome in order of frequency?**
   - Extrinsic compression by bronchogenic carcinoma (most common cause)
   - Indwelling intravenous catheters and pacer wires with thrombosis (*see* Figs. 19-1 and 19-2)
   - Other mediastinal tumors (lymphoma, thymoma, germ cell tumors) or metastatic disease (Fig. 19-4)
   - Granulomatous mediastinitis/fibrosing mediastinitis (histoplasmosis, sarcoidosis, tuberculosis)

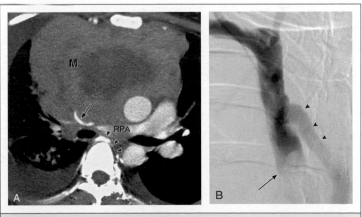

Figure 19-4. *A*, Axial CT shows a large anterior mediastinal tumor mass (M) in a patient with lymphoma. There is severe compression and displacement of the SVC *(arrow)*. The adjacent right pulmonary artery (RPA) is also severely compressed. Multiple paravertebral collaterals *(arrowheads)* are present. *B*, The physiologic effect is better shown by venography, in which the contrast is diverted retrograde down the azygous *(arrowheads)* and the SVC appears completely obstructed *(arrow)*.

- Arterial aneurysms (thoracic aorta or innominate artery)
- Substernal goiter
- Constrictive pericarditis

8. **Why should one evaluate the SVC syndrome by CT?**
   CT determines the level, extent, and length of the obstruction and may depict the cause, particularly if it is extramural (e.g., lung mass or mediastinal fibrosis). CT may show concomitant encasement or obstruction of other vessels and/or structures (pulmonary vessels, esophagus, or airways) (*see* Fig. 19-4).

9. **What are the common collateral pathways in patients with SVC syndrome?**
   - Internal mammary/chest wall varices (Fig. 19-5)
   - Azygous and hemiazygos veins (Fig. 19-6)
   - Accessory hemiazygos and superior intercostal veins
   - Lateral thoracic veins and umbilical veins (Fig. 19-7)
   - Paravertebral venous plexus (Fig. 19-8)

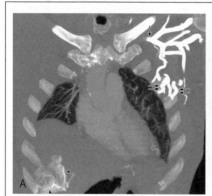 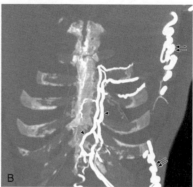

Figure 19-5. *A,* Coronal reformat shows the obstructed left brachiocephalic vein *(arrow),* the beginning chest wall collaterals *(double arrows),* and the abnormal focal retrograde venous enhancement of the liver *(arrowheads)* in the right lobe. *B,* Blood reaches the liver via the internal mammary vein collaterals *(arrowheads)* anteriorly. (The *double arrows* indicate chest wall collaterals.)

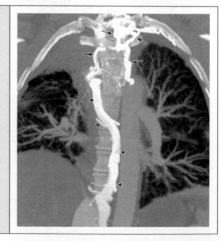

Figure 19-6. Coronal reformat shows dilated contrast filled azygous vein *(arrowheads)* as well as upper paravertebral veins *(arrows).*

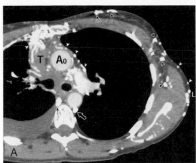

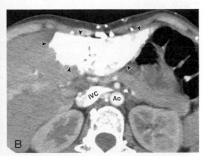

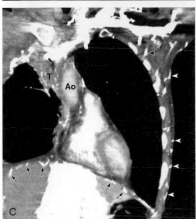

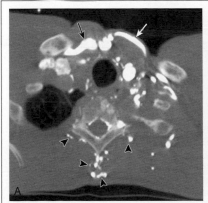

Figure 19-7. *A*, Axial CT just below the carina shows a soft tissue mass (T) to the right of the aorta. There are numerous collaterals *(arrowheads)* in the mediastinum and in the anterior chest wall. The azygous *(arrow)* and hemiazygous *(open arrow)* are also opacified. All veins are brighter than the adjacent aorta (Ao), indicating reflux from injection, not returning opacified blood. ***B*,** The axial image at the level of the liver shows the classic "hot liver" *(arrowheads)* with intense parenchymal enhancement of the left lobe due to collateral pathway through the liver from the chest wall and diaphragmatic veins to the IVC. The inferior vena cava (IVC) is brighter than the aorta (Ao) due to refluxed contrast. ***C*,** The coronal reconstruction illustrates the diaphragmatic *(arrows)* and left chest wall collaterals *(arrowheads)*.

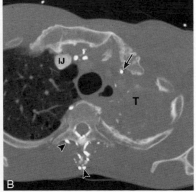

Figure 19-8. *A*, Axial image from a left-sided injection shows multiple anterior collaterals *(arrows)*, which cross the midline, and posterior paravertebral collaterals *(arrowheads)*. ***B*,** More caudally, the left subclavian is focally narrowed *(arrow)* and difficult to identify. The right internal jugular (IJ) is opacified more intensely than the aortic arch vessels due to the contrast reflux across the midline. Note the treated, partially calcified tumor mass (T) in the left lung apex. (The *arrowheads* indicate posterior paravertebral collaterals.)

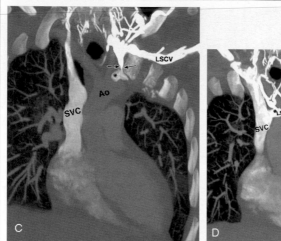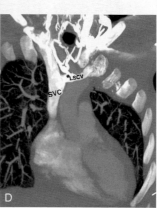

Figure 19-8.—cont'd *C,* Coronal reconstruction demonstrates the extremely narrow focal stenosis *(arrows)* and the innumerable neck collaterals *(arrowheads),* which fill the contralateral (right) internal jugular vein and the SVC. Note the relatively minimal opacification of the aorta (Ao) and the branch arteries. The proximal left brachiocephalic vein *(asterisk)* is less opacified than the left subclavian, which should supply it. *D,* More anteriorly we see the left brachiocephalic vein *(asterisk)* actually fills retrograde from the SVC, not from the left subclavian. LSCV = left subclavian vein.

Contrast-filled collateral venous pathways also include many small unnamed veins in the shoulder, chest wall, and superior mediastinum. Lakes of contrast-enhanced blood in the upper esophagus (upper esophageal varices) are occasionally also present.

10. **What is the "hot liver" sign?**
    Originally described in nuclear medicine scans as an area of increased uptake in the anterior left lobe, this is an area of liver parenchyma that bridges the systemic anterior chest wall venous collaterals and the hepatic veins draining into the inferior vena cava (IVC). It is a sharply defined polygonal area of high attenuation in the anterior liver, either the left or right lobe. It is nearly pathognomonic of SVC obstruction (*see* Fig. 19-7).

11. **Are contrast-filled small veins of the shoulder, axilla, and upper mediastinum diagnostic of SVC syndrome?**
    No. An occluded ipsilateral brachiocephalic, subclavian, or axillary vein can also give these findings. Furthermore, collaterals are not always abnormal because they can fill due to relative obstruction from arm positioning during injection. Higher injection rates (i.e., >3 cc/sec) can cause retrograde filling of veins without a stenosis (Fig. 19-9).

12. **What are the causes of stenosis or occlusion of the brachiocephalic veins in order of frequency?**
    - Indwelling venous catheters and pacemaker wires (most common overall)
    - Effort thrombosis/thoracic inlet syndrome (most common in young healthy individuals)
    - Tumors of the thoracic inlet/radiation therapy
    - Less common causes of SVC syndrome

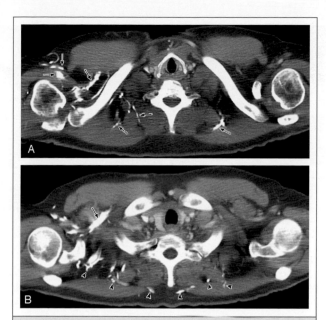

Figure 19-9. Axial images from a right-sided injection in a normal patient with arms overhead. **A,** Note filling of normal veins *(arrows)* in the arm, around the right shoulder, and posterior to the clavicle. **B,** More caudally at the level of the clavicular heads and ribs, the subclavian vein is opacified *(arrow)* and numerous posterior chest wall collaterals *(arrowheads)* extend across the midline to the left side. These collateral pathways fill retrograde from the high pressure of injection into a relatively obstructed vessel due to the arm position above the patient's head.

13. **What is the differential diagnosis of dilated and tortuous subcutaneous chest wall venous collaterals?**
    This may be due to the SVC syndrome (flow moving from thorax to abdomen to IVC), IVC obstruction (flow moving from abdomen to thorax to SVC), or occasionally severe congestive heart failure.

14. **What are the CT features of the esophageal varices?**
    These contrast-filled lakes of blood in the wall of the esophagus are seen on delayed venous phase acquisitions (usually 70–90 seconds after injection). They can be in the upper two thirds of the esophagus (downhill varices) or in the lower one third of the esophagus (uphill varices) (Fig. 19-10).

15. **What are the causes of upper esophageal varices?**
    In addition to SVC syndrome, these may result from highly vascular tumors in the mediastinum (e.g., medullary thyroid carcinoma) or a high-volume vascular anomaly in the mediastinum (arteriovenous malformation [AVM]).

16. **What causes lower esophageal varices?**
    The most common cause is cirrhosis with portal hypertension (*see* Fig. 19-10). Budd-Chiari syndrome can also cause esophageal varices due to IVC obstruction with resultant portal hypertension.

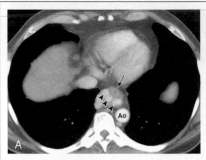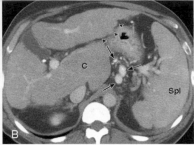

Figure 19-10. *A,* Esophageal varices *(arrowheads)* around the esophagus *(arrow)* adjacent to the aorta (Ao). *B,* More caudally in the upper abdomen note the cirrhotic nodular liver *(arrowheads)* with a large caudate lobe (C), large spleen (Spl), and dilated contrast-filled coronary vein collaterals *(arrows),* which divert the portal venous blood from the portal to the systemic system.

17. **What is Lemierre's syndrome?**
    This is an infection in the pharynx that extends to the parapharyngeal space and from there to the jugular vein, causing jugular vein thrombosis. Patients are usually young adults and present with fever, cough, and hemoptysis.

18. **What are the CT findings in Lemierre's syndrome?**
    The key finding is the association of jugular vein thrombosis with septic pulmonary emboli (multiple nodules, often cavitary with rim-like peripheral enhancement, usually located at the ends of vessels) (Fig. 19-11).

19. **What are the two extracardiac thoracic vascular findings that suggest poor cardiac function?**
    - Reflux of IV contrast from an arm injected through the SVC, right atrium, and IVC and filling the hepatic veins is always abnormal (Fig. 19-12).
    - A contrast-blood fluid level in the aorta with the contrast (higher specific gravity) layering in the dependent portion of the aorta is a sign of absent cardiac activity. Check the pulse and call a code!

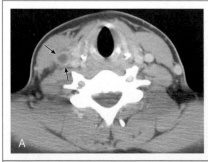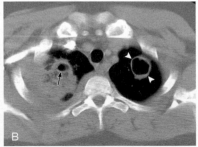

Figure 19-11. *A,* Axial image at the thoracic inlet shows the classical jugular vein thrombosis *(arrows),* which should suggest pharyngeal infection as the etiology of the septic pulmonary emboli shown in B. *B,* Image through the lung apices shows consolidation in the right upper lobe with a small cavity forming *(arrow).* A more mature cavitary lesion *(arrowheads)* is seen in the left apex.

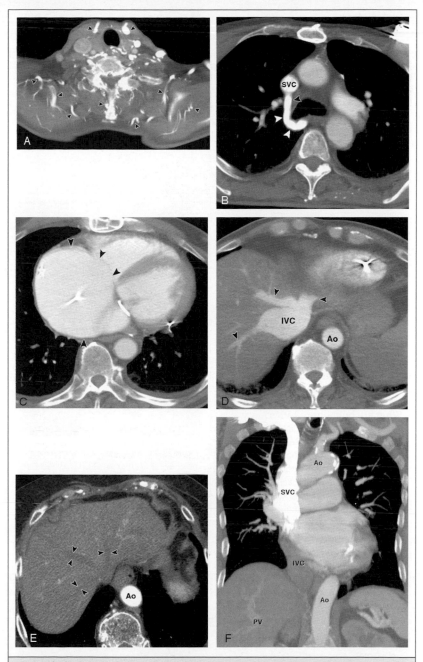

Figure 19-12. ***A,*** Axial image at the thoracic inlet shows numerous paravertebral and shoulder collaterals bilaterally *(arrowheads)* independent of the side of injection. ***B,*** At the level of the carina the azygous *(arrowheads)* and superior vena cava (SVC) are enhanced equally, whereas normally the azygous should not be enhanced. ***C,*** The heart is enlarged, particularly the right atrium *(arrowheads).* ***D,*** At the level of the diaphragm, the inferior vena cava (IVC) is enlarged and is equal in contrast enhancement to the adjacent aorta (Ao). Note the enhanced hepatic veins *(arrowheads)* while the liver parenchyma is unenhanced. ***E,*** Axial image of a normal patient for comparison at the diaphragm shows the normal enhancement relationship of the aorta (Ao) to the hepatic veins *(arrowheads).* ***F,*** Coronal reformat in the same patient shows the normal contrast relationships between the densest SVC, next dense aorta (Ao), followed by the portal vein (PV). Note the IVC is relatively unenhanced.

20. How do you decide whether the contrast in the hepatic veins is due to SVC-IVC reflux and not just normal antegrade filling of the hepatic veins?

With reflux, the high-attenuation hepatic vein contrast level is the same as that in the IVC and SVC. There is no hepatic parenchymal enhancement and the acquisition is obtained early (arterial phase: 25–30 seconds after injection). The kidneys may show early cortical enhancement. Normally in patients without reflux, the SVC shows the greatest enhancement, followed by the aorta and then the portal vein. The IVC and hepatic veins should not be enhanced in the early arterial phase of scanning (*see* Fig. 19-12).

21. What causes venous aneurysms in the thorax?

These may be congenital or acquired due to interruption of thoracic venous drainage. They can also be associated with developmental vascular anomalies, such as lymphangiomas. Vein bypass graft (saphenous vein) aneurysms can be due to infections (Fig. 19-13).

22. What is a pulmonary varix?

This is an asymptomatic dilation of a pulmonary vein, often incidentally found on chest radiographs as a pulmonary nodule. It can be distinguished from an arteriovenous (AV) fistula by its lack of enhancement during the arterial phase of contrast administration.

23. What are pulmonary AVMs?

These are abnormal vascular communications between pulmonary arteries and pulmonary veins. They range in size from microscopic to several centimeters. Ninety percent are simple with a single feeding artery and draining vein, and 10% are complex with two or more feeding arteries and draining veins. These abnormal vessels may communicate with the lung segments or with the chest wall.

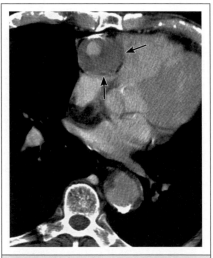

Figure 19-13. An 83-year-old man after three-vessel coronary artery bypass graft presented with dyspnea. Axial image at the level of the right atrioventricular groove reveals a 3-cm round mass *(arrows)* with a high-attenuation central lumen. This is the characteristic location for a saphenous vein coronary bypass graft. This aneurysm requires repair.

KEY POINTS: VENOUS CT OF THE CHEST

1. Incomplete mixing of opacified blood from the side of the injection with unopacified blood from the contralateral side and/or the azygous vein mimics SVC thrombosis.

2. Venous collaterals usually indicate obstruction, but retrograde filling of peripheral veins can occur with high injection rates and poor cardiac function and dependently due to gravity.

---

24. Are pulmonary AVMs associated with other malformations?

Approximately 70% of patients have associated AVMs in the skin, mucous membranes, or other organs.

25. **What is the name of the syndrome of multiple AVMs involving the lung and other sites?**

    This is known as hereditary hemorrhagic telangiectasia or Rendu-Osler-Weber disease. It has an autosomal dominance inheritance pattern and patients usually present in adulthood with hemoptysis.

26. **What are the CT characteristics of a pulmonary AVM?**

    This is a round or oval well-circumscribed mass, usually in the lower lobes, multiple in 30%. The mass is connected with enlarged serpiginous blood vessels, with enhancement similar to the pulmonary artery, and an early appearing enlarged draining vein directed toward the left atrium (Fig. 19-14).

27. **What are the some treatable causes of hemoptysis?**

    Most hemoptysis arises from chronic or recurring disease processes, including the following:

    Inflammation
    - Chronic bronchitis (most common cause of hemoptysis from blood streaking to gross bleeding)
    - Tuberculosis (most common in developing world)
    - Bronchiectasis (most common bronchial artery bleeding source)

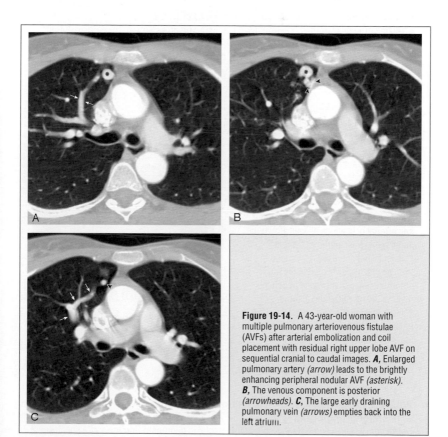

Figure 19-14. A 43-year-old woman with multiple pulmonary arteriovenous fistulae (AVFs) after arterial embolization and coil placement with residual right upper lobe AVF on sequential cranial to caudal images. *A,* Enlarged pulmonary artery *(arrow)* leads to the brightly enhancing peripheral nodular AVF *(asterisk)*. *B,* The venous component is posterior *(arrowheads)*. *C,* The large early draining pulmonary vein *(arrows)* empties back into the left atrium.

- Cystic fibrosis
- Aspergilloma complicating sarcoidosis
- Lung abscess/septic pulmonary emboli
- Pneumonia (particularly *Klebsiella*)

Neoplasia
- Bronchogenic carcinoma
- Bronchial adenoma

Vasculitis (rare)
- Wegener's granulomatosis
- Goodpasture syndrome
- Connective tissue disorders

28. **Why should hemoptysis be assessed by contrast-enhanced CT?**
    CT identifies lung pathology (parenchymal findings and/or dilated bronchial arteries) that may cause the hemoptysis. CT localizes the lesion permitting a focused bronchoscopic biopsy (while avoiding dilated adjacent arteries). CT permits a focused angiographic evaluation for diagnosis and/or embolization, saving time and reducing morbidity.

29. **What do abnormal bronchial arteries look like on CT?**
    - Dilated bronchial arteries (>2 mm). May receive as much as 30% of the cardiac output!
    - Bronchial artery tortuosity
    - Bronchial arteries leading to airway and/or parenchymal pathology, such as bronchiectasis, cavitating lesions, and lung malignancies
      (Note that normal bronchial arteries are visible on thin-slice multidetector CT.)

30. **What is the significance of pulmonary artery aneurysms?**
    These are relatively rare and usually are acquired due to infection or associated with cystic medial necrosis, atherosclerosis, hereditary telangiectasia (Rendu-Osler-Weber syndrome), trauma, or vasculitis (Behçet disease) (Fig. 19-15).

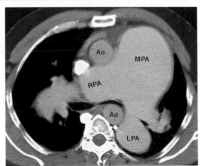

31. **What is Behçet disease?**
    A systemic disease that causes venous and arterial occlusions as well as arterial aneurysms. Vascular involvement ("vasculo-Behçet disease") is seen in only 25% of cases; however, it is the most common cause of mortality in Behçet disease. Vasculo-Behçet disease is venous in 88% of cases, arterial in 12% of cases. Arterial lesions develop in the aorta, pulmonary artery, or their major branches. Sixty-five percent of these lesions are aneurysms; 35% are occlusive.

Figure 19-15. Aneurysms of the main, left, and right pulmonary arteries. MPA = main pulmonary artery, RPA = right pulmonary artery, LPA = left pulmonary artery, Ao = aorta.

32. **What are the advantages of evaluating Behçet patients with CT compared with conventional angiography?**
    Unlike conventional angiography, spiral CT is useful in demonstrating the entire spectrum of thoracic manifestations of Behçet disease which include arterial and venous pathology. Spiral CT

is noninvasive and provides excellent delineation of the vessel lumen and wall and perivascular tissues as well as detailed information concerning the lung parenchyma, pleura, and mediastinal structures.

33. What is the significance of a pulmonary artery aneurysm in patients with Behçet disease?

Behçet disease is the most common cause of pulmonary artery aneurysm and indicates a poor prognosis: 30% mortality within 2 years. Hemoptysis is the most common presenting symptom and is one of the leading causes of death. Possible causes for hemoptysis include rupture of an aneurysm with erosion into a bronchus and thrombosis of pulmonary vessels.

BIBLIOGRAPHY

1. Chasen MH, Charnsangavej C: Venous chest anatomy: clinical implications. In Green R, Muhm JR (eds): Syllabus: A Categorical Course in Diagnostic Radiology—Chest Radiology. Oak Brook, IL, Radiological Society of North America, 1992, pp 121–134.

2. Chiles C, Davis KW, Williams DW III: Navigating the thoracic inlet. Radiographics 19:1161–1176, 1999.

3. Do KH, Goo JM, Im JG, et al: Systemic arterial supply to the lungs in adults: Spiral CT findings. Radiographics 21:387–402, 2001.

4. Fraser RS, Pare, Peter JA: Pulmonary abnormalities of developmental origin. In Fraser RS, Pare Peter JA, Fraser RG, Pared PD (eds): Synopsis of Diseases of the Chest, 2nd ed. Philadelphia, W.B. Saunders, 1994, pp 256–283.

5. Gilkeson RC, Goodman PC, McAdams HP: Anomalous azygous-hemiazygous anastomosis: Radiographic findings. Am J Roentgenol 168:285–286, 1997.

6. Glazer HS, Semenkovich JW, Guitierrez FR: Medistinum. In Lee JKT, Sagel SS, Stanley RJ, Heiken JP (eds): Computed Body Tomography with MRI Correlation, 3rd ed. Philadelphia, Lippincott-Raven, 1998, pp 261–349.

7. Haramati LB, Glickstein JS, Issenberg HJ, et al: MR imaging and CT of vascular anomalies and connections in patients with congenital heart disease: Significance in surgical planning. Radiographics 22:337–349, 2002.

8. Naidich DP, Webb WR, Muller NL, et al: Aorta, arch vessels, and great veins. In Naidich DP, Webb WR, Muller NL, et al (eds): Computed Tomography and Magnetic Resonance of the Thorax, 3rd ed. Philadelphia, Lippincott-Raven, 1999, pp 505–602.

9. Naidich DP, Webb WR, Muller NL, et al: Hilum and pulmonary arteries. In Naidich DP, Webb WR, Muller NL, et al (eds): Computed Tomography and Magnetic Resonance of the Thorax, 3rd ed. Philadelphia, Lippincott-Raven, 1999, pp 603–656.

10. Parikh SR, Prasad K, Lyer RN, et al: Prospective angiographic study of systemic venous connections in congenital and acquired heart disease. Cathet Cardiovasc Diagn 38:379–386, 1996.

11. Rossi SE, McAdams HP, Rosado-de-Christenson ML, et al: Fibrosing mediastinitis. Radiographics 21:737–757, 2001.

12. Seline TH, Gross BH, Francis IR: CT and MR imaging of mediastinal hemangiomas. J Comput Assist Tomogr 14:766–768, 1990.

13. Shaffer K, Rosado-de-Christenson ML, Patz EF Jr, et al: Thoracic lymphangioma in adults: CT and MR imaging features. Am J Roentgenol 162:283–289, 1994.

14. Trigaux J-P, Van Beers B: Thoracic collateral venous channels: Normal and pathologic CT findings. J Comput Assist Tomogr 14:769–773, 1990.

CHAPTER 20

CT OF THORACIC ARTERIAL DISEASE

Nael E. A. Saad, MBBCh, Wael E. A. Saad, MBBCh, and Deborah Rubens, MD

1. **Which medical emergencies involve the thoracic aorta?**
   The acute medical aortic emergencies are dissection, intramural hematoma (IMH), penetrating aortic ulcers, and leaking or rupturing aneurysms. Although these diagnoses can be made on routine CT, CT angiography (CTA) is more sensitive and depicts them better for surgical planning.

KEY POINTS: FIVE INGREDIENTS OF A GOOD COMPUTED TOMOGRAPHY ARTERIOGRAM

1. **High arterial opacification:** Use a fast injection rate.

2. **Cover the region of interest:** Sometimes it is not as easy as it sounds.

3. **Image while the contrast bolus is there:** Time the imaging to the bolus correctly.

4. **Minimize patient motion:** Image in a short breath-hold and buy a modern multislice scanner.

5. **Use thin slices:** Buy a modern multislice scanner.

2. **Which determines the degree of vessel opacification in CTA: the volume of contrast injected or the rate of injection?**
   The rate of injection. Iodinated contrast agents are extracellular agents. CTA images in the first pass, while the contrast is intra-arterial before it is diluted in the capillary beds. Therefore, the density is determined by the rate of contrast injection, relative to the patient's cardiac output. If you inject at 5 cc/sec and the patient's cardiac output is 3 L/minute (50 cc/sec), the arterial blood will be approximately 10% contrast during the first-pass bolus.

3. **But I thought the more contrast you give, the more you enhance things!**
   That rule is true for routine CT but not for CTA. Routine imaging does not image the first-pass bolus. Contrast equilibrates in the extracellular space, so opacification is determined by the amount of contrast divided by the size of the extracellular space. CTA is first-pass imaging, and opacification is determined by the rate of injection divided by the cardiac output.

4. **If the amount of contrast injected does not determine opacification, what does the amount injected determine?**
   The amount of contrast injected, divided by the injection rate, determines the length of time of the first-pass bolus. For example, if you inject 150 cc at 5 cc/sec, there is approximately a 30-second long bolus of contrast. You have to image the arteries during that first-pass time window, while the bolus goes through the region of interest.

5. **I have a patient with renal insufficiency so I am going to cut the contrast dose in half. What else do I need to think about?**
Reducing the rate of contrast and/or carefully timing the bolus. If you reduce the amount administered but do not reduce the rate of injection, you will shorten the length of time of the bolus. Of course, reducing the rate will give you less opacification. This is usually fine in the small, older patient but inadequate in the younger, larger patient (with higher cardiac output). This is another advantage of faster scanners.

6. **How do you time when to start scanning to get arterial enhancement?**
There are three methods: fixed timing delay, automatic bolus detection, and a test bolus. Each has its advantages.
   - A **fixed delay** is the simplest but can cause one to start scanning before the bolus arrives if there is slow transit time (i.e., superior vena cava occlusion or congestive heart failure).
   - **Automated bolus** detection (take low-dose scan over the aorta until bolus arrives, then trigger the diagnostic scan) takes more time to set up and has the risk of misplacing the location for the low-dose scan, but you do not risk scanning too early. There is also a delay between detection of the bolus and starting the scan, resulting in use of more contrast.
   - A **test bolus** (inject a small amount of contrast, scan repetitively over region of interest, determine the time to arrival, then inject the remainder of the contrast and scan with the determined delay) is very accurate but very labor-intensive.
   We usually do automated bolus detection.

7. **On which patient is it harder to get arterial opacification: the 20-year-old, 180-pound tachycardic trauma patient or the 90-year-old, 90-pound, beta-blocked patient with aortic stenosis?**
The large, healthy young patient. The lower the cardiac output, the greater the opacification. Low cardiac output is often associated with long transit times. Thus, it takes longer for the contrast bolus to arrive, but when it arrives, it will look like chalk. High cardiac output dilutes the contrast. The older patient is harder to time but easier to opacify strongly.

8. **What are the advantages of multislice CT when performing thoracic CTA?**
Newer, faster scanners have shorter scan time, which covers more territory with less respiratory motion artifact while acquiring thinner slices. Thinner slices with near isotropic voxels make for better coronal or sagittal reconstructed images.

9. **Are there any limitations to CT in the evaluation of the aorta?**
Evaluation of the aortic root can be limited by motion, especially motion artifacts at the aortic root near the valve cusps at the 12–1 o'clock and 6–7 o'clock positions. However, the newer multislice scanners enable cardiac-gated techniques, which reduce this problem. For imaging most of the thoracic aorta, however, gating is not necessary.

10. **How does electrocardiographic gating work to reduce motion artifacts?**
The heart and aorta rotate, distend, and contract with each heartbeat. Prospective electrocardiography (ECG)-assisted multidetector row CT can acquire each scan during diastole, which effectively places the image of the aorta and heart in a constant position in the chest with a uniform degree of chamber filling. Retrospective gating acquires throughout the cardiac cycle, then the data are broken up into phases. The price of multiple phases is increased radiation dose.

11. **So how do you image the acute aorta?**
We start with noncontrasted images from the arch to the diaphragm. Then we inject hypoosmolar contrast with 300 mg iodine/mL at a 3.5–5 cc/sec injection rate for a total of 150 cc to opacify the entire thoracic and abdominal aorta. We use a 30-cc saline flush at the end of injection to clear the contrast from the intravenous (IV) line and the patient's arm. We use a bolus tracker to trigger the start of the scan.

12. **What is the benefit of the noncontrast CT?**
An unenhanced CT makes it easier to detect an IMH or displaced intimal calcifications, which may be obscured by bright contrast within the lumen. The hematoma precontrast is brighter than the adjacent lumen (Fig. 20-1). After contrast it may be very difficult to tell the hematoma from atheroma or from a thrombosed false lumen (Fig. 20-2). An IMH will not enhance after contrast administration, whereas a false lumen, if patent, will enhance.

13. **What is an aortic dissection?**
A dissection shears the aortic wall longitudinally and divides the aortic lumen into two or more channels (Fig. 20-3). The normal aortic wall (from lumen to the periphery) is composed of three layers, the intima, media, and adventitia. Dissection splits the media. Dissections usual start at a focal intimal disruption. The dissecting blood creates a false lumen that continues antegrade and/or retrograde and may or may not thrombose.

14. **What is an IMH?**
Simplistically, this is an aortic dissection that lacks an intimomedial flap. Localized hemorrhage into the wall is caused by hypertension or by an intimal fracture. Bleeding is confined to the

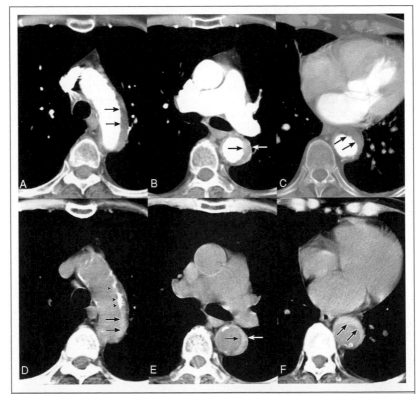

Figure 20-1. Elderly patient presents with chest pain radiating to the back. *A–C,* Contrasted images of the descending aorta from arch to the mid-descending aorta show apparent atheroma *(arrows)* on the left lateral side of the aorta. The elevated CT attenuation of this intramural hematoma is not apparent after contrast but is readily seen on the corresponding precontrast images *(D–F).* The displaced intimal calcifications *(arrowheads* in *D)* are also more apparent precontrast.

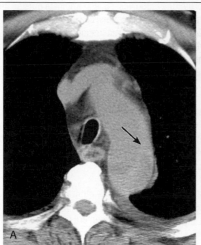
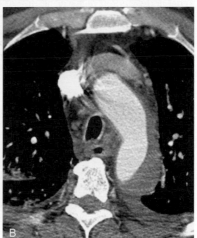
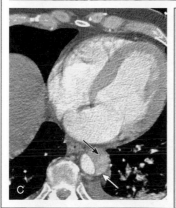

Figure 20-2. Type B dissection with thrombosed false lumen at the arch (*A* and *B*) and in the descending aorta (*C*). The higher density thrombus in the unenhanced lumen (*arrow* in *A*) at the level of the aortic arch is difficult to distinguish from atheroma on the enhanced image (*B*). Some flow (*arrows* in *C*) is reestablished caudally in the larger false lumen.

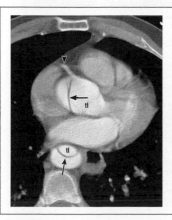

Figure 20-3. Type A aortic dissection with intimomedial flap *(arrows)* in the ascending and descending aorta with complete opacification of the true and false lumens. Note the position of the right coronary artery *(arrowhead)*, which arises from the true lumen (tl) in this instance but could easily be occluded or compromised by the flap.

media and results from rupture of the vasa vasorum, the blood vessels that originate outside the aorta and penetrate the outer half of the media to supply the aortic wall.

15. What are the potential consequences of an IMH?

IMH weakens the aorta and may result in aneurysm with risk of rupture or may disrupt the intima permitting aortic dissection with the development of a false lumen.

16. How do I detect IMH on CT?

On unenhanced images, the hematoma is high attenuation due to the increased iron attenuation in the thrombus, often brighter than the adjacent lumen. After contrast administration, the hematoma does not enhance (unlike dissection), but this may be very difficult to perceive next to the bright contrast in the aortic lumen (*see* Fig. 20-1).

17. How do I diagnose aortic dissection?

By seeing the intimomedial flap, a nonenhancing, thin, curvilinear band within a contrast-filled lumen (Figs. 20-3 and 20-4). The flap can be suggested on noncontrast CT if you see displaced intimal calcifications (Fig. 20-5). Other findings include delayed enhancement of the false lumen (*see* Fig. 20-2), widening of the aorta (*see* Fig. 20-4), and mediastinal, pleural, or pericardial hematoma (*see* Fig. 20-5).

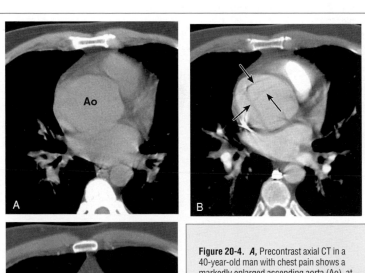

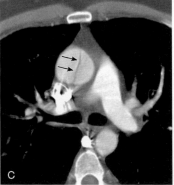

Figure 20-4. *A,* Precontrast axial CT in a 40-year-old man with chest pain shows a markedly enlarged ascending aorta (Ao), at least twice the size of the adjacent vertebral body, indicating an aneurysm. Note the lack of atheroma or calcification. *B,* Postcontrast image at the same level reveals multiple angulated filamentous lines *(arrows),* indicating shreds of intima-media, not a single flap. They could be misinterpreted as artifact, except they are multiple. Artifacts should arise from a visible displaced surface and there is no corresponding anatomic structure to generate these lines. *C,* A single dissection flap *(arrows)* can be identified in the distal ascending aorta.

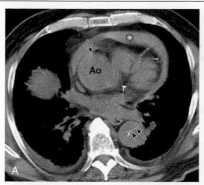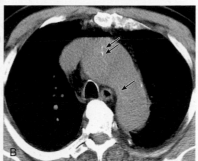

Figure 20-5. **A,** Initial images of a noncontrast abdominal CT performed in a hypotensive patient for suspected abdominal aortic aneurysm shows high-attenuation fluid in the pericardium *(asterisk)* indicating hemopericardium with potential cardiac tamponade. Note the dilated aortic root (Ao) with abnormal contour anteriorly *(arrow)* and displaced intimal calcification in the descending aorta *(paired arrows).* **B,** Subsequent chest CT confirms the irregular calcified intimal flap *(arrows)* involving the aortic arch. Displaced intimal calcification is the key finding of dissection in the unenhanced aorta.

18. **What is the "intimal flap" of aortic dissection?**
    The old term "intimal flap" is misleading because the cleavage plane is actually between the inner one third (luminal side) of the media and the outer two thirds of the media (i.e., the flap is made up of the intima + one third of the media). The proper terminology is an intimomedial flap.

KEY POINTS: DISEASES ASSOCIATED WITH AORTIC DISSECTION   ✓

1. Hypertension

2. Connective tissue disorders, such as Marfan's syndrome, cystic medial necrosis, and Ehlers-Danlos syndrome

3. Turner's syndrome

4. Other aortic abnormalities such as aortic stenosis, bicuspid aortic valve, and aortic coarctation

5. Cocaine abuse

19. **What is the Stanford classification of aortic dissections?**
    ■ **Stanford type A** is any dissection flap involving the ascending aorta and/or aortic arch (just proximal to the normal take-off of the left subclavian artery) (*see* Figs. 20-3, 20-4, and 20-5). Sixty to 75% of cases are type A. Type A dissection may extend into the great vessels of the neck (Fig. 20-6).
    ■ **Stanford type B** is a dissection flap involving the descending aorta only, typically starting at the aortic isthmus (just distal to the normal take-off of the left subclavian artery) (Fig. 20-7).

20. **Why is the Stanford classification clinically important?**
    Type A requires surgical management (an aortic graft with aortic valve replacement and rarely replacement of arch itself), whereas type B dissection can usually be managed with antihypertensive medication.

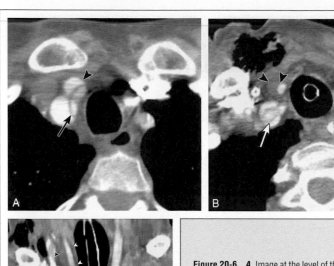

Figure 20-6. *A,* Image at the level of the great vessels shows dissection flap spanning the origins of the right carotid *(arrowhead)* and right subclavian *(arrow)* as they arise from the brachiocephalic artery. *B,* Higher in the neck, axial image shows the complex dissection in the subclavian *(arrow)*. The right common carotid is narrowed at least 50% by the thrombosed false lumen *(arrowheads)*. *C,* The extent of the narrowing of the right common carotid artery *(arrowheads)* is more easily appreciated on the coronal reconstruction in comparison to the normal left common carotid artery. Image A is from a 2-month follow-up, whereas images B and C are from the immediate postoperative period.

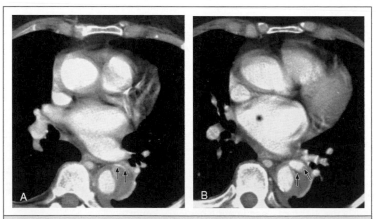

Figure 20-7. Sequential images from proximal to distal through the descending aorta show the dissection beginning anteriorly as a slit (*A*), with the false lumen *(arrows)* enlarging gradually (*B*) to be come greater diameter than the true lumen.

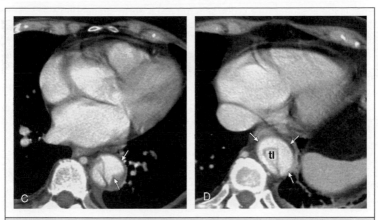

Figure 20-7.—cont'd (*C*) and eventually surrounding the true lumen (tl) (*D*). Note that there is a large amount of thrombus in the false lumen proximally and that the thrombus diminishes in sequential images.

21. **Why does Stanford type A dissection require surgical management?**
Type A dissection may propagate proximally toward the aortic root, dissecting the coronary arteries (resulting in cardiac ischemia and possible myocardial infarction). It may cause aortic valve insufficiency and lead to intrapericardial rupture, tamponade, and death (*see* Fig. 20-5).

22. **How effective is CT in detecting type A aortic dissection and its associated findings?**
The sensitivity, specificity, and accuracy of helical CT are reported to be 100%. The sensitivity, specificity, and accuracy are as follows:
- **An entry tear:** 82%, 100%, and 84%, respectively
- **Arch branch vessel involvement:** 95%, 100%, and 98%, respectively
- **Pericardial effusion:** 83%, 100%, and 91%, respectively

23. **How common are the branch vessels involved in type A dissection? What is the significance of branch vessel dissection?**
In one study, branch vessel involvement was found in 19 of 45 patients (42%), and in 63% (*n* = 12) of these patients more than one vessel was involved. Frequency of particular involvement was as follows:
- **Brachiocephalic artery:** 89%
- **Left common carotid artery:** 53%
- **Left subclavian artery:** 63%
Fortunately, despite the frequency of extension, acute neurologic deficits are rare, affecting only 5% of patients (*see* Fig. 20-6).

24. **Which coronary artery is usually supplied by the false lumen of a type-A aortic dissection (board question)?**
The right coronary artery (*see* Fig. 20-3) is usually supplied by this type of dissection.

25. **What is the prognosis for patients with type A aortic dissection who do not undergo surgery?**
The mortality rate is reported to be 38%, 50%, and 70% within 1, 2, and 7 days, respectively.

26. **What is the postoperative prognosis of type A aortic dissection?**
The 5-year survival rate is as follows:
- 95% when the false lumen is thrombosed
- 76% when the false lumen is patent

At 10 years, 15–30% of patients require surgery for life-threatening conditions, such as dilatation of the dissected region with risk of rupture. Elective resection is advisable if a false lumen aneurysm exceeds 5–6 cm in diameter or symptoms are present.

KEY POINTS: INDICATIONS FOR SURGERY WITH TYPE B DISSECTION

1. Propagation of dissection in the aortic arch (becomes type A dissection)

2. Visceral arterial compromise

3. Ruptured aorta

4. Descending aortic diameter greater than 6 cm

5. Pseudocoarctation syndrome with uncontrollable hypertension

27. **What are the technical pitfalls in the diagnosis of aortic dissection?**
- **Poor aortic enhancement** may be insufficient for visualization of the intimomedial flap, yielding a false-negative diagnosis. Poor aortic contrast levels result from scanning too early or too late (missing the peak enhancement) or from a slow rate of IV contrast injection.
- **Streak artifacts** create lines in the image, which may mimic a dissection flap. These artifacts are generated by high-attenuation material such as surgical clips, calcifications, and pacemaker leads and high contrast from adjacent venous blood (injection) in the left brachiocephalic vein or the superior vena cava.
- **Physiologic motion of the aortic root and pulmonary artery** commonly result in an artifact in the proximal ascending aorta (Figs. 20-8 and 20-9).

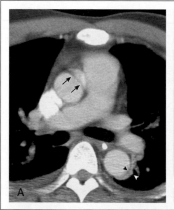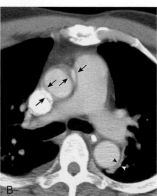

Figure 20-8. *A,* Motion of the aorta and pulmonary artery produces a ghost image with resulting pseudoflap *(arrows)* on the medial wall of the aorta. Enhancing atelectasis *(arrowheads)* adjacent to the descending aorta mimics a dissection here as well. *B,* Image superior to A confirms the motion artifact *(arrows)* of the ascending aorta now projecting over the pulmonary artery and the superior vena cava. Atelectasis *(arrowheads)* is again noted.

28. **How can streak/beam artifacts be differentiated from a true aortic dissection? How can they be reduced?**
Streaks are straight lines, typically varying from section to section, and extend beyond the confines of the aortic wall. In addition, they usually have an atypical orientation. Intimal flaps are contiguous from slice to slice. They may be curved, especially if the intima is fragmented (Fig. 20-10).

29. **Which extra-aortic structures may mimic dissection?**
   - **Periaortic vascular structures,** such as the origin of the aortic arch vessels and the left brachiocephalic, superior intercostal, and pulmonary veins may be misinterpreted as double lumina or intimal flaps (Fig. 20-11).
   - **Periaortic nonvascular structures,** such as residual thymus, atelectasis (Fig. 20-12), pleural thickening, pleural effusion, or the superior pericardial recess (Fig. 20-13) may also be misinterpreted as aortic dissection.

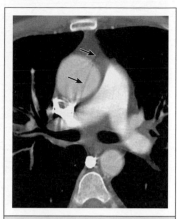

Figure 20-9. Note the thin line within the aorta that extends beyond the aortic margin into the anterior mediastinum *(arrows)*. This probably arises from the motion of the adjacent pulmonary artery.

30. **Where does the superior pericardial recess lie? What type of aortic dissection does it simulate?**
The retroaortic portion of a superior pericardial recess forms a semilunar area along the right posterior wall of the ascending thoracic aorta, whereas the preaortic portion is seen anterior to the ascending aorta. These recesses occur just above or at the level of the left pulmonary artery and can be recognized by their water attenuation, focal nature, and typical anatomic location. The superior pericardial recess can be misinterpreted as a Stanford type A dissection (*see* Fig. 20-13).

31. **What are the benefits of CT in the evaluation of aortic dissection?**
   - CT triages patients to surgical (type A) versus medical (type B) management.
   - CT identifies complications of dissection, including pericardial rupture, ruptured type B dissection, or ischemia of branch vessels (especially abdominal).
   - Follow-up with CT identifies progression or regression of the flap, aneurysm development, and perfusion status of the false lumen (Fig. 20-14).

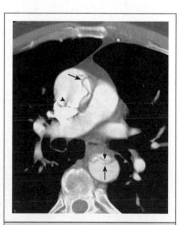

Figure 20-10. Small linear streak artifact *(arrowhead)* arises from the high contrast in the superior vena cava (SVC) and projects into the ascending aorta, not to be confused with the true wavy curving intimomedial flaps *(arrows)* in the ascending and descending aorta. Note multiple flaps in the descending aorta. This is not uncommon and reflects multiple shreds of the media.

32. **Is it important to differentiate between the false and true lumens?**
Accurate differentiation of the true and the false lumen was relatively unimportant because surgery was the main interventional therapy. However, with the recent advent of endograft repair, this distinction has become particularly important because the endograft needs to be placed in the true lumen.

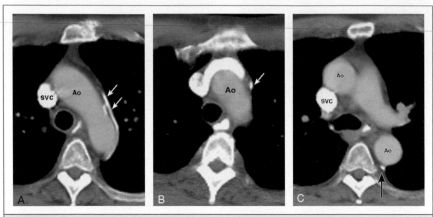

Figure 20-11. *A,* Linear vascular structure (the left superior intercostal vein) to the left and parallel to the aortic arch *(arrows)* mimics aortic dissection. Ao = aorta, SVC = superior vena cava. *B,* One clue to this normal variant is its origin *(arrow)* above the aorta at the left brachiocephalic vein. *C,* Another clue is its continuation *(arrow)* caudal and posterior to the aorta. Also note that the enhancement level is venous and matches that of the SVC, greater than the adjacent aorta.

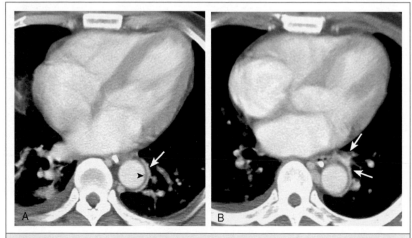

Figure 20-12. *A,* Brightly enhancing sliver of lung *(arrow)* lateral to the descending aorta causes the native aortic wall *(arrowhead)* to mimic a dissection flap. *B,* Adjacent more proximal image confirms the triangular atelectatic lung with its vessels *(arrows)* extending out from the hilum.

33. **What factors can help distinguish the false lumen from the true lumen?**
    - The true lumen is continuous with an undissected portion of the aorta (*see* Fig. 20-3).
    - When the dissection involves the entire aorta, the false lumen is usually on the right side of the ascending aorta and then spirals in the arch to involve the left side of the descending aorta (*see* Fig. 20-3).
    - The false lumen is usually larger in its cross-sectional area (*see* Fig. 20-14).
    - If the media is shredded and incompletely sheared away during the dissection, it results in multiple thin linear fragments. This process is relatively specific to the false lumen and has been termed the cobweb sign (*see* Fig. 20-10).

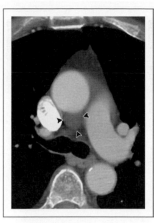

Figure 20-13. Axial CT image demonstrates the normal fluid-filled superior pericardial recess *(arrowheads)*, not to be mistaken for an aortic dissection or an abnormal lymph node. The amount of fluid here is normal.

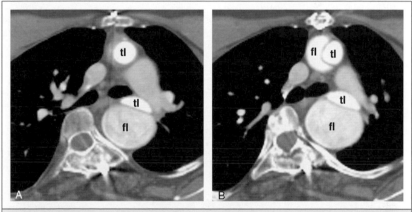

Figure 20-14. Patient with type A dissection following graft repair in the ascending aorta. **A,** At the level of the ascending aorta the graft is intact (true lumen, tl). The descending aorta is aneurysmal with an enlarged false lumen (fl), which has decreased opacification as compared with the true lumen. **B,** Slightly more cranial slice just beyond the end of the graft shows the persistent dissection in the arch. Here the proximal false lumen is well opacified.

- The false lumen may thrombose peripherally (*see* Fig. 20-6C) or may be thrombosed in one portion of the dissection and patent in another (*see* Fig. 20-2).
  Even with all this, sometimes it is difficult to be sure.

34. **When is there danger of ischemia?**
    When the intimal flap has a "C" shape (deep curvilinear) that is concave toward the false lumen (the false lumen is round and the true lumen is an adjacent crescent.). This appearance is associated with a higher risk of branch vessel ischemia (often in the abdomen involving renal or mesenteric arteries) (Fig. 20-15).

35. **What is a penetrating aortic ulcer? How does it differ from ulcerated atheroma?**
    A penetrating atherosclerotic ulcer is an atheromatous lesion that penetrates the internal elastic lamina and extends into the media. It commonly results in intramural hemorrhage and has an

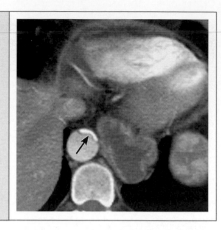

Figure 20-15. Axial image of the descending aorta of a patient with a type A dissection. The true lumen is compressed anteriorly *(arrow)* with a concave margin to the false lumen, indicating that the false lumen potentially has higher pressure than the true lumen. Lower in the abdomen the compressed true lumen gave off the celiac and superior mesenteric arteries, which are potentially at risk for ischemia should the blood flow through the true lumen become inadequate. Note that the false lumen has decreased contrast attenuation, in part due to dilution by more stagnant flow.

associated hematoma, which indicates its aggressive nature. It frequently results in a focal bulge of the aortic contour (Fig. 20-16).

Atheromatous ulceration is superficial erosion of an atheromatous plaque. It does not extend to the media and usually does not extend through multiple axial slices. If calcification is present in the intima, the atheromatous ulcer does not extend beyond it. The difference is one of degree. They are part of a continuum of disease (Fig. 20-17).

36. **How commonly do penetrating ulcers progress?**
    - Thirty percent progress within 18 months.
    - Most (70%) of these lesions grow eventually and are incorporated within a dilating aorta.
    - Almost all lead to some degree of aortic dilation.
    - Twenty to 30% of ulcers develop saccular aortic aneurysms.

    Overall, the natural history is of aortic enlargement with development of saccular or fusiform aneurysms or pseudoaneurysms. Therefore, these patients require surveillance (*see* Fig. 20-16).

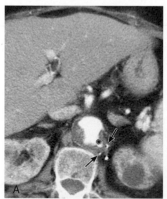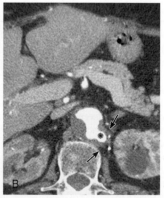

Figure 20-16. *A,* Initial study from an elderly hypertensive but otherwise asymptomatic patient shows focal contrast extension into the aortic wall *(asterisk)* with associated contour deformity of the aortic wall *(arrows)*. *B,* Subsequent study 2 years later with image at the same level as A shows increasing size of the ulcer *(asterisk)* and greater outpouching of the adjacent aortic wall *(arrows)*.

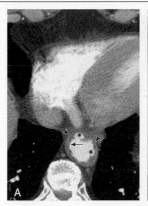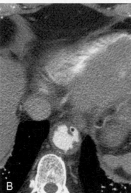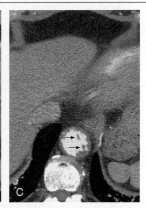

Figure 20-17. *A,* Asymptomatic patient with multiple atheromatous ulcers *(asterisks).* Note the low-attenuation of the cholesterol-laden atheroma *(arrow).* The wall thickness is relatively even *(arrowheads)* and the wall contour intact, which helps differentiate the atheromatous ulcer from a penetrating ulcer. The edges of the ulcer overhang the crater *(B)* and mimic dissection flaps *(arrows)* in the more caudal section *(C).* However, the aorta is not dilated as one would expect with dissection.

37. **Which penetrating ulcers are most dangerous?**
    Lesions in the ascending aorta and the aortic arch are more likely to progress than those located in the descending thoracic aorta. This is due to the higher wall pressures and mechanical/hydraulic stress in this portion of the aorta. For this reason, surgical therapy is recommended for patients with ulcers and hematoma in the ascending aorta, whereas descending ulcers are managed with antihypertensive medication.

38. **How do you differentiate a penetrating atherosclerotic ulcer from a classic (true) aortic dissection?**
    Extensive atherosclerosis is associated with the ulcer, and there is no compression of the aortic lumen (a hallmark of dissection). Penetrating ulcers are common in the elderly, and although patients may present with chest or back pain, many ulcers are discovered incidentally in asymptomatic patients.

39. **What are the common features of aortic atherosclerosis?**
    - Thickening of the aortic wall
    - Atheroma (or plaque) in the aortic wall that has fatty attenuation; may be surface irregularity including ulceration in the atheroma
    - Aortic dilation/ectasia (lengthening and meandering of the aorta)
    - Aneurysms
    - Penetrating ulcers
    - Wall calcifications (*see* Fig. 20-18)

40. **Can endoluminal calcification differentiate between dissection and aneurysm formation?**
    Unfortunately, no. Although calcification in the displaced intimomedial flap is common in aortic dissection (75% of cases), approximately 25% of thoracic aneurysms have dystrophic calcification that may mimic dissection with a thrombosed false lumen.

41. **Are thoracic aortic calcifications active by positron emission tomography (PET)?**
   Sometimes. Calcifications in the thoracic aorta usually do not correlate with areas of increased activity by fluoro-2-deoxy-D-glucose (FDG) PET. Fourteen percent of patients with calcifications on CT do have FDG uptake at the same site. Increased FDG uptake most likely represents areas of active atherosclerotic disease.

42. **What is an aneurysm?**
   A thoracic aortic aneurysm is defined as dilation of the aorta to twice its normal diameter with all three layers of the wall (intima, media, and adventitia) present. The ascending aorta and arch are usually 1 cm greater in diameter than the descending aorta. The normal aorta should continually taper (*see* Fig. 20-18).

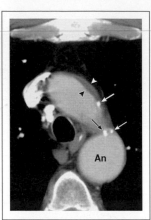

Figure 20-18. Axial CT image at the level of the aortic arch shows a normal-caliber ascending aorta and dilating descending aorta with aneurysm (An) originating just beyond the arch. Note associated atheroma *(arrowheads)* and calcifications *(arrows)*, indicative of atherosclerosis.

43. **What is aortic ectasia?**
   With age and advanced atherosclerotic disease, the aorta dilates but also lengthens, causing aortic tortuosity or even apparent kinking. It does not dilate focally. This differentiates ectasia from aneurysm. Once the descending aorta reaches 4 cm in diameter, it is considered ectatic. With aortic lengthening, the descending thoracic aorta may shift from the left paravertebral location to the right paravertebral location and then return close to midline at the diaphragmatic hiatus. Ectasia is often used loosely for dilated aortas that are not quite aneurysmal.

44. **What is a pseudoaneurysm?**
   This is a focal (saccular) dilation of the aorta and does not contain all three layers of the wall. It usually is caused by a penetrating ulcer, infection, trauma, or surgery (Figs. 20-19 and 20-20).

45. **What causes an aortic aneurysm?**
   Atherosclerosis is most common, followed by degeneration (including Marfan and Ehlers-Danlos syndromes and cystic medial necrosis), infection, inflammation (Takayasu's arteritis), and trauma.

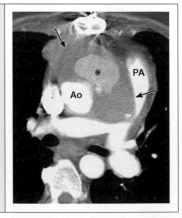

Figure 20-19. Large saccular pseudoaneurysm originated from the anterior aorta (Ao) in a patient 6 months after aortic valve replacement. This patient developed symptoms of right heart failure due to outflow obstruction of the adjacent pulmonary artery (PA) from compression by the largely thrombosed mass *(arrows)*. On echocardiography this mass was believed to arise from the pulmonary artery; however, on CT the epicenter of the mass is between the aorta and pulmonary artery, and the enhancing residual lumen *(asterisk)* connects to the aorta.

CT OF THORACIC ARTERIAL DISEASE

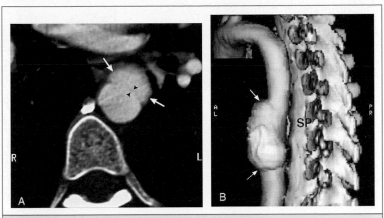

Figure 20-20. A young patient had spine surgery several months ago and has recurrent back pain. **A,** Transverse CT image shows a subtle contour deformity of the left anterolateral aortic margin *(arrows)*. The overhanging edge of the pseudoaneurysm *(arrowheads)* could be misinterpreted as a dissection. **B,** The sagittal reconstruction clearly defines the saccular shape of the pseudoaneurysm *(arrows)* and its proximity to the spine (SP) posteriorly.

46. **What are the primary features of atherosclerotic aneurysms?**
They are fusiform and contain mural atheroma. About 85% have calcification in the wall or in the atheroma itself. The atheroma (or thrombus) may be crescentic or circumferential (*see* Fig. 20-18). *Atheroma* (which comes from the Greek word for gruel) is a better term for the mix of cholesterol, fibroblasts, calcification, and hemorrhage than *thrombus*.

47. **How do the causes and sites relate to the morphology of thoracic aortic aneurysms?**
See Table 20-1.

48. **What percent of patients with nontraumatic thoracic aneurysms have disease elsewhere?**
Up to 28% of patients with thoracic aortic aneurysms also have abdominal aortic aneurysms. Therefore, complete screening and continued surveillance are important.

TABLE 20-1. RELATIONSHIP OF CAUSE AND SITE TO MORPHOLOGY OF THORACIC AORTIC ANEURYSMS

Etiology	Site	Morphology
Atherosclerotic	Proximal descending	Fusiform
Atherosclerotic	Mid to distal descending	Saccular
Degenerative	Ascending	Fusiform
Mycotic	Ascending	Saccular
Aortitis	Ascending	Saccular
Traumatic	Aortic isthmus	Saccular

49. **Which grows faster: thoracic or abdominal aneurysms?**
    In general, the more proximal the aortic aneurysm, the faster it is likely to grow. This may be due to increased intraluminal pressure. The following are average growth rates in different parts of the aorta:
    - Aortic arch: 0.56 cm/year
    - Thoracic aorta: 0.42 cm/year
    - Abdominal aorta: 0.28 cm/year

50. **When are thoracic aortas considered at risk for rupture?**
    Median size for rupture or dissection of the ascending aorta is 6 cm; median size for rupture or dissection of the descending aorta is 7.2 cm. Therefore, ascending aneurysms are usually repaired at 5–5.5 cm and descending aneurysms at 5.5–6.5 cm.

51. **What are the signs of rupture?**
    These include mediastinal hematoma and/or high-attenuation pleural effusion (Fig. 20-21).

52. **Into which thoracic compartments do thoracic aortic aneurysms rupture?**
    The left hemithorax is most common (especially the left pleural space). The mediastinum and right hemithorax are less often involved (*see* Fig. 20-21).

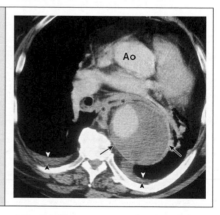

Figure 20-21. Axial image at the level of the aortic root (Ao) shows markedly enlarged descending aortic aneurysm *(arrows)* with large atheroma in the lumen. Rupture is indicated by the mediastinal hemorrhage anteriorly and to the right *(asterisks)*. Bilateral high-attenuation (greater than water density) pleural effusions *(arrowheads)* also confirm rupture.

53. **Which findings indicate impending aneurysm rupture?**
    These include a rapid increase in aortic diameter, a high-attenuation crescent in the aortic thrombus (acute bleeding in the aortic thrombus), a high-attenuation periaortic hematoma (aortic leak), and the "aortic drape sign" (Fig. 20-22).

54. **What is an "aortic drape sign"?**
    The posterior aortic wall becomes indistinct and cannot be differentiated from adjacent structures. The posterior aorta "drapes" over the spine and follows the contour of the vertebra on at least one side. This finding suggests a contained aortic leak.

55. **How is CT used for surgical planning?**
    CT maps the location and extent of the aneurysm, its diameter, and the amount of mural disease. The proximal extent dictates the type of repair (including aortic valve). Thoracoabdominal aneurysms need complete evaluation of the abdominal aorta and may require a two-stage repair.

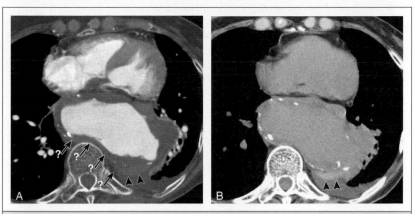

Figure 20-22. **A,** Postcontrast image of large thoracic aneurysm with loss of the posterior wall *(arrows and question marks).* The hematoma *(arrowheads)* is difficult to discern within the small left pleural effusion on the postcontrast image. **B,** The precontrast image clearly demonstrates the contained hematoma *(arrowheads),* which may be within the wall or outside the aorta.

56. **Which types of aortitis cause aneurysms?**
    Syphilis is the classic infectious cause of aortitis resulting in aneurysms. Inflammatory aortitis is far more common in the Western world and includes Takayasu's arteritis, Behçet disease, ankylosing spondylitis, and giant cell arteritis.

57. **What diseases cause mycotic aneurysms?**
    These are the result of disseminated hematologic infections. The common causes include IV drug abuse (*Candida, Streptococcus viridans, Staphylococcus aureus*), endocarditis, and iatrogenic (catheter, surgery).

58. **What imaging findings suggest an infected aneurysm?**
    Ninety-three percent of infected aneurysms have a saccular shape versus the fusiform shape of atherosclerotic or degenerative aneurysms. Specific features include a paraaortic soft tissue mass, stranding, and/or fluid (48% of cases), rapid aneurysm progression (nearly 100% of cases), adjacent vertebral body destruction (4%), and periaortic gas (7%).

59. **What types of open aortic graft repair are performed?**
    The diseased segment can be excised and an interposition graft is sewn to the remaining aortic ends with a full-thickness attachment. If the diseased segment is not removed, an inclusion graft is placed in the lumen and tacked down to the inner layers of the aorta. This leaves potential space between the graft and native aorta for persistent blood flow, which may exacerbate the remaining dissection, or for pseudoaneurysm formation, which occurs in 4% of patients.

60. **What is the significance of low-attenuation collections adjacent to the postoperative aorta?**
    From 52% to 82% of postoperative aortas have associated soft tissue attenuation collections, which decrease in size with time. Approximately 50–60% of patients have persistent low-attenuation collections more than 1 year after operation.

61. **What are the indications for endoluminal stent graft repair of thoracic aortic aneurysms?**
    Patients with atherosclerotic aneurysms, traumatic pseudoaneurysms, and dissections (type B) who have contraindications to open surgery may be considered candidates for stent-graft thoracic aortic repair, as long as the aorta is not infected. (You cannot currently put a graft into an infected bed.) The long-term outcomes—reduction in aneurysm size and prevention of rupture—are less well-established than for abdominal procedures. The criterion for success is reduction of the aneurysm sac size (Fig. 20-23).

62. **What findings are commonly seen on CT following endoluminal stent graft repair?**
    - **Pleural effusion:** 73%
    - **Periaortic changes:** 33% (*see* Fig. 20-23)
    - **Perigraft leak:** 3–21%
    - **Atelectasis:** 10%
    - **Mural thrombus within the stent-graft:** 3%
    - **New aortic dissection:** 2%
    - **Aortic rupture:** 3%

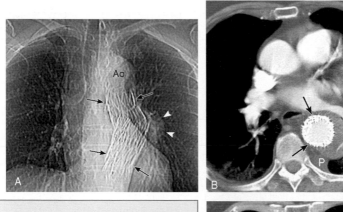

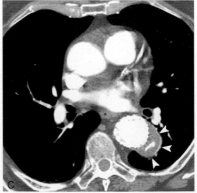

Figure 20-23. *A,* Scout CT image in a patient after recent endograft repair. Note the two wire mesh components of the endograft *(arrows)* beginning just below the aortic arch (Ao) and ending above the diaphragm. The contour of the residual aneurysm sac *(arrowheads)* is still visible. *B,* Axial CT through the aneurysm sac shows endograft *(arrows)* with contrast in the lumen. A linear calcification is noted in the residual aneurysm sac *(arrowheads)* and a small pleural effusion (P) is present. *C,* One year later the sac size *(arrowheads)* is smaller, indicating a good repair. The calcification is unchanged, and the pleural fluid has resolved.

63. **What is the classification of stent-graft endoleaks? How are they identified?**
Endoleaks are identified as an area of contrast enhancement within the residual aneurysm sac and outside the endograft lumen. They may be seen in the early arterial phase of enhancement or occasionally as delayed enhancement of the sac (slow leak). Persistent calcification within the sac may mimic a leak; therefore, a precontrast scan is useful to distinguish calcification from leak. The following classification was developed for abdominal aortic aneurysms; however, it can be applied to thoracic aneurysms.
- **Type I:** Leak from the cuff at either end of the graft
- **Type II:** Back flow leak from collateral circulation (side branches)
- **Type III:** Leak from a breach in the fabric of the graft (structural failure of the graft)
- **Type IV:** Leak from increased porosity of the graft without structural failure of graft
- **Type V:** Also-known as "endotension"; the aneurysm sac continues to grow despite no demonstrable leak or structural failure of the graft

64. **What is the significance of the artery of Adamkiewicz in open thoracic aorta repair?**
This vessel is the feeding vessel of the anterior spinal artery and arises at the T9-T10 level. Patients who undergo surgical descending aortic repairs are at risk for ischemic spinal cord injury and paraplegia. These complications are caused by ischemia while cross-clamped and occur in 5–10% of patients.

65. **What is the importance of the artery of Adamkiewicz in patients who undergo endoluminal (stent-graft) repair?**
Evaluating the artery of Adamkiewicz for endoluminal management per se is not very important because paraplegia is almost unheard of after stent-graft placement. However, should the endoluminal procedure be a technical failure and converted to an open surgical repair, then the status of the artery of Adamkiewicz becomes important.

66. **What are the restrictive (stenotic) disease processes that involve the aorta?**
These include true coarctation, pseudocoarctation, midaortic dysplastic syndrome, atherosclerotic aortic occlusive disease, chronic vasculitis, aortic dissection (due to compression of the true lumen), postoperative stenosis, and stenosis from periaortic disease (extrinsic or mural).

67. **What causes periaortic stenosis?**
Extrinsic compression may be cause by neurofibromatosis and aggressive mediastinal tumors. (Lymphomas that encase the aorta usually do not obstruct the aorta.) Mural tumors, such as fibrous histiocytoma, fibrosarcoma, giant cell sarcoma, leiomyosarcoma, and angiosarcoma, involve the aortic wall with resultant narrowing and outflow obstruction.

68. **What is Takayasu's arteritis?**
Also known as pulseless arteritis, this is the most common aortitis, usually affecting young women.

69. **How does Takayasu's arteritis affect the aorta?**
Takayasu's involves the vessel wall, causing stenosis, occlusion, dilation, and/or aneurysm. Any or all may occur in an individual patient (Fig. 20-24).

70. **What other vessels are affected by Takayasu's arteritis?**
In addition to the aorta, Takayasu's may involve the aortic arch vessels, the pulmonary arteries, or any of the visceral aortic branches in the abdomen.

71. **How does Takayasu's arteritis present clinically?**
Acutely, patients present with fever, night sweats, arthralgia, muscle pain, anemia, and an elevated erythrocyte sedimentation rate. On CT, the vessel walls are thickened from inflammation.

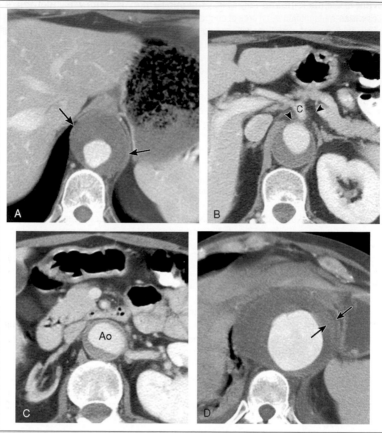

Figure 20-24. *A,* Descending thoracic aortic aneurysm *(arrows)* in a 33-year-old woman begins in the mid chest and continues in a fusiform fashion through the hiatus and into the abdomen. *B,* Note the abnormal soft tissue *(arrowheads)* adjacent to and narrowing the celiac axis (C) origin. *C,* Also note the profound atrophy of the right kidney due to prior stenosis of the right renal artery. Ao = aorta. *D,* Three months later the aneurysm has markedly enlarged. Note the wall enhancement *(arrows)* indicating inflammatory disease. The concomitant aneurysm and stenosis in a young patient should suggest Takayasu's arteritis, which is the case here.

72. **What are the advantages of CT assessment of Takayasu's arteritis?**
    CT depicts mural changes (thickening, thrombosis, and calcifications) more than conventional angiography and is especially useful as a noninvasive assessment of the thoracoabdominal vascular tree in this systemic disease.

73. **What are the mural findings in Takayasu's disease by CT?**
    High-attenuation aortic wall thickening on precontrast CT (range: 47–82 HU) is seen in up to 80–85% of Takayasu's disease patients, regardless of disease activity. Arterial phase heterogeneous wall enhancement was found to be 75% sensitive and 100% specific for disease activity (*see* Fig. 20-24). Delayed phase wall enhancement is 88% sensitive and 75% specific for disease activity. Mural calcifications are seen in 75% of patients. Measuring wall enhancement is not always straightforward however.

74. **How common is pulmonary artery involvement in patients with Takayasu's disease?**
Seventeen percent of patients have pulmonary artery mural findings including wall thickening and early and delayed wall enhancement.

75. **What is the anatomic classification of pulseless (Takayasu's) arteritis?**
The Numano classification is as follows:
- **Type I:** Involves the branches of the aortic arch only.
- **Type IIa:** Involves the ascending aorta and/or at the aortic arch. The branches of the aortic arch may be involved as well. The rest of the aorta is not affected.
- **Type IIb:** Affects the descending thoracic aorta with or without involvement of the ascending aorta or the aortic arch with its branches. The abdominal aorta is not involved.
- **Type III:** Involves the descending thoracic aorta, the abdominal aorta, and/or the renal arteries. The ascending aorta and the aortic arch and its branches are not involved.
- **Type IV:** Involves the abdominal aorta and/or the renal arteries only.
- **Type V:** Is the generalized type, with combined features of the other types.
    Note that involvement of the coronary and pulmonary arteries should be indicated as C(+) or P(+), respectively.

76. **Which vascular abnormalities of Ehlers-Danlos syndrome are detected by CT?**
These include aneurysms of the great vessels or the aortic arch, aortic dissection, tortuosity and ectasia of the aortic arch, and ectasia of the pulmonary arteries.

77. **What are the vascular findings of Marfan's syndrome in the chest?**
Marfan's syndrome may result in aortic annulus and sinuses of Valsalva dilation ("tulip bulb" sign by angiography or reconstructed CTA, which gives rise to aortic valve insufficiency). It also may cause aortic aneurysm and/or dissection and/or pulmonary artery aneurysm.

78. **How does Turner's syndrome affect the aorta?**
Fifteen percent of patients with Turner's syndrome have coarctation of the aorta. They may also have dissecting aneurysms of the aorta and/or a bicuspid aortic valve (not detectable by CT).

BIBLIOGRAPHY

1. Macura KJ, Corl FM, Fishman EK, et al: Pathogenesis in acute aortic syndromes: Aortic dissection, intramural hematoma, and penetrating atherosclerotic aortic ulcer. Am J Roentgenol 181:309–316, 2003. Available at http://www.ajronline.org/cgi/content/full/181/2/309.

2. Anagnostopoulos CE, Prabhakar MJ, Kittle CF: Aortic dissections and dissecting aneurysms. Am J Cardiol 30:263–273, 1972.

3. Batra P, Bigoni B, Manning J, et al: Pitfalls in the diagnosis of thoracic aortic dissection at CT angiography. Radiographics 20:309–320, 2000.

4. Castañer E, Andreu M, Gallardo X, et al: CT in nontraumatic acute thoracic aortic disease: Typical and atypical features and complications. Radiographics 23:93–110, 2003.

5. Ergin MA, Phillipps RA, Galla JD, et al: Significance of distal false lumen after type A dissection repair. Ann Thorac Surg 57:820–825, 1994.

6. Fattori R, Napoli G, Lovato L, et al: Descending thoracic aortic diseases: Stent-graft repair. Radiology 229:176–183, 2003.

7. Halliday KE, Al-Kutoubi A: Draped aorta: CT sign of contained leak of aortic aneurysms. Radiology 199:41–43, 1996.

8. Harris J, Bis K, Glover J, et al: Penetrating atherosclerotic ulcers of the aorta. J Vasc Surg 19:90–99, 1994.

9. Hayashi H, Matsuoka Y, Sakamoto I, et al: Penetrating atherosclerotic ulcer of the aorta: Imaging features and disease concept. Radiographics 20:995–1005, 2000.

10. Heiberg E, Wolverson MK, Sundaram M, et al: Characteristics of aortic atherosclerotic aneurysm versus aortic dissection. J Comput Assist Tomogr 9:78–83, 1985.

11. Hiller N, Lieberman S, Chajek-Shaul T, et al: Thoracic manifestations of Behçet disease at CT. Radiographics 24:801–808, 2004.

12. Kouchoukos NT, Dougenis D: Surgery of the thoracic aorta. N Engl J Med 336:1876–1886, 1997.

13. Ledbetter S, Stuk JL, Kaufman JA: Helical (spiral) CT in the evaluation of emergent thoracic aortic syndromes: Traumatic aortic rupture, aortic aneurysm, aortic dissection, intramural hematoma, and penetrating atherosclerotic ulcer. Radiol Clin North Am 37:575–589, 1999.

14. Macedo TA, Stanson AW, Oderich GS, et al: Infected aortic aneurysms: Imaging findings. Radiology 231:250–257, 2004.

15. Morgan-Hughes GJ, Owens PE, Marshall AJ, et al: Thoracic aorta at multi-detector row CT: Motion artifact with various reconstruction windows. Radiology 228:583–588, 2003.

16. Naidich DP, Webb WR, Muller NL, et al: Aorta, arch vessels, and great veins. In Naidich DP, Webb WR, Muller NL, et al (eds): Computed Tomography and Magnetic Resonance of the Thorax, 3rd ed. Philadelphia, Lippincott-Raven, pp 505–602.

17. Park JH, Chung JW, Im JG, et al: Takayasu arteritis: Evaluation of mural changes in the aorta and pulmonary artery with CT angiography. Radiology 196:89–93, 1995.

18. Quint LE, Williams DM, Francis IR, et al: Ulcerlike lesions of the aorta: Imaging features and natural history. Radiology 218:719–723, 2001.

19. Roos J, Willmann J, Weishaupt D, et al: Thoracic aorta: motion artifact reduction with retrospective and prospective electrocardiography-assisted multi-detector row CT. Radiology 222:271–277, 2002.

20. Rubin GD, Shiau MC, Leung AN, et al: Aorta and iliac arteries: Single versus multiple detector-row helical CT angiography. Radiology 215:670–676, 2000.

21. Sakai T, Dake MD, Semba CP, et al: Descending thoracic aortic aneurysm: Thoracic CT findings after endovascular stent-graft placement. Radiology 212:169–174, 1999.

22. Sebastià C, Pallisa E, Quiroga S, et al: Aortic dissection: Diagnosis and follow-up with helical CT. Radiographics 19:45–60, 1999.

23. Sebastià C, Quiroga S, Boyé R, et al: Aortic stenosis: Spectrum of diseases depicted at multisection CT. Radiographics 23:79–91, 2003.

24. Sueyoshi E, Matsuoka Y, Imada T, et al: New development of an ulcerlike projection in aortic intramural hematoma: CT evaluation. Radiology 224:536–541, 2002.

25. Tatsumi M, Cohade C, Nakamoto Y, et al: Fluorodeoxyglucose uptake in the aortic wall at PET/CT: Possible finding for active atherosclerosis. Radiology 229:831–837, 2003.

26. Ugolini P, Mousseaux E, Hernigou A, et al: Infectious pseudoaneurysms suspected at echocardiography: Electron-beam CT findings. Radiology 217:263–269, 2000.

27. Williams DM, Lee DY, Hamilton BH, et al: The dissected aorta: Percutaneous treatment of ischemic complications—principles and results. J Vasc Interv Radiol 8:605–625, 1997.

28. Yamada I, Nakagawa T, Himeno Y, et al: Takayasu arteritis: Evaluation of the thoracic aorta with CT angiography. Radiology 209:103–109, 1998.

29. Yoshida S, Akiba H, Tamakawa M, et al: Thoracic involvement of type A aortic dissection and intramural hematoma: Diagnostic accuracy—Comparison of emergency helical CT and surgical findings. Radiology 228:430–435, 2003.

30. Yoshioka K, Niinuma H, Ohira A, et al: MR angiography and CT angiography of the artery of Adamkiewicz: Noninvasive preoperative assessment of thoracoabdominal aortic aneurysm. Radiographics 23:1215–1225, 2003.

KIDNEY

Shweta Bhatt, MD, Suleman Merchant, MD, and Vikram Dogra, MD

1. **Describe the anatomic features of the kidneys on unenhanced multislice CT.**
   On CT, the transverse contour of the kidney is smooth and oval, with an anteromedial break in the renal outline at the hilus where the vascular pedicle enters (Fig. 21-1). The renal sinus is a potential space contained by the renal parenchyma, filled with fatty tissue and contains the renal arteries, veins, lymphatics, and pelvicalyces.

   On unenhanced CT scans, the normal renal parenchyma has an attenuation value of 30–40 Hounsfield units (HU), depending on patient hydration. The cortex and medulla show no visible density differences.

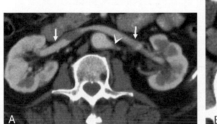 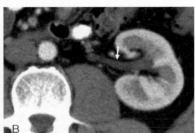

Figure 21-1. Normal kidney. *A,* Normal renal hilum of the kidney. Renal veins are seen *(arrows)* draining into the inferior vena cava (IVC). Origin of the left renal artery from the aorta is also demonstrated *(arrowhead)*. *B,* Renal hilum of the left kidney showing the origin of the ureter *(arrow)*.

2. **Describe the CT technique for imaging the kidneys.**
   - The technique should be tailored according to the specific clinical problem involved. However, there are some common aspects to all dedicated renal CT studies.
   - Patients undergoing renal CT should receive oral contrast medium, because unopacified bowel loops may simulate perinephric masses and retroperitoneal adenopathy.
   - Examination should be performed in suspended respiration.
   - Same peak kV, mA-sec setting, section thickness, and field of view (FOV) should be used for both pre- and postcontrast study.
   The parameters in Table 21-1 are used for imaging the kidneys with the Philips 16 detector multislice CT. These parameters vary with different manufacturers.

3. **What is the protocol used for triple-phase CT in kidney evaluation?**
   - Patients should be given oral contrast to opacify the bowel.
   - Area scanned is from the dome of the liver to the level of the iliac crest.
   - Noncontrast scan is done prior to injection of intravenous (IV) contrast.
   - IV contrast (90 mL) is injected at the rate of 1.5–2.0 mL/sec.
   - Corticomedullary phase is at 20- to 30-second delay.
   - Nephrographic phase is at 75- to 85-second delay.

TABLE 21-1. PARAMETERS FOR IMAGING THE KIDNEYS WITH THE PHILIPS 16 DETECTOR MULTSLICE CT

Resolution	Ultra-Fast
Collimation	16×1.5
Slice thickness (mm)	5.0
Increment (mm)	5.0
Pitch	0.5
Rotation time (sec)	0.5
kV	120
mAs/slice	250

- Excretory phase is at 180-second delay.
- The slice thickness of 3 mm at slice interval of 1.5 mm.

4. **What is the advantage of multidetector spiral CT over single-detector CT in the renal studies?**
   Multislice scanners allow 1- to 2.5-mm slices through the region of interest in a single breath-hold, allowing rapid image acquisition, with almost no motion artifact.

5. **What is the significance of doing unenhanced scans along with the contrast-enhanced renal scans?**
   - Unenhanced scans permit contrast enhancement of a renal lesion to be measured.
   - They ensure that renal parenchymal calcifications, renal calculi, renal and perinephric hemorrhage and fat, and calcification in a renal mass are not obscured by contrast medium.
   - They help differentiate a hyperdense cyst from a renal solid tumor.

6. **Describe the various phases of contrast-enhanced renal scans.**
   There are three phases of contrast-enhanced renal scans:
   - **Corticomedullary phase** (Fig. 21-2A): This phase occurs between 25 and 70 seconds after initiating IV contrast administration as the contrast enters the cortical capillaries and the peritubular spaces and filters into the proximal cortical tubules. At this stage, the renal cortex can be differentiated from the medulla, because of greater vascularity of the cortex compared with the medulla.
   - **Nephrographic phase** (Fig. 21-2B): This phase begins at about 80 seconds and lasts up to 180 seconds after the start of injection, as contrast material proceeds into the loops of Henle and collecting tubules. A homogeneous nephrogram results, in which corticomedullary differentiation is lost.
   - **Excretory phase** (Fig. 21-2C): This phase begins approximately 180 seconds after the start of contrast injection. After contrast is excreted into the collecting system, the attenuation of the nephrogram progressively decreases.

7. **Describe the clinical significance of each of these phases in a contrast-enhanced renal scan.**
   - The **corticomedullary phase** is important in assessing renal vasculature. This phase is important in detecting renal artery stenosis, renal artery aneurysm, arteriovenous malformation, or a fistula. It also allows confident diagnosis of tumor extension to the renal vein. This is the single most important phase in the evaluation of renal artery stenosis.

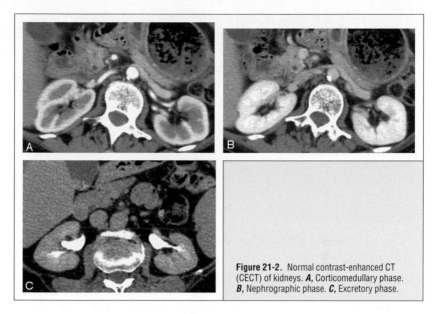

Figure 21-2. Normal contrast-enhanced CT (CECT) of kidneys. **A,** Corticomedullary phase. **B,** Nephrographic phase. **C,** Excretory phase.

- The **nephrographic phase** is the best phase for discrimination between the normal renal medulla and a renal mass. This phase is most valuable for detecting renal masses and characterizing indeterminate lesions.
- The **excretory phase** is helpful to delineate the relationship of a centrally located mass within the collecting system. This phase is also helpful for evaluating urothelial masses.

8. **What are the CT criteria for the diagnosis of a simple renal cyst?**
    - Sharp margination and demarcation from the surrounding renal parenchyma
    - A smooth, thin wall
    - Homogeneous, water density contents with an attenuation value of 0–20 HU
    - No enhancement after IV administration of contrast medium (*see* Fig. 21-3)

KEY POINTS: CT OF THE KIDNEY

1. Patients undergoing renal CT should receive oral contrast medium, because unopacified bowel loops may simulate perinephric masses and retroperitoneal adenopathy.

2. Same peak kV, mA-sec setting, section thickness, and FOV should be used for both pre- and postcontrast study.

3. There are three phases of contrast-enhanced renal scans: corticomedullary phase (between 25 and 70 seconds after initiating IV contrast administration); nephrographic phase (begins at about 80 seconds and lasts up to 180 seconds after the start of injection); and excretory phase (begins approximately 180 seconds after the start of contrast injection).

9. **What is the Bosniak classification of renal cysts?**
    See Table 21-2 and Figures 21-3 and 21-4.

TABLE 21-2.　BOSNIAK CLASSIFICATION OF RENAL CYSTS

Category I (benign)	Classic simple cyst (*see* Fig. 21-3)
	Sharp margination and interface
	Smooth thin wall
	Homogeneous water density (0–20 HU)
	No enhancement
Category II (probably benign)	Minimally complicated cysts (Fig. 21-4A)
	Thin <1 mm septa
	Fine linear calcification in wall or septa
	High-density cysts (40–100 HU) on unenhanced scans (Fig. 21-4B)
	CT criteria: smooth, round, sharply marginated, homogenous
	<3 cm
	Nonenhancing
	At least one-fourth of circumference extends outside the kidney
Category IIF (F stands for follow-up)	More complex cysts (Fig. 21-4C)
	> 3 cm
	Increased number of septa
	Increased calcification, thicker and nodular
Category III (probably malignant)	True indeterminate cystic masses requiring surgical evaluation (Fig. 21-4D)
	Uniform wall thickening and nodularity
	Thick or irregular peripheral calcification
	Multilocular with multiple enhancing, > 1 mm thick, septa
Category IV (malignant)	Clearly malignant lesions (Fig. 21-4E)
	Nonuniform, enhancing thick wall
	Enhancing, large nodules in the wall
	Clearly solid components in the cystic lesion

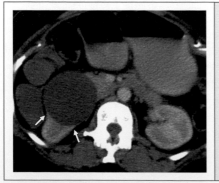

Figure 21-3. Simple renal cyst (Bosniak I cyst). Contrast-enhanced CT demonstrates features of a simple renal cyst as an imperceptible wall, absence of septa or calcification, and nonenhancing contents of the cyst with a fluid density (15 HU). Claw sign *(arrows)* confirms the origin of the cyst from right kidney.

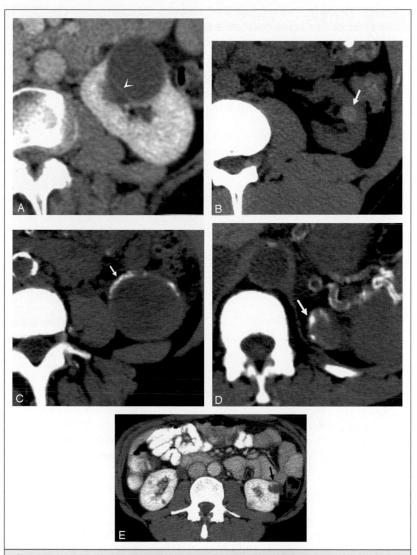

Figure 21-4. *A,* Bosniak II cyst with a thin (<1 mm) septa *(arrowhead). B,* Bosniak II cyst. A hyperdense (hemorrhagic) cyst *(arrow)* in the left kidney on a nonenhanced CT (NECT) scan. *C,* Bosniak II F cyst. NECT image of the left kidney reveals a 4.8-cm cystic lesion with thick, peripheral calcification *(arrow).* Size > 3 cm and presence of thick peripheral calcification rule out a Bosniak II category. *D,* Bosniak III cyst. Cystic lesion arising from the superior pole of the left kidney with thicker and nodular calcification *(arrow). E,* Bosniak IV cyst. A patient with known history of von Hippel-Landau disease with multiple bilateral renal lesions. A cystic lesion in the left renal midpolar region with an enhancing mural nodule *(arrow)* is suggestive of renal cell carcinoma.

10. **Describe the category IIF lesions.**

Category IIF consists of minimally complicated cysts that need follow-up. This is a group not well defined by Bosniak but consists of lesions that do not neatly fall into category II or III. These lesions have some suspicious features that deserve follow-up up to detect any change in character. These cysts differ from type II cysts in being > 3 cm. These cysts may contain an increased number of septa and an increased amount of calcification, which may be thicker and nodular (*see* Fig. 21-4C). As in category II cysts, these lesions may demonstrate minimal enhancement of a hairline-thin, smooth septum or wall but no enhancement of the tissues in which calcification is present.

11. **What are renal sinus cysts?**

Renal sinus (parapelvic) cysts are benign extraparenchymal cysts located in the renal sinus (Fig 21-5). They are not true renal cysts but are probably lymphatic in origin. They may be unilocular or multilocular and are often bilateral. They do not communicate with the renal collecting system. On CT, the characteristic feature of a renal sinus cyst is a surrounding halo of renal sinus fat, indicating its non-parenchymal origin.

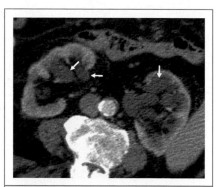

Figure 21-5. Parapelvic cysts. CECT image of the kidneys in an 80-year-old woman demonstrates multiple cystic structures in the renal pelvis on both sides *(arrows)*.

12. **What is a multicystic dysplastic kidney (MDK)?**

MDK is the most common form of cystic disease in infants, usually presenting as an asymptomatic flank mass, associated with intrauterine ureteral obstruction or atresia. The renal artery may also be hypoplastic or atretic. Contralateral renal anomalies are detected in 41% of patients with MDK and include obstruction of the ureteropelvic junction (UPJ), renal agenesis, renal hypoplasia, vesicoureteral reflux, and bilateral MDK. Bilateral MDK is seen in 19% and contralateral agenesis is seen in 11% of patients.

13. **What are the types of MDK ?**

There are two types:

- The **classic type (pelvoinfundibular atresia)** has no discernible renal pelvis on imaging. The kidney may be small, normal in size, or enlarged and contains multiple variable-sized non-communicating renal cysts. There is no perfusion of the affected kidney on renal scintigraphy, and contrast-enhanced CT (CECT) shows no evidence of contrast excretion by the affected kidney.
- The **hydronephrotic form** of MDK is characterized by dilatation of the renal pelvis and calyces (identification of parenchymal cysts that do not communicate with the collecting system helps to differentiate from simple hydronephrosis).

14. **What is multilocular cystic nephroma?**

It has a bimodal distribution and affects females younger than 20 years or after the fifth decade. The average size of the lesion, which is single and unilateral and involves only part of the kidney, is 8–10 cm in diameter. The lesion frequently herniates into the renal pelvis, causing a filling defect. Septa in the lesion may enhance.

15. **Describe the CT findings in autosomal recessive polycystic kidney disease (ARPKD).**

    ARPKD is characterized by ectasia of the renal collecting ducts, interstitial fibrosis, and variable degrees of portal hepatic fibrosis (congenital hepatic fibrosis), often causing portal hypertension. On noncontrast CT examination, the kidneys are smooth, enlarged, and low in attenuation, likely to be due to a reflection of the large fluid volume in the dilated ducts. On administration of contrast, a striated nephrogram is seen, representing accumulation of contrast in the dilated tubules. Tubular ectasia is confined mainly to the renal medulla with macrocysts noted only occasionally. The renal cortex is less severely affected. CT may also show evidence of associated congenital hepatic fibrosis and portal hypertension.

16. **Describe the features of autosomal dominant polycystic kidney disease (ADPKD).**

    ADPKD disease is one of the most commonly inherited diseases in the United States and accounts for 5–10% of patients with end-stage renal disease (ESRD). ADPKD is a systemic disorder; cysts appear with decreasing frequency in the kidneys (Fig. 21-6A), liver, pancreas, brain, spleen, ovaries, and testis. Cardiac valvular disorders, abdominal and inguinal hernias, and aneurysms of cerebral (Berry aneurysms) and coronary arteries and aorta are also associated with ADPKD. Seventy percent of patients with ADPKD have hepatic cysts (Fig. 21-6B). Colonic diverticula occur in about 80% of patients with ADPKD.

17. **What are Bear's criteria for the diagnosis of ADPKD?**
    - Family history of ADPKD
    - Three or more renal cysts
    - Of the three cysts, at least one cyst in each kidney

18. **What are the most common causes of pain in ADPKD? What is the role of CT in its identification?**

    Flank pain and hematuria are the most common symptoms of ADPKD. Hemorrhagic cysts, the most common cause of pain in ADPKD, have attenuation values of 40–100 HU on unenhanced scans (*see* Fig. 21-6A), do not enhance after IV contrast administration, and are homogeneously hyperdense and well defined. Pseudoenhancement of 10 HU can be seen in cysts smaller than

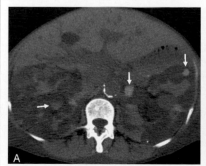
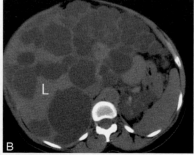

Figure 21-6. Autosomal dominant polycystic kidney disease (ADPKD). *A,* Nonenhanced CT (NECT) of the kidneys demonstrates bilaterally enlarged kidneys with multiple cysts. Few cysts are hyperdense *(arrows),* suggestive of hemorrhage. *B,* NECT in another patient with ADPKD demonstrates multiple cysts in the liver (L). Hepatic cysts are seen in 70% of patients with ADPKD.

2 cm. Renal calculi are another cause of flank pain in ADPKD and occur in 20–36% of patients with ADPKD. Fifty-seven percent of calculi in ADPKD are composed predominantly of uric acid, which are radiolucent on conventional tomography, and therefore such calculi are best evaluated by CT.

19. **What is pseudoenhancement? What are its causes?**

Renal cystic pseudoenhancement refers to the artifactual increase in CT attenuation value of a simple cyst after the administration of iodinated contrast material. It is commonly seen in small cysts (less than 2 cm). Enhancement of 10 HU has been widely accepted as the threshold value. An attenuation increase of less than 10 HU is considered to be within the limits of artifactual pseudoenhancement. A host of technical factors, including beam hardening and partial volume averaging, can possibly cause pseudoenhancement. Additionally, an increase in background attenuation by contrast medium may possibly cause pseudoenhancement.

20. **What are the complications associated with ADPKD?**

The most common complication is end-stage renal disease (ESRD) seen in about 35–48% of patients. Average age at ESRD is 55 years. Pain and hematuria resulting from hemorrhage into the cysts (*see* Fig 21-6A) or, less commonly, from renal calculi are less frequent complications of ADPKD. The cysts may rupture into the perinephric space, causing large hematomas. Hemorrhagic cysts often develop mural calcification over a long period of time.

Cyst infection is difficult to diagnose on CT. Its presence is suggested by a cyst larger than the surrounding cysts, with thickening and irregularity of its wall, increase in attenuation value of its contents, and localized thickening of the adjacent renal fascia.

21. **What is the risk of renal cell carcinoma (RCC) in patients with ADPKD?**

The risk of renal cancer in ADPKD patients not on dialysis is probably not increased; however, when on prolonged dialysis (more than 3 years) they have an increased risk of developing renal malignancy relative to the general population.

22. **How is acquired cystic kidney disease (ACKD) diagnosed?**

The radiologic diagnosis of ACKD is best established by CECT. The diagnosis is based on detection of at least three to five cysts in each kidney in a patient with chronic renal failure not due to hereditary renal cystic disease (Fig. 21-7). The affected kidneys are usually small; nephromegaly may eventually develop.

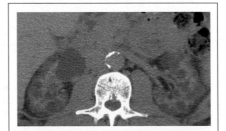

Figure 21-7. Acquired cystic kidney disease (ACKD) with end-stage renal disease. NECT image of the kidneys demonstrates bilateral, small-sized kidneys with multiple cysts.

23. **Why is it important to identify ACKD?**

The significance of diagnosing ACKD is because of the increased incidence of renal cell carcinoma (RCC). The incidence is about 12–18 times higher than that in the general population and these cancers may be asymptomatic.

24. **What are the various hereditary syndromes associated with renal cystic involvement?**

- von Hippel-Lindau disease (VHLD)
- Tuberous sclerosis complex (TSC)
- Renal lymphangiectasia

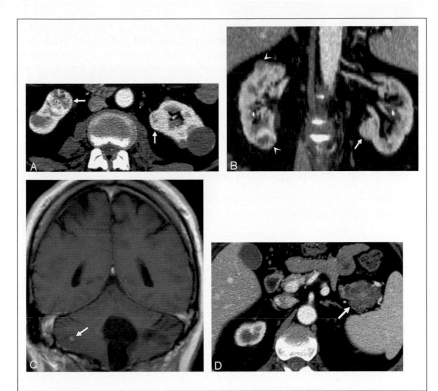

Figure 21-8. von Hippel-Lindau disease. *A,* CECT image of the kidneys demonstrates multiple cysts in both kidneys with two enhancing solid renal masses *(arrows)* consistent with RCC. *B,* Corresponding coronal image demonstrates cystic *(arrowheads)* and solid *(arrow)* renal neoplasms. *C,* Associated tumors in von Hippel-Lindau disease. Gadolinium-enhanced image of the brain through the posterior fossa reveals an enhancing mass in the right cerebellar hemisphere *(arrow)* consistent with hemangioblastoma. *D,* CECT image through the pancreas demonstrates an associated cystic-solid neoplasm of the tail of the pancreas *(arrow).*

25. Describe the characteristic renal features in VHLD.

Multiple bilateral renal cysts and cystic and solid neoplasms are the most common manifestations of VHLD (Fig. 21-8). Predominantly cystic lesions with solid components are characteristic lesions of VHLD. The solid component usually represents RCC. RCC is reported to develop in 24–45% of VHLD patients and is often multifocal and bilateral.

26. Describe the renal features in the TSC.

Renal lesions are seen in 50% of patients with TSC. They include multiple cysts, angiomyolipomas (AMLs), and perirenal cystic collections, or lymphangiomas. Multiple renal AMLs are sine qua non of TSC and are usually bilateral and occur in about 15%, mostly female patients. Renal cystic disease in TSC may sometimes be the earliest and only clinical manifestation of the disorder in infancy and childhood. The combination of renal cysts and AMLs is strongly suggestive of tuberous sclerosis. Patients with TSC have high incidence of RCC.

27. Describe the CT findings in renal lymphangiectasia.

There is bilateral nephromegaly, with large lymphatic cysts in the renal sinuses, perinephric spaces, and the central retroperitoneum, as well as diffuse intrarenal lymphangiectasia. Renal lymphangiectasia may be complicated during pregnancy by large perinephric lymph collections and ascites, usually secondary to lymphatic rupture due to increased renal lymph flow during pregnancy, in the presence of lymphatic obstruction.

KEY POINTS: CYSTIC DISEASE

1. Multicystic dysplastic kidney is the most common form of cystic disease in infants, usually presenting as an asymptomatic flank mass, associated with intrauterine ureteral obstruction or atresia.

2. Autosomal recessive polycystic kidney disease is characterized by ectasia of the renal collecting ducts, interstitial fibrosis, and variable degrees of portal hepatic fibrosis (congenital hepatic fibrosis), often causing portal hypertension.

3. Autosomal dominant polycystic kidney disease is one of the most commonly inherited diseases in the United States and accounts for 5–10% of patients with end-stage renal disease.

4. The radiologic diagnosis of acquired cystic kidney disease is best established by contrast-enhanced CT.

5. Hereditary syndromes associated with renal cystic involvement include von Hippel-Lindau disease, tuberous sclerosis complex, and renal lymphangiectasia.

28. **What is the best imaging modality for diagnosing urinary tract calculi?**
Helical unenhanced CT is superior to all other imaging modalities in diagnosing urinary tract calculi (Fig. 21-9). The CT parameters below are usually used for the Philips 16 detector multislice CT. These parameters vary with different manufacturers.

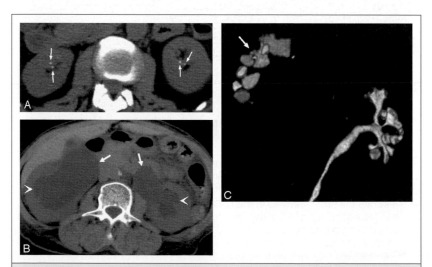

Figure 21-9. Renal calculi. *A,* Nonenhanced multidetector CT of the kidneys demonstrates presence of small, nonobstructive calculi *(arrows). B,* Nonenhanced CT (NECT) image of the kidneys in another patient demonstrates presence of bilateral hydronephrosis *(arrowheads)* and hydroureter *(arrows). C,* Volume-rendered CT urography demonstrates right hydronephrosis *(arrow).* Right renal pelvis and ureter are not opacified. Left pelvocalyceal system is normal.

- **Resolution:** Ultra-fast
- **Collimation:** 16 × 1.5 mm
- **Slice thickness:** 3.0 mm
- **Increment:** 3.0 mm
- **Pitch:** 0.74
- **Rotation time:** 0.5 sec
- **kV:** 120
- **mAs/slice:** 245

29. **Which stones may not be visible on CT?**

    Virtually all stones (including uric acid stones) are of sufficient x-ray attenuation to be readily visible on CT, except for stones associated with protease inhibitor (indinavir) used for treating human immunodeficiency virus (HIV) and matrix stones, which refer to aggregates of mucus that may form within the urinary tract of both healthy and immuno-suppressed individuals (they tend to have soft tissue attenuation at unenhanced CT, unless mixed with calcified impurities).

30. **What are the CT features of urinary tract obstruction?**

    Presence of a calculus is the most definitive sign for the presence of urinary tract obstruction. Other associated features that may be seen on CT include ureteral dilatation, perinephric strand-ing (Fig. 21-10), and unilateral absence of white pyramids.

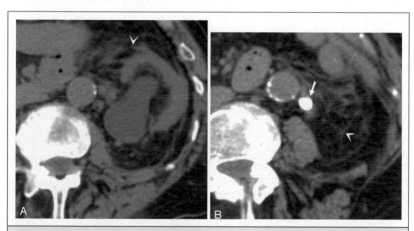

Figure 21-10. Urinary tract obstruction. **A,** Nonenhanced CT (NECT) image of the left kidney reveals hydronephrosis, hydroureter, and perinephric stranding *(arrowhead).* **B,** A 5-mm calculus *(arrow)* is seen within the left mid ureter, resulting in the changes described in A. The *arrowhead* indicates perinephric stranding.

31. **What is a staghorn calculus?**

    A staghorn calculus is a calculus occurring in the renal pelvis, with branches extending into the infundibula and calices (Fig. 21-11). It is also called a coral calculus or a dendritic calculus because of its appearance. Staghorn stones are usually made up of triple ammonium phosphate compounds.

32. What is a "white pyramids" sign?

Bilateral high-attenuation renal pyramids are an occasional incidental finding. The presence of bilateral white pyramids excludes the presence of an obstruction and is called the white pyramids sign (Fig. 21-12). Unilateral ureteral obstruction may result in decreased attenuation of the medullary pyramid on the obstructed side so that the pyramids have high attenuation on only the unobstructed side. This unilateral absence of the white pyramid has been described as an additional secondary sign of urinary tract obstruction.

33. What are the common sites of impaction of urinary tract calculi?

The most common sites of impaction include uretro-pelvic junction (UPJ) (35%), mid ureter (7%), distal ureter (33%), and the ureterovesical junction (18%) (Fig. 21-13).

34. What is nephrocalcinosis?

Nephrocalcinosis is defined as the presence of calcification within the kidney. It is of two forms: cortical (5%) and medullary (95%).

- **Cortical nephrocalcinosis** may arise as a result of vascular insult, glomerulonephritis, and hyperoxaluria. It is also seen in patients with Alport syndrome (hereditary nephritis and deafness).
- **Medullary nephrocalcinosis** (Fig. 21-14) is the presence of calcifications within the medullary region of the kidney and is frequently seen in medullary sponge kidney, hyperparathyroidism, and renal tubular acidosis (type I).

35. What is the "soft tissue rim sign"?

The "soft tissue rim sign" represents edema of the ureteral wall at the level where a stone has become impacted (Fig. 21-15). A positive tissue rim sign is specific for the diagnosis of ureterolithiasis. However, a negative tissue rim sign does not preclude such a diagnosis. The soft tissue rim sign may be absent with stones larger than 4 mm (*see*

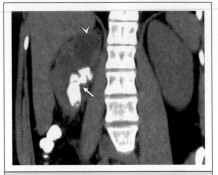

Figure 21-11. Staghorn calculus. Coronal nonenhanced CT (NECT) image of the kidneys demonstrates a large calculus *(arrow)* occupying the right renal pelvis. Associated hydronephrosis *(arrowhead)* is seen.

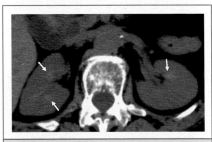

Figure 21-12. White pyramids sign. Nonenhanced CT (NECT) of the kidneys demonstrates presence of high-attenuation renal pyramids *(arrows)* bilaterally. Unilateral absence of white pyramids is a secondary sign of urinary tract obstruction.

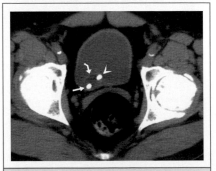

Figure 21-13. Ureterovesical junction calculi. Nonenhanced CT (NECT) of the pelvis demonstrates presence of two calculi. The proximal calculus lies at the right ureterovesical junction *(arrow)*, whereas the distal calculus *(arrowhead)* appears to lie within the right ureterocele *(curved arrow)*.

Fig. 21-10A) or when a stone is impacted at the ureterovesical junction.

36. **What are the mimics of renal colic that need to be considered on unenhanced CT in the absence of urinary tract calculi?**
    - **Urinary tract disease unrelated to calculi:** Pyelonephritis, renal, and transitional carcinomas in elderly patients, congenital UPJ obstruction, and ureteral obstruction from compressive lymphadenopathy and cystitis
    - **Extraurinary/gynecologic:** Hemorrhagic ovarian cysts, tubo-ovarian abscesses, dermoid cysts, endometriomas, ovarian neoplasms, degenerated or twisted fibroids, and ectopic pregnancy
    - **Gastrointestinal:** Appendicitis, diverticulitis; less commonly: abdominal hernias, small bowel obstruction, intussusceptions, and inflammatory bowel disease
    - **Hepatobiliary:** Stones within the gallbladder and within the bile duct
    - **Vascular:** Ruptured abdominal aortic aneurysms and aortic dissection
    - **Musculoskeletal:** Metastasis to bones, psoas hematomas
    - **Miscellaneous:** Focal intraperitoneal fatty infarctions, such as epiploic appendicitis and focal omental infarctions

37. **How is a phlebolith differentiated from a ureteric calculus?**
    A phlebolith has the "comet tail sign." Presence of an adjacent, eccentric, tapering, soft tissue density corresponding to the noncalcified portion of a pelvic vein is called the comet tail sign. This helps differentiate between a ureteric calculus and a phlebolith (Fig. 21-16). On a plain radiograph, the presence of a central lucency may also help in identifying a phlebolith.

38. **What is the growing calculus sign?**
    The growing calculus sign refers to the apparent enlargement of stones between the preliminary image and the image obtained after contrast administration as the contrast material fills the ectatic tubules harboring the stones.

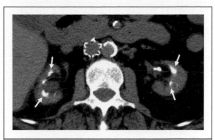

Figure 21-14. Medullary nephrocalcinosis. Nonenhanced CT (NECT) of the kidneys demonstrates multiple calcifications in the medullary region *(arrows)*.

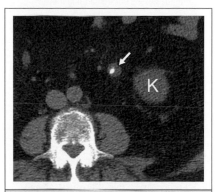

Figure 21-15. Soft tissue rim sign. Nonenhanced CT (NECT) image of the ureter demonstrates an impacted ureteric calculus with edematous ureteric wall *(arrow)*. K = inferior pole of the left kidney.

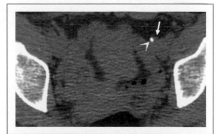

Figure 21-16. Comet tail sign. Nonenhanced CT (NECT) image of the pelvis demonstrates a phlebolith (calcific focus) *(arrowhead)* with an associated noncalcified soft tissue density *(arrow)* representing the noncalcified portion of the vein.

39. **What do perirenal cobwebs on CT suggest?**
Perirenal cobwebs refer to the visualization of the perirenal septa. These are most frequently encountered during CT evaluation of urinary tract obstruction from stone disease (Fig. 21-17).

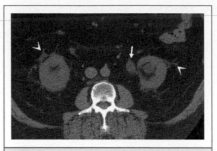

Figure 21-17. Perirenal cobweb sign (perinephric stranding) *(arrowheads)*. Associated left hydronephrosis and hydroureter *(arrow)* is seen.

40. **Describe a congenital UPJ obstruction.**
Congenital UPJ obstruction is most likely secondary to abnormal musculature that prevents relaxation and filling of the ureter (Fig. 21-18). It is more common in males. It has high association of abnormalities in the contralateral kidney in 27% of patients. Associated anomalies include renal agenesis, vesicoureteric reflux, ureteral duplication, and nonfunctioning kidney. In 11–39% of patients with UPJ obstruction, an accessory renal artery crosses the UPJ, and this ureterovascular tangle may be considered a secondary cause of obstruction.

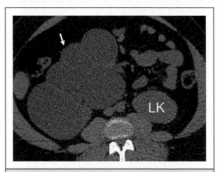

Figure 21-18. Congenital ureteropelvic junction (UPJ) obstruction. Nonenhanced CT (NECT) image of the kidneys demonstrates a grossly enlarged right kidney secondary to marked hydronephrosis *(arrow)* resulting from right UPJ obstruction. The left kidney (LK) is normal.

41. **What are the main etiologic agents causing acute bacterial infection?**
Escherichia coli typically causes ascending acute renal infection, whereas hematogenous disease is often caused by *Staphylococcus aureus*.

KEY POINTS: RENAL CALCULI

1. Helical unenhanced CT is superior to all other imaging modalities in diagnosing urinary tract calculi.

2. A staghorn calculus is a calculus occurring in the renal pelvis, with branches extending into the infundibula and calices.

3. The most common sites of impaction of urinary tract calculi include ureteropelvic junction (35%), mid ureter (7%), distal ureter (33%), and ureterovesical junction (18%).

4. The soft tissue rim sign represents edema of the ureteral wall at the level where a stone has become impacted.

5. Perirenal cobwebs refer to the visualization of the perirenal septa, which are most frequently encountered during CT evaluation of urinary tract obstruction from stone disease.

42. **Describe CT features of pyelonephritis.**
A striated nephrogram may be seen in patients with pyelonephritis (Fig. 21-19A). Some patients show unifocal or multifocal renal abnormalities with extensive areas of apparently uninvolved renal parenchyma; this is seen on CECT scans as wedge-shaped zones of decreased attenuation (Fig. 21-19B).

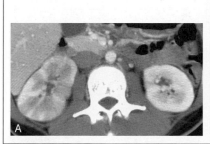

Figure 21-19. *A,* Acute pyelonephritis (striated nephrogram). Nephrographic phase demonstrates an enlarged right kidney with a striated nephrogram. *B,* Focal pyelonephritis. Nephrographic phase in another patient reveals a focal wedge-shaped area of decreased attenuation *(arrow)*.

43. **How are renal abscesses differentiated from renal cysts?**
On CECT scans, renal abscesses usually have attenuation values of about 30 HU; this distinguishes them from fluid-density renal cysts. Their contents do not enhance. They may have distinct, rounded margins and thick enhancing walls (Fig. 21-20, compared with Fig. 21-3). Gas is occasionally found in renal abscesses. Focal thickening of the adjacent renal fascia and stranding in the adjacent perinephric fat are also associated with an abscess.

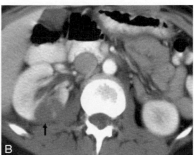

Figure 21-20. Renal abscess. Nephrographic phase of the left kidney demonstrates an enhancing thick-walled cystic lesion *(arrow)*.

44. **What are the etiologic agents in emphysematous pyelonephritis (EPN)?**
E. coli are the most common bacteria associated with emphysematous nephritis. *Klebsiella, Pseudomonas,* and *Proteus* spp. are the other bacteria associated with this entity.

45. **What is the most common predisposing factor in the development of EPN?**
Diabetes mellitus is the most common predisposing factor for EPN. Ninety percent of patients with EPN have diabetes mellitus.

46. What are the CT features of EPN?

EPN is a severe necrotizing infection of the renal parenchyma, with formation of gas within the renal parenchyma that may extend to collecting system and perirenal spaces (Fig. 21-21A). CT scan is the most sensitive and definitive modality to diagnose EPN. Several patterns have been described, including streaky, streaky and mottled, and streaky and bubbly. Gas can be rim-like or crescent-shaped in the perinephric area. Gas can also be seen in the renal vein or inferior vena cava. Gas can be seen along the psoas muscle. Gas in the renal pelvis alone, without parenchymal gas, is often referred to as emphysematous pyelitis (Fig. 21-21B).

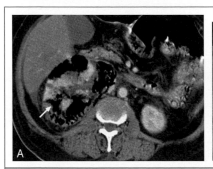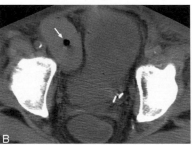

Figure 21-21. *A,* Emphysematous pyelonephritis. Nephrographic phase demonstrates an enlarged right kidney with air within the renal parenchyma *(arrow).* *B,* Air within the right renal pelvis *(arrow)* of a transplant kidney consistent with emphysematous pyelitis.

47. What is pyonephrosis? How is it diagnosed?

Pyonephrosis is the accumulation of pus in an obstructed pelvocaliceal system. It represents a true urologic emergency requiring either urgent percutaneous nephrostomy or passage of a ureteral stent to bypass the obstruction. Increased pelvic wall thickness, inflammatory changes in the perinephric fat, and in rare cases, layering of intravenously injected contrast material anterior to the pus in the dilated renal pelvis are the findings seen on contrast enhanced CT (known as inversion sign). However, the presence of clinical signs of infection in the presence of hydronephrosis is an indicator more sensitive than CT findings of pyonephrosis.

48. What is the pathogenesis of xanthogranulomatous pyelonephritis?

Xanthogranulomatous pyelonephritis is a sequela of chronic infection occurring in an obstructed kidney. It is an inflammatory process that begins in the renal pelvis and later extends into the medulla and cortex, which are gradually destroyed and replaced by lipid-laden macrophages (xanthoma cells).

49. What are the CT findings in xanthogranulomatous pyelonephritis?

CT findings of diffuse reniform enlargement with ill defined central low-attenuation areas (Fig. 21-22), apparent cortical thinning, and a staghorn calculus (in 70%), along with unilaterally decreased or (more commonly) absent renal excretion are pathognomonic in most cases.

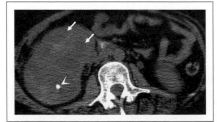

Figure 21-22. Xanthogranulomatous pyelonephritis. Nonenhanced CT (NECT) of the kidneys demonstrates an enlarged right kidney with low-attenuation areas *(arrows)* and a calculus *(arrowhead).*

50. What is the imaging triad of xanthogranulomatous pyelonephritis?
- Renal enlargement
- Presence of an obstructing stone
- Nonfunctional kidney

51. What is the "bear paw sign"?
The replacement of renal parenchyma by the indolent infectious process in the diffuse form of xanthogranulomatous pyelonephritis produces hypoattenuation masses arranged in a "hydronephrotic pattern," which replaces the renal parenchyma; with enhancement in the margins of these masses after contrast administration. This appearance on CT is termed the bear paw sign.

52. Describe the CT features of renal tuberculosis (TB).
Renal TB may present as follows:
- Focal caliectasis, diffuse caliectasis without pelvic dilatation, and generalized hydronephrosis, depending on the site of scarring or stricture
- Low-density parenchymal lesions, probably representing areas of caseous necrosis (Fig. 21-23A)

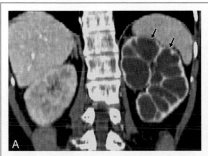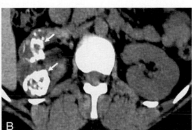

Figure 21-23. Renal tuberculosis. *A,* Coronal CECT image of the kidneys demonstrates an enlarged left kidney with low-attenuation areas *(arrows)* representing caseous necrosis. *B,* Nonenhanced CT (NECT) of the kidneys in another patient demonstrates lobar type of calcifications *(arrows)* within the renal parenchyma suggestive of putty kidney.

53. What are the causes of TB autonephrectomy?
1. Obstructive: Dense strictures (usually renal pelvis or ureter) causing hydronephrosis
2. Replacement of parenchyma by caseous tissue
3. A combination of 1 and 2

54. What is a putty kidney?
Putty (clay-like) kidney refers to the end-stage tuberculous kidney, which is replaced by caseous areas (hence soft clay-like). Such a kidney may show scattered calcification and an overall ground-glass appearance on the topogram and/or may subsequently reveal a peripheral "lobar" type of calcification, which is pathognomic for TB (Fig. 21-23B). It is seen in end-stage renal TB and represents an autonephrectomized kidney.

KEY POINTS: KIDNEY INFECTIONS

1. *Escherichia coli* typically causes ascending acute renal infection, whereas hematogenous disease is often caused by *Staphylococcus aureus*.

2. *E. coli* are the most common bacteria associated with emphysematous nephritis. Others include *Klebsiella, Pseudomonas,* and *Proteus* spp.

3. Pyonephrosis—the accumulation of pus in an obstructed pelvocalyceal system—represents a true urologic emergency, requiring either urgent percutaneous nephrostomy or passage of a ureteral stent to bypass the obstruction.

4. Xanthogranulomatous pyelonephritis, a sequela of chronic infection in an obstructed kidney, is an inflammatory process which begins in the renal pelvis and later extends into the medulla and cortex, which are gradually destroyed and replaced by lipid-laden macrophages (xanthoma cells).

5. Putty (clay-like) kidney refers to the end-stage tuberculous kidney, which is replaced by caseous areas (hence soft clay-like).

55. **What is a thimble bladder?**
Chronic tuberculous involvement of the bladder may be accompanied by marked cicatrization in the wall, which may become thick and reduce the capacity of the bladder. The resultant, very small bladder has been referred to as a thimble bladder. Calcification may be noted but is a more common feature in schistosomiasis.

56. **Describe the radiologic appearances of a renal hydatid cyst.**
Renal involvement occurs in 3% of cases. It usually remains asymptomatic for many years. The most common signs and symptoms are flank mass, pain, and dysuria. Cysts are frequently solitary and located in the cortex, and they may reach 10 cm before any clinical symptoms are noted.

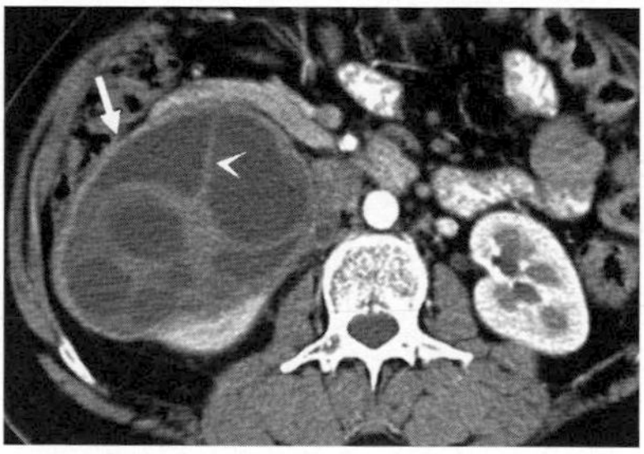

Hydatid cysts are classified into four types on the basis of their appearance:

Figure 21-24. Renal hydatid cyst. CECT of the kidneys demonstrates a large, multiloculated, septate mass within the right kidney *(arrow)*. The *arrowhead* points to the septa.

- **Type I:** Simple cyst with no internal architecture, appearing as a well-defined water attenuation mass
- **Type II:** Cyst with daughter cyst(s) and matrix. At CT, type II hydatid cysts can be visualized in three stages:
  1. **Type IA:** Round daughter cysts arranged at the periphery. The average CT attenuation of the mother cyst—higher than that of daughter cysts
  2. **Type IIB:** Larger, irregularly shaped daughter cysts that occupy almost the entire volume of the mother cyst, creating a rosette appearance (Fig. 21-24)
  3. **Type IIC:** Relatively high-attenuation round or oval masses with scattered calcifications and occasional daughter cysts
- **Type III:** Dead cysts with calcification
- **Type IV:** Complicated cysts including rupture and superinfection

57. **What are the types of renal neoplasms and their respective incidence?**
    RCC is the most common primary renal cancer, accounting for about 86% of all primary malignant renal parenchymal neoplasms. Of the remainder, 12% are Wilms tumors and 2% are renal sarcomas. Secondary neoplasms of the renal parenchyma include malignant lymphoma and metastases. The most common renal neoplasm overall is metastases.

58. **What are the predisposing factors for RCC?**
    Cigarette smoking, exposure to petroleum products, obesity, ACKD, VHL, TSC, and hereditary papillary renal cancer (HPRC) are common risk factors for development of RCC.

59. **Where does the RCC arise from in the kidney?**
    RCC arises from the proximal tubules.

60. **What are the pathologic subtypes of RCC?**
    - **Conventional (garden variety):** 70–80%
    - **Papillary (multicentricity):** 10–15%
    - **Chromophobe:** 4–5%
    - **Oncocytoma (benign):** 3–5%
    - **Collecting duct (poor prognosis):** <1%
    - **Medullary cell (poor prognosis):** <1%

61. **Describe the CT findings in a case of RCC.**
    The nonenhanced CT (NECT) appearance varies and can be hypodense, isodense, or hyperdense compared with normal renal parenchyma. Most RCCs are solid lesions with attenuation values of 20 HU or greater at unenhanced CT. After IV contrast administration, RCC enhances less than the surrounding renal parenchyma on nephrographic phase.

62. **Which phase of contrast-enhanced study is best for the detection of venous extension of RCC?**
    Venous extension of RCC is best detected in the corticomedullary phase (Fig. 21-25).

63. **What is the characteristic feature of RCC on contrast-enhanced study?**
    Nephrographic phase is the best phase for the detection of RCC. The RCC enhances less than the surrounding parenchyma in this phase (Fig. 21-26).

64. **What is the Robson's staging of RCCs?**
    See Table 21-3.

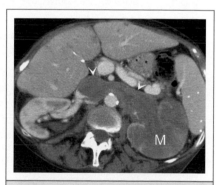

Figure 21-25. RCC extending into renal vein (stage III). Corticomedullary phase demonstrates a left kidney mass (M) with extension into the left renal vein *(arrowheads)* up to the inferior vena cava (IVC). Right renal vein is normal.

65. **Which tumor is associated with sickle cell trait?**
    Renal medullary carcinoma is a rare tumor of the kidney, occurring exclusively in young black patients with sickle cell trait.

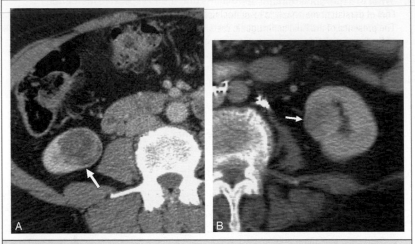

Figure 21-26. RCC. Nephrographic phase in two different patients demonstrates RCC *(arrows)* in the right kidney *(A)* and RCC in the left kidney *(B)* showing decreased enhancement of the RCC relative to the normal renal parenchyma.

TABLE 21-3.	ROBSON'S STAGING OF RENAL CELL CARCINOMA
Stage I	Tumor confined within the renal capsule
Stage II	Perinephric extension including the ipsilateral adrenal gland
Stage IIIA	Venous invasion (renal vein that may extend into the inferior vena cava)
Stage IIIB	Regional lymph node metastases
Stage IIIC	Both tumor venous extension and regional lymph node metastases
Stage IVA	Extension through the Gerota's fascia to involve adjacent organs
Stage IVB	Distant metastases

66. **What is the radiologic appearance of renal medullary carcinoma?**
    The radiologic appearance of renal medullary carcinoma is that of a prototypical infiltrative lesion. An ill-defined mass centered in the renal medulla with extension into the renal sinus and cortex is characteristic; caliectasis may be seen, the reniform shape being maintained. The heterogeneous appearance is typically seen, because of characteristic tumor necrosis.

67. **What is the CT appearance of a typical Wilms tumor?**
    Wilms tumor usually presents as a large, spherical, intrarenal tumor, very often with a well-defined rim of compressed renal parenchyma or pseudocapsule surrounding it. The tumor is less dense than normal renal parenchyma on CECT scans, with areas of low attenuation, which coincide with tumor necrosis and/or fat deposition. Renal vein and inferior vena caval tumor extension may be seen as a low-density intraluminal-filling defect.

68. **What is nephroblastomatosis?**
Foci of persistent metanephric blastemal tissue are designated as nephrogenic rests. The presence of multiple nephrogenic rests is termed nephroblastomatosis. It may be of the "superficial" (multifocal perilobar or diffuse perilobar, with subcapsular foci), "deep" (usually intralobar, commonly with solitary foci), or "generalize" type (panlobar—the entire kidney is affected). It is widely accepted as a premalignant lesion and a precursor to Wilms tumor.

69. **What are the types of renal sarcomas?**
Subtypes of renal sarcoma include leiomyosarcoma, angiosarcomas, hemangiopericytoma, rhabdomyosarcoma, fibrosarcoma, and osteosarcoma. Leiomyosarcoma is the most common renal sarcoma, accounting for about 58% of all sarcomas. Capsular localization is a feature of more than 50% of these tumors.

70. **What are the CT patterns of renal lymphoma?**
Five CT patterns of renal lymphoma include the following:
- Multiple renal masses
- Solitary mass
- Renal invasion from contiguous retroperitoneal disease
- Perirenal disease
- Diffuse renal infiltration (Fig. 21-27)

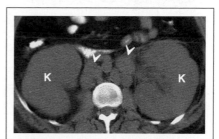

Figure 21-27. Renal lymphoma. Nonenhanced CT (NECT) demonstrates bilaterally enlarged kidneys (K) with associated retroperitoneal lymphadenopathy *(arrowheads).*

71. **What is the most common CT manifestation of renal lymphoma?**
Multiple renal nodules are the most common CT manifestation of renal lymphoma, occurring in about 59% of cases. The nodules range from 1–3 cm, are less dense than normal renal parenchyma on CECT scans, and typically show a homogeneous appearance.

72. **What are the primary sources of renal metastasis?**
The kidney is the fifth most common site of metastases in the body after lung, liver, bone, and adrenals. The three neoplasms with the highest frequency of renal metastases are lung carcinoma, breast carcinoma, and carcinoma of the opposite kidney.

73. **Enumerate the benign neoplasms involving the kidney.**
The benign tumors of the kidneys include adenoma, oncocytoma, reninoma (juxtaglomerular neoplasm), multilocular cystic renal tumor, and AML.

74. **Describe CT features of an oncocytoma.**
On CT, oncocytomas are typically well-defined masses with smooth, rounded margins. A central, sharply defined stellate scar is present in 25–33% of large oncocytomas and strongly suggests the diagnosis. The classic angiographic findings of an oncocytoma include a spoke-wheel pattern, a homogeneous nephrogram, and a sharp, smooth rim. Calcification has also been noted in oncocytomas.

75. **How is an AML diagnosed on CT?**
The presence of intratumoral fat is almost diagnostic of AML. The presence of fat is best shown by CT (preferably using thin-section [3–5 mm] technique) (Fig. 21-28). Fatty tissue

is considered to be present in a tumor if a region-of-interest measurement of −10 HU or lower is found within the tumor.

76. **Does the presence of fat in a renal tumor always imply an AML?**

Generally speaking, fat in a renal tumor usually indicates an AML. However, fat can also be seen occasionally (although in much lesser quantity) in RCCs. Unusual fat-containing renal tumors include oncocytomas, liposarcomas, and other rarer lesions, such as intrarenal teratomas/dermoids.

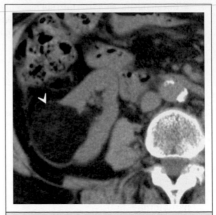

Figure 21-28. Angiomyolipoma. Nonenhanced CT (NECT) demonstrates a fat-density (−60 HU) lesion *(arrowhead)* arising from the right kidney.

KEY POINTS: RENAL NEOPLASMS

1. Renal cell carcinoma (RCC) is the most common primary renal cancer, accounting for about 86% of all primary malignant renal parenchymal neoplasms. Of the remainder, 12% are Wilms tumors and 2% are renal sarcomas.

2. Secondary neoplasms of the renal parenchyma include malignant lymphoma and metastases. The most common renal neoplasm overall is metastases.

3. Renal medullary carcinoma is a rare tumor of the kidney, occurring exclusively in young black patients with sickle cell trait.

4. The benign tumors of the kidneys include adenoma, oncocytoma, reninoma (juxtaglomerular neoplasm), multilocular cystic renal tumor, and angiomyolipoma.

77. **What are the various hereditary renal cancers?**
    - VHLD
    - Tuberous sclerosis
    - Hereditary papillary renal cancer (HPRC)
    - Hereditary leiomyoma renal cell carcinoma (HLRCC)
    - Birt-Hogg-Dube (BHD) syndrome
    - Familial renal oncocytoma

78. **What is HPRC?**

HPRC is inherited in an autosomal dominant manner and affects patients in the fifth decade. It is usually bilateral and multiple papillary type I renal cancer. The tumor is usually hypovascular.

79. **What is BHD syndrome?**

BHD is an autosomal dominant disorder with the following characteristics:
    - Fibrofolliculomas of face and trunk
    - Pulmonary cysts, usually in the lower lobes

- Pneumothoraces, which may not be symptomatic and are resistant to pleurodesis
- RCC—chromophobe or oncocytomas—in 15–30% of patients with BHD
- Higher rate of colonic polyps in some families

80. **What is HLRCC?**

HLRCC is an autosomal dominant genodermatosis associated with cutaneous leiomyomas, uterine leiomyomas, and type II papillary renal tumors. Reed's syndrome consists of cutaneous leiomyoma and uterine leiomyomas. HLRCC was initially described in Finland but has since been described in the United States and other parts of Europe. Seventeen percent of patients with HLRCC have papillary cancer. Uterine fibroids occur in more than 90% of women with HLRCC.

81. **Which is the most common type of pelvocaliceal tumor?**

Transitional cell carcinoma is the most common pelvocaliceal tumor (almost 90%) (Fig. 21-29). Of the remaining, 9% are squamous cell carcinomas (Fig. 21-30), and less than 1% are adeno-carcinomas.

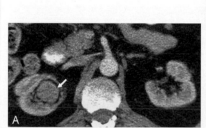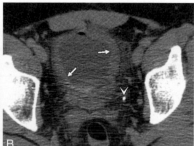

Figure 21-29. Transitional cell carcinoma of the kidney and bladder. *A,* Nephrographic phase reveals an enhancing mass *(arrow)* in the right renal pelvis. *B,* CECT of the bladder in the same patient reveals a significantly thickened and irregular bladder wall *(arrows)* consistent with transitional cell carcinoma. Incidentally seen is a left-sided phlebolith *(arrowhead).*

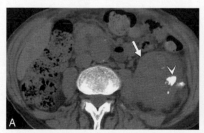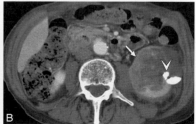

Figure 21-30. Squamous cell carcinoma. *A,* Nonenhanced CT (NECT) of the left kidney demonstrates a left renal mass *(arrow)* with chunky calcification *(arrowhead).* *B,* Corresponding CECT demonstrates heterogeneous enhancement.

82. **What are the predisposing factors for the development of transitional carcinomas?**

Occupational exposure to industrial dyes, phenacetin abuse, cigarette smoking, prior cyclophosphamide therapy, and urinary stasis associated with horseshoe kidneys predispose an individual to the development of transitional cell carcinomas.

83. **Describe the role of CT in ureteral neoplasms.**

Ureteral neoplasms present on CT as soft tissue intraluminal filling defects, often with ureteral widening, or thickening of the ureteral wall. CT helps by confirming that a ureteric filling defect seen on urography represents a neoplasm and not a radiolucent calculus or blood clot. CT also helps to determine whether a ureteral neoplasm has extended outside the muscularis to involve the retroperitoneal fat and surrounding structures or whether it has metastasized to regional lymph nodes. An important use of CT is in determining whether ureteral obstruction is due to an intrinsic neoplasm or extrinsic disease, when excretory urography and retrograde pyelography are indeterminate. CT is particularly useful in detecting such causes of extrinsic ureteric obstruction as idiopathic and malignant retroperitoneal fibrosis, inflammatory aortic aneurysms, and lymphomatous and metastatic retroperitoneal adenopathy.

84. **How are renal injuries classified on imaging?**

See Table 21-4.

TABLE 21-4.	CT CLASSIFICATION OF RENAL INJURIES
Category I	Contusions and small corticomedullary lacerations not communicating with the collecting system
Category II	Major lacerations through the cortex extending to the medulla or collecting systems, with or without urinary extravasation
Category III	Shattered kidney (multiple deep lacerations) and injury to the renal pedicle
Category IV	Ureteropelvic junction avulsion and laceration of the renal pelvis

85. **Which is the best imaging modality in cases of abdominal trauma?**

CECT-triple phase is the preferred modality for evaluation of patients with blunt or penetrating abdominal trauma (Fig. 21-31). CECT is obtained at 70 seconds and 3 minutes after initiation of contrast material administration. Usually 125–150 mL of low osmolar contrast is injected at a rate of 2–4 mL/sec.

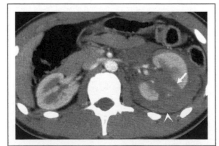

Figure 21-31. Shattered kidney. Corticomedullary phase in this patient with blunt abdominal trauma demonstrates complete laceration *(arrow)* of the left kidney. Associated perinephric hematoma *(arrowhead)* is seen.

86. **What are the causes of renal hemorrhage?**

The most common cause of renal hemorrhage is trauma, either blunt or penetrating. Spontaneous (nontraumatic) renal hemorrhage may be caused by anticoagulation, blood dyscrasias, renal infarction, polyarteritis nodosa, renal aneurysms and arteriovenous malformations, RCC, renal AML, renal abscess, renal vein thrombosis, and rupture of hemorrhagic solitary cysts, or of hemorrhagic cysts in renal cystic disease. Perinephric hematomas may also arise iatrogenically following a renal biopsy (Fig. 21-32).

87. What is Page kidney?
Page kidney is a clinical entity caused by chronic subcapsular hematomas that compress the renal parenchyma. This, in turn, may cause hypertension by reducing renal blood flow; ischemia triggers the renin-angiotensin aldosterone mechanism.

88. What are the causes of renal infarction? How is it diagnosed?
Renal infarction may be due to renal artery thrombosis or embolism, vasculitis (as in polyarteritis nodosa), trauma, sickle cell disease, and aortic dissection. The most common cause is thromboembolism from cardiovascular disease. On CECT scans, the affected kidney shows lack of enhancement, apart from a high-density cortical rim reflecting perfusion of the preserved outer rim of the cortex by collateral vessels (cortical "rim" sign).

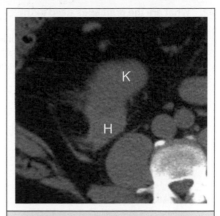

Figure 21-32. Perinephric hematoma Nonenhanced CT (NECT) of the right kidney demonstrates a small hematoma (H) near the inferior pole of the kidney (K). This hematoma is secondary to a renal biopsy.

89. What is the main CT differential diagnosis of renal infarction?
The main CT differential diagnosis of acute renal infarction is acute pyelonephritis, because both conditions often show wedge-shaped, low-attenuation renal lesions on CT and because both often present with an acute onset of flank pain and fever. A cortical rim sign, as described previously, should strongly suggest the diagnosis of renal infarction, because it is usually not seen in acute pyelonephritis (see Fig. 21-19B).

90. Describe the protocol used for the CT angiography of the renal artery.
CT angiography of the renal arteries is done using bolus tracking for acquiring the images in arterial phase; venous phase images are acquired after a delay of 75 seconds after injection of IV contrast. The following parameters are used for the acquisition of both these phases with the Philips 16 detector multislice CT. These parameters vary with different manufacturers.
- **Resolution:** Ultra-fast
- **Collimation:** 16×1.5
- **Slice thickness:** 2.0 mm
- **Increment:** 1.0 mm
- **Pitch:** 0.5
- **Rotation time:** 0.5 sec
- **kV:** 120
- **mAs/slice:** 250

91. What are the indications for performing a CT angiography of the renal artery?
- Suspected renal artery stenosis
- Stent planning and follow-up
- Renal donor evaluation and renal graft follow-up
- Preoperative staging of RCC
- Evaluation of UPJ obstruction

92. **What are the principles used in the reconstruction of images of CT angiography of renal arteries?**
Images should be reconstructed with 50% overlap to improve renal artery stenosis detection and three-dimensional (3D) reconstruction. Commonly used 3D visualization techniques include surface rendering, maximum intensity projection (MIP), and volume rendering. Volume rendering is superior to MIP and surface rendering because it uses the volume data and can provide life-like images (Fig. 21-33). This permits multiplanar reconstruction (MPR) in any plane. This technique is very useful in the evaluation of pretransplant renal donor evaluation and in presurgical planning.

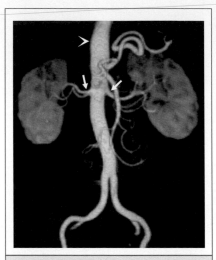

Figure 21-33. Normal CT angiography. Three-dimensional CT angiography depicts the origin of the renal arteries *(arrows)* from the aorta *(arrowhead).*

93. **What are the causes of renal artery aneurysms?**
Atherosclerosis is the commonest cause of renal artery aneurysms. Other causes include medial fibrodysplasia, pregnancy, neurofibromatosis, and Ehlers-Danlos syndrome. Multiple small intrarenal aneurysms are usually associated with polyarteritis nodosa, Wegener's granulomatosis, and fungal infections (mycotic aneurysms in IV drug abusers)

94. **Describe the CT features of renal vein thrombosis.**
In acute and subacute cases, an enlarged, swollen kidney is seen on CT. The nephrogram is delayed and persistent. Perinephric fat stranding and enlarged perirenal collateral veins are noted; the renal vein is often enlarged and may show a filling defect due to a thrombus (*see* Fig. 21-25). Thrombosis of the inferior vena cava at or near the renal vein orifices occurs in about 40–50% of patients with renal vein thrombosis.

95. **Describe the rim sign of vascular compromise.**
This sign is most commonly seen with renal artery obstruction from thrombosis, embolus, or dissection (also seen with renal vein thrombosis and acute tubular necrosis), which causes a 1- to 3-mm rim of subcapsular enhancement at CECT imaging, paralleling the renal margin; this is seen as a result of preserved perfusion of the outer renal cortex by capsular perforating vessels.

96. **What is the modality of choice in the evaluation of a renal transplant?**
Radiologic evaluation of the transplanted kidney and its complications, such as peritransplant fluid collections, including hematomas, lymphoceles, abscesses, and urinomas, and evaluation of kidney function is best done by using renal scintigraphy and sonography. NECT is used in cases where sonography fails. CECT should be avoided because of the potential for nephrotoxicity.

97. **What is CT urography?**
The application of multidetector row CT in the evaluation of the urinary tract has been termed CT urography (Fig. 21-34).

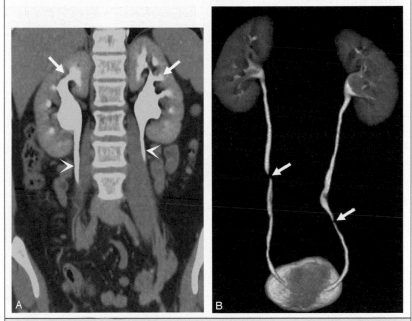

Figure 21-34. CT urography. *A,* Coronal excretory phase image demonstrates normal pelvocalyceal system *(arrows)* and normal proximal ureters *(arrowheads).* *B,* Three-dimensional normal CT urography (posterior view) shows the normal pelvocalyceal system with normal insertions of the ureters in the bladder. Focal areas of narrowing in the ureters *(arrows)* are due to normal peristalsis.

98. **What are the advantages of CT urography over conventional excretory urography?**
    - Both the renal parenchyma and the urothelium can be evaluated with a single comprehensive examination.
    - The overall duration of the patient's schedule for diagnostic evaluation is shortened considerably.
    - Characterization of the renal mass can be done in the same examination.

99. **Describe the protocol for CT urography.**
    The following protocol is used at our institution for CT urography:
    1. **Unenhanced CT images from kidneys through bladder:** 3-mm section thickness
    2. **IV contrast:** 100 mL (300 mg I/mL) at a rate of 3 mL/sec, immediately followed by rapid infusion of 250-mL normal IV saline
    3. **CT images acquired from kidneys to bladder 100 seconds after IV contrast (nephrographic phase):** 3-mm section thickness
    4. **CT images acquired from kidneys to bladder 10 minutes after IV contrast (excretory phase):** 1- to 2-mm section thickness
    5. **3D reconstruction of the excretory phase images with volume rendering or MIP**
    6. **Optional features**
        - Prone position for better delineation of distal ureter
        - Compression device for delineation of renal collecting system and proximal ureter. Postdecompression images of distal ureter and bladder
        - CT topogram after excretory phase

100. What is the reverse rim sign?

The reverse rim sign refers to a hypoattenuating renal cortex visualized at CT, seen against a background of intact medullary perfusion after contrast material is given. This sign implies severe derangement of cortical blood flow with development of cortical necrosis.

101. What causes the spotted nephrogram?

Spotted nephrogram refers to irregular, patchy enhancement in the renal parenchyma, which occurs as a result of small vessel occlusion, seen with necrotizing vasculitis (periarteritis nodosa), scleroderma, and hypertensive nephrosclerosis.

102. What is faceless kidney?

Faceless kidney includes any process that obliterates the normal renal sinus appearance. Thus, edema from inflammatory conditions or a more "sinister" infiltrative process, such as lymphoma or transitional cell carcinoma, may render the kidney faceless.

103. What are the types of CT nephrogram?

- **Global absence** is nearly always unilateral and is most often seen with blunt abdominal trauma with renal pedicle injury.
- **Segmental absence** is attributable to focal renal infarction, most likely due to arterial emboli.
- **Global persistence** may be unilateral (caused by renal artery stenosis, renal vein thrombosis, or urinary tract obstruction) (Fig. 21-35) or bilateral (due to systemic hypotension, intratubular obstruction, or abnormalities in tubular function).
- **Striated nephrogram** may be unilateral or bilateral and is caused by ureteric obstruction, acute pyelonephritis (*see* Fig. 21-19A), contusion, renal vein thrombosis, tubular obstruction, hypotension, and ARPKD.
- The **rim pattern** is most often associated with renal infarction and occasionally with acute tubular necrosis and renal vein thrombosis.

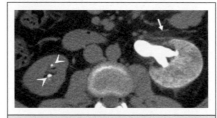

Figure 21-35. Unilateral persistent nephrogram. CECT of the kidneys scanned 25 minutes after IV contrast injection demonstrates a case of distal UPJ obstruction with persistence of the nephrogram in the left kidney and contrast in the dilated pelvocalyceal system. Associated perinephric stranding *(arrow)* is seen. In contrast to left kidney, there is complete excretion of radiographic contrast from the right kidney. Two nonobstructive calculi *(arrowheads)* are seen.

104. What are the future concepts in the CT imaging of kidneys?

Future concept in the imaging of kidneys includes image plate detector technology in CT. It may greatly improve the spatial resolution of CT for imaging of very small structures. Characterization of smaller feeding vessels will be possible. Less volume averaging or pixilation of the images will result in improved image quality.

BIBLIOGRAPHY

1. Bae KT, Heiken JP, Siegel CL, Bennett HF: Renal cysts: Is attenuation artifactually increased on contrast-enhanced CT images? Radiology 216:792–796, 2000.
2. Dogra VS, Levine E: The kidney. In Haaga JR, Lanzieri CF, Gilkeson RC (eds): Computed Tomography and Magnetic Resonance Imaging of the Whole body, 4th ed. St. Louis, Mosby, 2003, pp 1537–1610.
3. Dyer RB, Chen MY, Zagoria RJ: Classic signs in uroradiology. Radiographics 24(Suppl 1):S247–S280, 2004.

4. Helenon O, Merran S, Paraf F, et al: Unusual fat-containing tumors of the kidney: A diagnostic dilemma. Radiographics 17:129–144, 1997.

5. Israel GM, Bosniak MA: Follow-up CT of moderately complex cystic lesions of the kidney (Bosniak category IIF). AJR 181:627–633, 2003.

6. Kawashima A, Vrtiska TJ, LeRoy AJ, et al: CT urography. Radiographics 24(Suppl 1):S35–S54; discussion, S55–S58, 2004.

7. Polat P, Kantarci M, Alper F, et al: Hydatid disease from head to toe. Radiographics 23:475–494, 2004.

8. Rucker CM, Menias CO, Bhalla S: Mimics of renal colic: Alternative diagnoses at unenhanced helical CT. Radiographics 24(Suppl 1):S11–28; discussion, S28–S33, 2004.

9. Saunders HS, Dyer RB, Shifrin RY, et al: The CT nephrogram: Implications for evaluation of urinary tract disease. Radiographics 15:1069–1085; discussion, 1086–1088, 1995.

CHAPTER 22

ADRENAL GLANDS

Sherif G. Nour, MD, and Shweta Bhatt, MD

1. **Describe the anatomy of the adrenal glands.**
   - The **right adrenal gland** may have the shape of a comma or the letter V or Y. It lies superior to the right kidney, medial to the right lobe of the liver, lateral to the right crus of the diaphragm, and posterior to inferior vena cava (IVC) (Fig. 22-1A).
   - The **left adrenal gland** may have the shape of an inverted V or Y or a reversed letter L. It is located superior to the left kidney in a triangle formed by the left lateral margin of the aorta, the posterior surface of the body and tail of pancreas, and the anterior superior medial surface of the upper pole of the left kidney (*see* Fig. 22-1B).

2. **Describe the arterial supply and venous drainage of the adrenal glands.**
   Each adrenal gland is supplied by three arteries and drained by one vein.
   Arterial supply
   - **Superior adrenal artery:** From the ipsilateral inferior phrenic artery
   - **Middle adrenal artery:** From the abdominal aorta
   - **Inferior adrenal artery:** From the ipsilateral renal artery
   Venous drainage
   - **Single adrenal vein drains**:
     - On the right into the IVC
     - On the left into left renal vein

3. **What hormones are secreted by the adrenal glands?**
   The adrenal gland consists of an outer cortex and inner medulla. The **adrenal cortex** consists of three separate histologic zones. From superficial to deep, these zones are as follows:

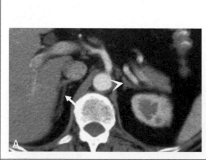
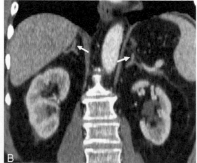

Figure 22-1. Normal adrenal glands. *A,* Contrast-enhanced CT scan shows the normal location and appearance of the adrenal glands. The right adrenal gland *(arrow)* is shaped like an inverted Y, and the left adrenal gland *(arrowhead)* is shaped like an inverted V. *B,* Coronal CT image demonstrates the normal adrenal glands with better visualization of the limbs of the adrenals *(arrows)* on both sides.

- **Zona glomerulosa:** Secretes aldosterone
- **Zona fasciculata:** Secretes cortisol
- **Zona reticularis:** Secretes sex hormones
The **adrenal medulla** secretes epinephrine and norepinephrine.

4. **Describe the multislice computed tomography (CT) protocol for adrenal glands.**
   - Breath-hold scans are obtained at 3-mm beam width, 4.5 pitch, and 3-mm slice thickness (5-mm scans may be performed for large masses).
   - First a noncontrast scan is performed. If no adrenal mass is seen, no further scanning is performed. If a mass is seen, CT density is measured. If it is less than 10 HU, an adrenal adenoma is diagnosed and no further imaging is needed. If the density is 10 HU or higher, then the mass is indeterminate. Proceed to a contrast-enhanced scan.
   - Nonionic contrast (150 mL) is administered intravenously (IV) at 2–3 cc/sec, and the scan is acquired at 70 seconds after injection.
   - If there is a question of a lipid-poor adenoma, a third (wash-out) scan is acquired at 10 minutes after contrast injection.

5. **What is an incidentaloma?**
   Any adrenal mass detected in a patient other than those undergoing imaging procedure for staging of known cancer.

6. **What are the diagnostic CT criteria for benign adrenal adenomas?**
   On noncontrast CT: An adrenal mass with CT density less than 10 HU is diagnostic of benign adenoma (Fig. 22-2).
   On contrast-enhanced CT scan: Several methods have been described:
   - If the absolute CT density after 15 minutes measures < 30 HU, benign adenoma is diagnosed.
   - Washout evaluation: Benign adrenal adenomas enhance moderately and wash out rapidly. On the other hand, malignant adrenal lesions demonstrate persistent intense enhancement.
   The percentage of enhancement washout can be calculated utilizing 150 cc of contrast at 2–3 cc/sec. The images are obtained at 70 seconds and 10 minutes after contrast injection. The formula is as follows:

   %washout = 1 − (delayed enhancement at 10 minutes HU value/ HU value at 70 seconds) × 100

   Using this equation:
   - A washout of 50% or more is a benign adenoma (Fig. 22-3).
   - A washout of <50% is suggestive of malignancy (Fig. 22-4).

7. **Describe the sensitivity and specificity of unenhanced CT in diagnosing adrenal adenomas.**
   CT has 73% sensitivity and 96% specificity for the diagnosis of adrenal adenoma using a threshold value of 10 HU.

8. **What are the major types of adrenal adenomas?**
   1. **Functioning adenomas:** Arise from the adrenal cortex and may have variable clinical presentation, depending on the histologic zone of origin:

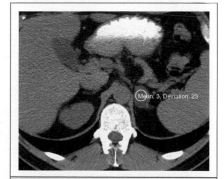

Figure 22-2 Adrenal adenoma. Nonenhanced CT image demonstrates a low-attenuation left adrenal mass (3 HU) consistent with an adenoma.

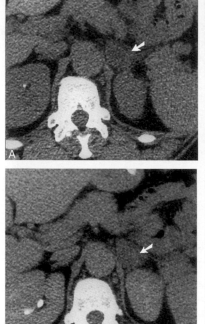

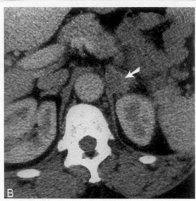

Figure 22-3. Washout phenomenon in adrenal adenoma. **A,** Nonenhanced CT image demonstrates a low-attenuation left adrenal mass *(arrow),* density of 4 HU. **B,** Corresponding portovenous phase demonstrates enhancement in the adrenal mass *(arrow)* with density of 54 HU. **C,** Delayed phase at 10 minutes demonstrates attenuation value of 23 HU (washout of > 50%) consistent with an adenoma *(arrow).* (From Mayo-Smith WW, Boland GW, Noto RB, Lee MJ: State-of-the-art adrenal imaging. Radiographics 21:995–1012, 2001, with permission.)

- **Zona glomerulosa:** Conn's adenoma → primary hyperaldosteronism (Fig. 22-5)
- **Zona fasciculata:** Cushing's syndrome
- **Zona reticularis:** Adrenogenital syndrome

2. **Nonfunctioning adenomas:** These are seen as incidental findings in approximately 1% of patients undergoing abdominal CT scans (and in approximately 3% at autopsy). The incidence of adenomas increases in patients with diabetes mellitus and hypertension and in old age. Nonfunctioning adenomas are characterized by their lipid-rich cells although approximately 10% of benign adenomas are lipid-poor. On CT imaging, adrenal adenomas appear as well-defined smooth round or ovoid homogeneous masses ranging in diameter between 1 and 5 cm. Calcification and cystic appearance is rare but possible. CT density and contrast washout criteria are used to confirm the diagnosis as explained previously.

9. **What is macronodular hyperplasia?**
   The pathogenesis of macronodular hyperplasia is unclear, and a number of theories have been proposed to explain the development of massive adrenal enlargement (Fig. 22-6). These adrenals have intracellular fat and have Hounsfield values equal to that of adrenal adenoma. Affected patients may have Cushing's disease secondary to increased cortisol secretion that is independent of adrenocorticotropic hormone (ACTH).

10. **What is the differential diagnosis for an adrenal mass associated with disturbed adrenal function?**
    1. **Masses associated with hyperfunction:**
       - **From adrenal cortex:** Functioning adenomas, carcinoma (50% functioning)
       - **From adrenal medulla:** Pheochromocytoma

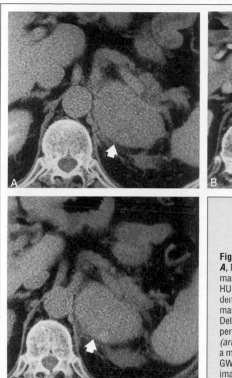

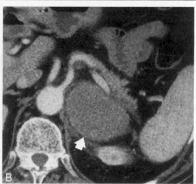

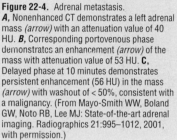

Figure 22-4. Adrenal metastasis.
A, Nonenhanced CT demonstrates a left adrenal mass *(arrow)* with an attenuation value of 40 HU. ***B,*** Corresponding portovenous phase demonstrates an enhancement *(arrow)* of the mass with attenuation value of 53 HU. ***C,*** Delayed phase at 10 minutes demonstrates persistent enhancement (56 HU) in the mass *(arrow)* with washout of < 50%, consistent with a malignancy. (From Mayo-Smith WW, Boland GW, Noto RB, Lee MJ: State-of-the-art adrenal imaging. Radiographics 21:995–1012, 2001, with permission.)

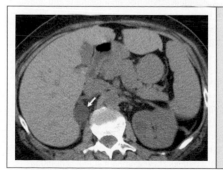

Figure 22-5. Aldosterone-producing adenoma. Nonenhanced CT image demonstrates a 1.5-cm low-attenuation (4 HU) right adrenal mass *(arrow)* consistent with an adenoma. Functioning and nonfunctioning adenomas cannot be differentiated radiologically.

2. **Masses associated with hypofunction:** Any nonfunctioning adrenal lesion such as tuberculosis (TB), histoplasmosis, or metastases that becomes large enough to cause sufficient destruction of the gland will result in hypofunction and manifest with Addison's disease.

11. **What is the differential diagnosis for an adrenal mass that is *not* associated with disturbed adrenal function?**
    From adrenal cortex
    - Hyperplasia
    - Nonfunctioning adenoma
    - Carcinoma (50% nonfunctioning)
    - Metastases
    - Myelolipoma
    - Others such as lymphoma, hemorrhage, cyst, and infection
    From adrenal medulla
    - Neuroblastoma
    - Ganglioneuroblastoma
    - Ganglioneuroma (rarely functioning)

12. **What is the differential diagnosis for bilateral adrenal masses?**
    - Bilateral adrenal hyperplasia
    - Bilateral adenomas
    - Metastases
    - Lymphoma
    - Hemorrhage
    - Infection (TB, histoplasmosis)
    - Pheochromocytoma (bilateral in 10%)

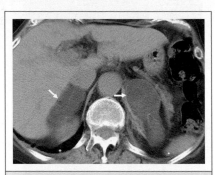

Figure 22-6. Macronodular hyperplasia. Nonenhanced CT image demonstrates bilaterally enlarged, low-attenuation adrenal glands (6 HU) *(arrows)*. MRI (not shown) revealed a drop in the signal on out-of-phase scan, confirming a lipid content and showed no enhancement on gadolinium injection.

13. **Can you administer iodinated contrast material IV in a patient with suspected pheochromocytoma?**
    Literature data addressing this issue are sparse and controversial. A small series demonstrated the elevation of catecholamine levels in patients with pheochromocytoma after ionic contrast administration. A more recent study demonstrated the safe application of nonionic contrast media in another small cohort of patients with pheochromocytoma in which none of the subjects had elevated catecholamine levels following contrast. To eliminate any potential patient risk of precipitating hypertensive crisis, the current recommendation is therefore to perform an unenhanced scan, to premedicate patients with an alpha-blocker, such as phentolamine and phenoxybenzamine, prior to injecting nonionic contrast, or to perform magnetic resonance imaging (MRI), which is considered superior for the evaluation of pheochromocytoma. Pharmacologic prophylaxis should also be provided prior to attempting percutaneous biopsy of suspected pheochromocytoma.

14. **Describe the CT findings of pheochromocytoma.**
    Pheochromocytomas (adrenal paragangliomas) are rare tumors of chromaffin tissue. They are typically imaged when they are 2–5 cm in diameter and appear as round or oval masses with attenuation similar to that of the liver (Fig. 22-7). Larger lesions are heterogeneous due to the frequent necrosis and hemorrhage and may demonstrate fluid-fluid levels. Cystic pheochromocytomas have also been reported. Large necrotic pheochromocytomas may mimic adrenal cortical carcinomas or metastasis. Calcification is rare (< 5%). Intense enhancement is noted if contrast is administered. CT is more than 93% sensitive for the detection and 95% specific in the diagnosis of pheochromocytomas.

15. **What is the "rule of 10" regarding pheochromocytoma?**
    - 10% are multiple or bilateral.
    - 10% are malignant.

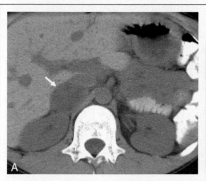
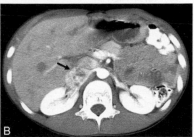

Figure 22-7. Pheochromocytoma. **A,** Nonenhanced CT demonstrates a low-attenuation right adrenal mass (37 HU) *(arrow).* **B,** Corresponding nonionic contrast-enhanced CT image demonstrates intense heterogeneous enhancement of the right adrenal mass *(arrow).*

- 10% are familial (familial pheochromocytomatosis).
- 10% present as adrenal incidentalomas.
- 10% recur after surgical removal.
- 10% occur in children.
- 10% are extra-adrenal.

16. **Where do extra-adrenal pheochromocytomas arise?**
    Extra adrenal pheochromocytomas are subdiaphragmatic in 98% of cases and usually arise from the organ of Zuckerkandl (Fig. 22-8), which is located around the aortic bifurcation or at the origin of the internal mammary artery. Other possible origins for extra-adrenal pheochromocytomas are anywhere along the sympathetic chain from the neck to sacrum, such as in the para-aortic region. Pheochromocytomas also arise in the urinary bladder and gonads.

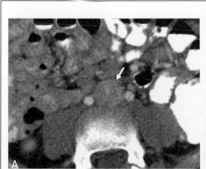
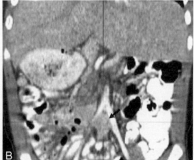

Figure 22-8. Extra-adrenal pheochromocytoma. Axial *(A)* and coronal *(B)* contrast-enhanced CT images demonstrate a 4.4-cm enhancing lesion *(arrows)* below the aortic bifurcation in the vicinity of the organ of Zuckerkandl. Positron emission tomography (PET) (not shown) demonstrated an increased uptake consistent with an extra-adrenal pheochromocytoma.

17. **What disease entities may be associated with pheochromocytomas?**
    - Multiple endocrine neoplasia (MEN type IIa or IIb). Patients with MEN syndromes may have atypical findings, such as thickened and nodular adrenal glands, without discrete large masses.
    - They are seen in 10% of patients with neurofibromatosis and 10% of patients with von Hippel-Lindau (VHL).
    - Pheochromocytomas are also found in Carney's syndrome (paraganglioma, gastric epithelioid leiomyosarcoma, pulmonary chondroma).

18. **What are paragangliomas? Do you know tumors that belong to this entity other than pheochromocytoma?**
    Paragangliomas are rare neuroendocrine tumors arising from paraganglionic tissues anywhere between the skull base and pelvic floor. Cells of paraganglioma belong to the amine precursor uptake and decarboxylation (APUD) system and are characterized by cytoplasmic vesicles containing catecholamines. Paragangliomas exist in three types:
    - **Adrenal paraganglioma (80%) = pheochromocytoma:** Hormonally active; they secrete epinephrine and norepinephrine.
    - **Aorticosympathetic paraganglioma (15%):** Arising from the sympathetic chain and the retroperitoneal ganglia and intermediately hormonally active, secreting norepinephrine but not epinephrine. Some paragangliomas also secrete dopamine.
    - **Parasympathetic paraganglioma (5%) = chemodectomas = nonchromaffin paraganglioma:** Usually hormonally nonactive. Examples include glomus jugulare, glomus tympanicum, glomus vagale, and carotid body tumor.

19. **What is the most common cause of adrenal calcification?**
    Adrenal calcification is most commonly a sequel of adrenal hemorrhage. Other causes in **children** include the following:
    - Adrenal cysts
    - Neuroblastoma
    - Ganglioneuroma
    - Wolman's disease
    Other causes in **adults** include the following:
    - Adrenal cysts
    - TB and histoplasmosis
    - Carcinoma
    - Pheochromocytoma
    - Ganglioneuroma

20. **How are adrenal cysts classified?**
    - **Pseudocysts (40%):** These are secondary to adrenal hemorrhage or infarction, lined by fibrous tissue, unilocular, and may have wall calcification.
    - **True cysts:** These are multilocular, may have septal calcification, and are lined by endothelium (40%; lymphangioma or hemangioma) or epithelium (10%; cystic adenoma, retention cyst, embryonal cyst). Parasitic cysts are most commonly echinococcal. Cystic degeneration may affect various tumors, such as carcinoma, metastasis, pheochromocytoma, schwannoma, and cystic adenomatoid tumor (*see* Fig. 22-9).

21. **What is Wolman's disease (primary familial xanthomatosis)?**
    This fatal autosomal recessive enzyme deficiency disorder results in accumulation of cholesterol esters and triglycerides in the liver, spleen, lymph nodes, adrenal cortex, and small bowel. It presents in neonates with malabsorption, failure to thrive, and steatorrhea. Radiologic findings include bilateral extensive punctate adrenal calcification (diagnostic), hepatosplenomegaly, enlarged fat-containing lymph nodes, small bowel wall thickening, and osteoporosis.

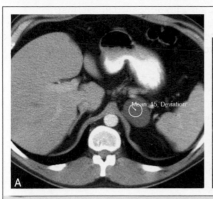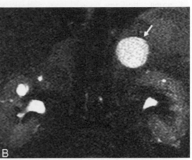

Figure 22-9. Adrenal cyst. *A,* Contrast-enhanced CT demonstrates a nonenhancing left adrenal lesion with HU of 15. *B,* Corresponding coronal haste MRI of the left adrenal gland further confirms the lesion *(arrow)* to be a cyst.

22. What are the most common causes of adrenal hemorrhage in children?

In children, adrenal hemorrhage is usually bilateral and is seen most commonly in the first week of life. Most common causes are hypoxia especially in premature infants, birth trauma, and septicemia. Adrenal hemorrhage may also occur in infants of diabetic mothers, infants with hemorrhagic disorders, and victims of child abuse.

23. What are the most common causes of adrenal hemorrhage in adults?

In adults, hemorrhage is usually unilateral. Most common causes are stress situations (such as sepsis and burns) and blunt abdominal trauma. Other causes include anticoagulant therapy (with adrenal hemorrhage occurring within the first month of treatment), orthotropic liver transplantation, adrenal venography and adrenal venous sampling (hemorrhage occurs in up to 10% of cases), and hemorrhage within an adrenal tumor.

24. Describe the CT findings of adrenal hematoma.

Acute adrenal hematoma demonstrates high attenuation (+ 30 HU) on unenhanced CT scan (Fig. 22-10). On postcontrast scans, it appears hypodense compared with the liver and spleen. As the hematoma ages, attenuation on unenhanced scans gradually decreases, liquefaction may occur, and fluid-fluid level can be seen. Calcification in adrenal hematoma may be seen within 1 week. Chronic hematoma may eventually evolve into a pseudocyst. Ancillary findings that may be seen with adrenal hematomas include downward displacement of the ipsilateral kidney, stranding of the adjacent fat, and thickening of pararenal (Gerota's) fascia.

25. What is Waterhouse-Friderichsen syndrome?

This is a fulminant variety of meningococcal infection in which organisms colonize the central nervous system, skin, adrenal glands, and serosal surfaces. The associated disseminated intravascular coagulopathy (DIC) results in diffuse bleeding in multiple organs. It has been postulated that adrenal hemorrhage in patients with Waterhouse-Friderichsen syndrome occurs because sepsis, as a state of stress, is associated with increased blood flow to the adrenal glands in an attempt to produce more cortisol. With its rich arterial supply (three arteries) and limited venous drainage (one vein), the gland becomes overwhelmed with blood flow and intraglandular hemorrhage ensues.

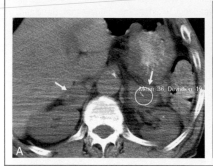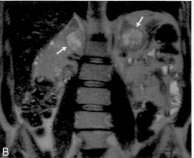

Figure 22-10. Adrenal hemorrhage. **A,** Nonenhanced CT image demonstrates bilaterally enlarged adrenal glands *(arrows)* with a mean attenuation value of 36 HU, which is suggestive of hemorrhage. **B,** Corresponding MRI (T1 sequence in coronal plane) reveals hyperintense signal *(arrows)* within both adrenal glands, confirming adrenal hemorrhage.

26. **What tumors arise from the adrenal medulla?**

These include neuroblastoma, ganglioneuroma, and ganglioneuroblastoma. Ganglioneuroma can viewed as the most benign and mature tumor entity on a spectrum of neurogenic tumors arising from sympathetic ganglia. On the other side of this spectrum lies neuroblastoma as the most malignant and immature entity. Ganglioneuroblastoma occupies an intermediate location on this spectrum. Although usually nonfunctioning, in rare cases ganglioneuromas may demonstrate hormone activity and are associated with diarrhea, sweating, hypertension, virilization, or myasthenia gravis.

27. **How frequently does ganglioneuroma arise in adrenal glands?**

Ganglioneuroma originates in the adrenal medulla (more often on the left side) in only 20% of cases. It demonstrates CT attenuation less than adjacent muscles and is a cause of adrenal calcification in children and adults. It has a tendency to surround blood vessels without compromising the lumen.

In general, common locations are the abdomen (50%) and posterior mediastinum (40%), where it may enlarge and cause local pressure and respiratory symptoms. Other locations include the pelvis and neck. Oral and intestinal ganglioneuromatosis are associated with MEN IIb (marfanoid patient with thyroid medullary carcinoma, adrenal pheochromocytoma, and multiple mucosal neuromas, including oral and intestinal ganglioneuromatosis).

28. **How frequently does neuroblastoma arise from the adrenal glands?**

Approximately 40% of neuroblastomas occur in the adrenal medulla. Outside the adrenals, neuroblastoma may arise along the sympathetic chains anywhere in the neck (5%), posterior mediastinum (15%), abdomen (25%), or pelvis (5%). Rare entities include cerebral, olfactory, and chest wall neuroblastomas.

29. **Describe the CT features of neuroblastoma.**

Neuroblastoma (Fig. 22-11) usually presents as a large retroperitoneal soft tissue mass that demonstrates fine granular or stippled calcification in approximately 90% of cases on CT scans (50% on plain radiographs). This is in contrast to Wilms tumor, which calcifies infrequently (5% or less). Neuroblastoma tends to cross the midline, where it becomes inseparable from the associated lymphadenopathy and may obstruct the contralateral renal hilum, resulting in hydronephrosis. The ipsilateral kidney is classically displaced laterally without distortion of the renal collecting system (the collecting system is usually deformed in Wilms tumor).

Neuroblastoma also tends to encase rather than displace major vessels (the opposite occurs with Wilms tumor). Neuroblastoma also has tendency to extend into spinal canal. Bone and lymph node metastases are common in neuroblastoma, whereas liver and lung deposits are more common in Wilms tumor.

30. **What is stage IVs of neuroblastoma? Does it carry a different prognosis compared with stage IV?**
    Neuroblastoma is classified as stage IVs when an undetectable primary or a stage I or II primary neuroblastoma is associated with skin, liver, and/or bone marrow involvement (<10% marrow involvement). The prognosis is more favorable compared with stage IV: The survival rate for patients with stage IVs is equivalent to that of patients with stage I or II, unless there is extensive bone marrow involvement.

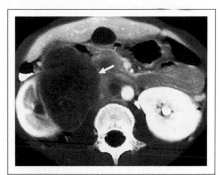

Figure 22-11. Surgically confirmed neuroblastoma. Contrast-enhanced CT image demonstrates a right adrenal mass *(arrow)* that displaces the right kidney laterally.

31. **From which part of the adrenal gland does carcinoma arise?**
    Adrenal carcinoma is a rare but lethal tumor that arises from the adrenal cortex.

32. **What is the usual size of adrenal carcinoma when first diagnosed on CT scan?**
    Adrenal carcinoma (Fig. 22-12) usually presents as a large heterogeneous mass, typically measuring 5–20 cm in diameter. CT scan demonstrates areas of hemorrhage and necrosis. Calcification is rare. Hepatic and lymph node metastases are common. It is important to look for associated tumor thrombosis in the renal vein or IVC.

33. **Summarize the size criteria for diagnosing adrenal carcinoma.**
    - **< 4 cm:** 2% are malignant.
    - **4.1–6 cm:** 6% are malignant.
    - **> 6 cm:** 25% are malignant.

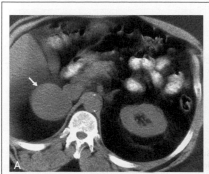 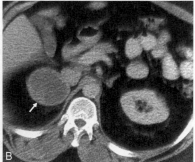

Figure 22-12. Adrenal cortical carcinoma. *A,* Nonenhanced CT demonstrates a 6-cm right adrenal mass *(arrow). B,* Corresponding contrast-enhanced CT demonstrates peripheral enhancement *(arrow).*

Sixty adrenalectomies have to be done to find one adrenal carcinoma if the size of >6 cm is considered diagnostic of adrenal carcinoma.

34. Can adrenal carcinoma present as a functioning tumor?

Fifty percent of adrenal carcinomas present as functioning tumors, usually secreting cortisol and presenting with Cushing's syndrome. Less commonly, it presents with symptoms of virilization or feminization. In children, adrenocortical carcinoma may be associated with hemihypertrophy, Beckwith-Wiedemann syndrome, or astrocytoma.

35. List the poor prognostic indicators of adrenal carcinoma.

- Mass greater than 12 cm
- High mitotic count
- Intratumoral hemorrhage

36. Describe the CT findings of adrenal myelolipoma.

Adrenal myelolipoma is a rare benign tumor that arises from bone marrow elements in adrenal glands. It is usually unilateral (10:1) and usually reaches large size, up to 30 cm, at time of diagnosis. CT evaluation demonstrates heterogeneous appearance with large areas of low attenuation due to fat (Fig. 22-13). The differential diagnosis of this appearance is liposarcoma, although myelolipoma itself does not have any malignant potential. Twenty-two percent of myelolipomas demonstrate evidence of calcification, 15% are associated with nonfunctioning adrenal adenoma, and 7% are associated with endocrine disorders, such as Cushing's syndrome or 21-hydroxylase deficiency. In 12% of cases, acute hemorrhage occurs and may cause increase in the size of tumor.

37. What plasma renin level would you expect in patients with hyperaldosteronism?

Hyperaldosteronism falls into two categories: primary and secondary.

- In **primary hyperaldosteronism,** the source for excess aldosterone is primary adrenal hyperfunction, which is caused by a cortical adenoma (Conn's adenoma) in approximately 70% of cases, adrenal hyperplasia in approximately 30%, or a functioning adrenocortical carcinoma in less than 1%. In all these cases, the increased aldosterone level exerts a negative feedback mechanism, resulting in decreased plasma renin level.

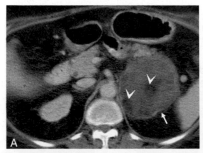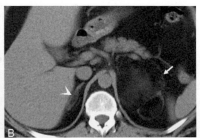

Figure 22-13. Adrenal myelolipoma. **A,** Contrast-enhanced CT image in a patient with surgically confirmed myelolipoma demonstrates a heterogeneous mass of the left adrenal gland *(arrow)* with areas of fat-density *(arrowheads)* within the mass. **B,** Nonenhanced CT image demonstrates a bilobed, left adrenal mass *(arrow)* with predominant fat density. A small myelolipoma *(arrowhead)* is also present in right adrenal gland.

- In **secondary hyperaldosteronism,** excess aldosterone is a reflection of elevated plasma renin level, which may be caused by a renin-secreting tumor, renal ischemia (e.g., due to renal artery stenosis), renal failure, congestive heart failure (CHF), or Barter's syndrome.

38. **Describe the CT findings in Conn's adenoma.**

    Conn's adenomas are small tumors that are usually smaller than 2 cm and rarely exceed 4 cm in diameter (*see* Fig. 22-5). The accuracy of CT to detect these small adenomas is higher than 80%. On unenhanced CT scan, the adenoma appears homogeneous and is usually isodense to the surrounding solid organs. Less frequently it may appear hypodense due to a small lipid content (up to 5% lipid content). Rarely, Conn's adenoma may appear hyperdense on unenhanced CT due to calcium content. On contrast-enhanced scans, an aldosterone-producing adenoma demonstrates less enhancement compared with the adjacent normal adrenal tissue.

KEY POINTS: ADRENAL GLANDS

1. On noncontrast CT, a homogeneous adrenal mass with CT density less than 10 HU is benign.

2. A contrast washout of 50% or more on the 10-minute postcontrast CT is suggestive of benign adrenal adenoma.

3. Premedicate patients with suspected pheochromocytoma with an alpha blocker before injecting iodinated contrast material and before attempting percutaneous biopsy. Pheochromocytoma with biochemical evidence is treated with surgery.

4. Tumors greater than 6 cm are treated with surgery, whereas tumors < 4 cm can be followed.

5. Adrenal calcification is most commonly a sequel of adrenal hemorrhage.

39. **What appearance do you expect in the adrenal glands in patients with Cushing's syndrome?**

    Imaging the adrenal glands in patients with Cushing's syndrome demonstrates adrenal hyperplasia in approximately 70%, adrenal adenoma in approximately 20%, or adrenal carcinoma in approximately 10% of cases. Functioning adrenal adenoma or carcinoma represents the cause of primary Cushing's syndrome, with the associated increase in cortisol secretion being responsible for feedback inhibition of pituitary ACTH. Adrenal hyperplasia represents the glandular response to elevated ACTH in cases of secondary Cushing's syndrome. In these cases, the elevated ACTH is most commonly iatrogenic. Intrinsically elevated ACTH results from either pituitary adenoma (90%) or an ectopic source (10%). The most common source for ectopic ACTH production is small cell lung carcinoma, although several other neoplasms, such as carcinoid tumors and pancreatic islet cell tumors, may also produce ACTH and cause Cushing's syndrome.

40. **What is primary pigmented nodular adrenocortical dysplasia?**

    This is a rare cause of ACTH-independent adrenal Cushing's syndrome in infants, children, and young adults. It exists either as an isolated abnormality or as a part of a familial syndrome called **Carney complex,** which consists of adrenal hyperplasia associated with spotty skin pigmentation, calcified Sertoli cell tumor of the testis, and cardiac and soft tissue myxomas. The nodular enlargement of the adrenal glands may mimic metastatic disease or granulomatous infection, such as TB or histoplasmosis.

41. **What are the causes of adrenogenital syndrome? How do they affect the CT appearance of the adrenal glands?**

    - **Congenital adrenogenital syndrome** is caused by enzyme deficiency and results in blocking the synthesis of glucocorticoids and mineralocorticoids. The resultant decrease in cortisol and aldosterone levels results in bilateral and symmetric feedback hyperplasia of the adrenal glands, and the associated accumulation of androgenic precursors leads to virilizing symptoms in the typically female patients. Patients may also be pseudohermaphrodites or males who present with precocious puberty as early as 2–3 years of age.

- **Acquired adrenogenital syndrome** results from a virilizing tumor, which may be an adrenal adenoma, carcinoma, or hyperplasia resulting in focal or diffuse enlargement of the gland, an ovarian or testicular tumor, or a gonadotropin-producing tumor, such as pineal or hypothalamic neoplasms or choriocarcinoma.

42. **Describe the causes and CT findings of Addison's disease.**

    Addison's disease is a primary adrenocortical insufficiency that results when a destructive process involves at least 90% of the adrenal cortex. Autoimmune destruction, as an isolated pathology or as a part of polyendocrine deficiency syndrome, is the etiology in approximately 70% of cases. Other causes include chronic granulomatous processes (e.g., TB, histoplasmosis, sarcoidosis), fungal infection (e.g., blastomycosis, coccidioidomycosis), amyloidosis, bilateral adrenal metastases, and, in rare cases, adrenal hemorrhage (e.g., secondary to trauma, sepsis, anticoagulation, or bleeding disorders). The appearance on CT scan depends on the etiology. Small adrenal glands are seen in cases of autoimmune atrophy and chronic inflammation, whereas gland enlargement is expected in case of a tumor mass, hemorrhage, or acute inflammation. Additionally, adrenal calcifications are seen in up to 25% of patients with chronic Addison's disease.

43. **What is the most common source for adrenal metastases?**

    Lung carcinoma is the most common source for adrenal metastatic disease. Other primary sources include the breast, kidney, bowel, ovary, and melanoma. It is to be noted that even in patients with known primary malignancy, up to 50% of small adrenal masses are benign adenomas rather than metastatic deposits.

44. **Describe the CT appearance of adrenal metastases.**

    Small metastatic lesions in the adrenal glands appear homogeneous and well defined. Larger lesions, especially when > 4 cm (Fig. 22-14), show features of malignant masses (e.g., heterogeneous density and enhancement, irregular outline, thick irregular rim, and even invasion of adjacent structures). Intense enhancement and slow washout are noted following contrast administration.

45. **What is collision tumor?**

    Metastasis that occurs in an adrenal gland with a preexisting adrenal adenoma is called collision tumor.

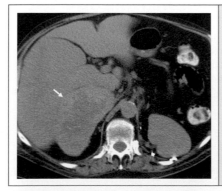

Figure 22-14. Adrenal metastasis. Nonenhanced CT image demonstrates a heterogeneous right adrenal mass *(arrow)* with low-attenuation areas in the center of the mass.

46. How long should you follow adrenal masses?

For tumors that remain stable on two imaging studies carried out at least 6 months apart and that do not exhibit hormonal hypersecretion over 4 years, further follow-up may not be warranted.

BIBLIOGRAPHY

1. Caoili EM, Korobkin M, Francis IR, et al: Delayed enhanced CT of lipid-poor adrenal adenomas. AJR 175:1411–1415, 2000.

2. Gold RE, Wisinger BM, Geraci AR, et al: Hypertensive crisis as a result of adrenal urography in a patient with pheochromocytoma. Radiology 102:597–580, 1972.

3. Korobkin M, Brodeur FJ, Francis IR, et al: CT time-attenuation washout curves of adrenal adenomas and nonadenomas. AJR 170:747–752, 1998.

4. Mayo-Smith WW, Boland GW, Noto RB, Lee MJ: State-of-the-art adrenal imaging. Radiographics 21:995–1012, 2001.

5. Mukherjee JJ, Peppercorn PD, Reznek RH, et al: Pheochromocytoma: Effect of nonionic contrast medium in CT on circulating catecholamine levels. Radiology 202:227–231, 1997.

6. National Institutes of Health Consensus Conference on Adrenal Glands, Bethesda, MD, 2004.

7. Raisanen J, Shapiro B, Glazer GM, et al: Plasma catecholamines in pheochromocytoma: Effect of urographic contrast media. AJR 143:43–46, 1984.

8. Welch TJ, Patrik F, Sheedy PF II: The adrenal glands. In Haaga JR, Lanzieri CF, Gilkeson RC (eds): Computed Tomography and Magnetic Resonance Imaging of the Whole Body, 4th ed. St. Louis, Mosby, 2003, pp 1511–1536.

CHAPTER 23

STOMACH AND INTESTINE

Baz Debaz, MD

1. **When is water-soluble oral contrast medium used? How is it prepared?**
   Water-soluble oral contrast is used to opacify the gastrointestinal (GI) tract when perforation is suspected, such as in the presence of free air, and to evaluate anastomosis sites. Ready-made water-soluble agents are commercially available. If needed, it can be prepared by mixing 20 mL of Gastrografin with 600 mL of water. Add flavor to taste, such as one packet of Kool-Aid.

2. **What is the protocol for a dedicated high-resolution multidetector CT scan of the stomach?**
   To obtain a good quality scan, three criteria should be fulfilled:
   - Proper gastric distention
   - Intravenous (IV) contrast timing
   - High-resolution scanning
   Patients should have fasted for at least 6 hours, and the following parameters should be observed:
   - **Oral contrast:** Use 1500 mL of water or three 450-mL bottles of Volumen (E-Z-EM), administered over 1 hour.
   - **Glucagon:** Use 1 mg IV prior to scan.
   - **Position:** Supine for lesions in the fundus and body. Scan in the prone position to evaluate lesions in the antrum and pylorus.
   - **IV contrast:** 120 mL at a rate of 4 mL/sec. Use saline flush if available.
   - **Scanning delay:** Use dual phase (arterial and portovenous) at 30 and 60 seconds. Scan at near isotropic resolution and view in MPR, three-dimensional (3D), and surface rendering, according to available software.

3. **What are the indications and advantages of dedicated high-resolution multidetector CT scans of the stomach?**
   They are used as an adjunct to endoscopy, but unlike endoscopy and double-contrast GI studies, high-resolution gastric CT provides information about both the gastric wall and the extragastric extent of disease as well as the status of other adjacent organs and lymph nodes. The most common indication is suspected gastric carcinoma. Other indications include lymphoma, carcinoid, metastases, and gastrointestinal stromal tumor (GIST) and other benign tumors. It is also valuable in gastric varices and gastric outlet obstruction.

4. **Name the benign gastric tumors.**
   Epithelial polyps may be hyperplastic or adenomatous. The **hyperplastic polyps** represent more than 85% of all benign gastric growths, but they are not true tumors. They are believed to develop from excessive regeneration of superficial epithelium. They are often multiple, and most are less than 1.5 cm in diameter.
   Most **adenomatous polyps (adenomas)** are larger in size. The CT appearance is improved with better gastric distention with contrast, water, or air. There are no reliable CT features to distinguish between benign and malignant lesions.
   Lipomas are rare, are submucosal in location, and occur in the antrum. They may ulcerate, resulting in hemorrhage. They are characterized on CT by their low-attenuation value.

Hemangiomas are rare, submucosal tumors. They may contain calcified phlebolites, which suggest the diagnosis on CT scanning.

Other tumors are **benign GIST, juvenile polyps**, and **pancreatic rests**.

5. What is GIST?

GIST is the most common nonepithelial neoplasm of the stomach and small bowel. It is rare in the colon and rectum. GISTs are GI mesenchymal tumors derived from either the interstitial cell of Cajal or from a more primitive stem cell. Tumors previously classified as leiomyoma, leiomyoblastoma, and leiomyosarcoma have been found to contain CD-117 and are now classified as GIST. GISTs may be benign or malignant, depending on cell type, and they may calcify. Lymphadenopathy is uncommon. GISTs have a heterogeneous enhancement on CT (Fig. 23-1).

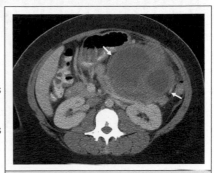

Figure 23-1. Malignant GIST of the stomach *(arrows)*. Note thick enhancing walls with invasion of the surrounding adipose tissue.

6. How does GIST involve the stomach?

- **Submucosal:** 60%
- **Subserosal:** 30%
- **Intramural:** 10%

Ninety percent of GISTs are in the fundus and body of the stomach.

7. List some important statistics and facts about gastric adenocarcinoma.

- There are 24,000 new cases diagnosed each year in the United States. About 700,000 new cases are diagnosed worldwide.
- The incidence is highest in Japan, South America, and Eastern Europe. In the United States it is 1.5–2.5 times more common in African-Americans, Hispanics, and Native Americans.
- The male-to-female ratio is 2:1.
- In recent years, it has become less common in the body and distal stomach and more prevalent in the gastroesophageal junction.
- Risk factors include *Helicobacter pylori* infection, adenomatous polyps, chronic atrophic gastritis, pernicious anemia, and partial gastrectomy for benign disease such as peptic ulcers (15–20 years latent period).

8. What are the pathways of spread of gastric adenocarcinoma?

- **Direct extension:** Depends on location in stomach; to gastrohepatic ligament, liver, spleen, lesser sac, pancreas, and esophagus (Fig. 23-2)
- **Lymphatic spread:** Regional lymph nodes, Virchow node (left supraclavicular) in 15% of cases
- **Hematogenous spread:** Liver, lung, and adrenal glands; ovaries in 10% of cases (Krukenberg's tumor, which often presents before the gastric primary tumor)
- **Peritoneal seeding:** In 40% of patients—the omentum, peritoneum, and serosa along the mesenteric side of the intestine

9. What are CT findings in gastric carcinoma?

Conventional CT scanning is not sensitive in early gastric cancer, with a reported sensitivity of about 50%. It may appear as focal wall thickening with mucosal enhancement in the early arteriovenous phase of contrast. Advanced cases appear as thickened enhancing gastric wall or a polypoid mass. Ulceration may be detected. Scirrhous carcinoma frequently involves the distal

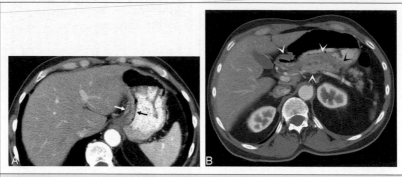

Figure 23-2. Carcinoma of the stomach. *A,* Invasion of the gastrohepatic ligament *(arrows). B,* Invasion of the pancreas *(arrowheads).*

half of the stomach and spreads predominantly in the submucosa and causes diffuse thickening of the gastric wall.

High-resolution CT of the stomach is more sensitive in detecting early cancer due to its 3D and virtual gastroscopy capability. Lesions that protrude more than 5 mm into the gastric lumen are better detected than those that are flat or depressed.

10. **Name CT features that may help differentiate gastric carcinoma from lymphoma.**
    - Gastric wall thickness is more impressive in lymphoma (mean = 4 cm) than in carcinoma (mean = 0.8 cm) (Fig. 23-3).
    - Mural thickening is more homogenous and the perigastric fat is more preserved with lymphoma.
    - Adenopathy in lymphoma is more pronounced and, unlike carcinoma, may extend below the level of the renal veins.
    - Lymph nodes in lymphoma are larger than those encountered with adenocarcinoma.

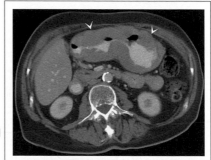

Figure 23-3. Gastric lymphoma with marked generalized mural thickening *(arrowheads).* Note the preservation of the perigastric fat.

11. **What is gastric volvulus? How it is classified?**
    Gastric volvulus is twisting of the stomach on itself. It may be transient with few symptoms or may cause obstruction, ischemia, and necrosis. It is classified according to its method of twisting and the location of the stomach:
    - **Organoaxial:** The stomach twists along its long axis. Organoaxial volvulus is usually associated with a diaphragmatic hernia and produces acute symptoms. Frequency of vascular compromise is reported to be between 5% and 28%.
    - **Mesenteroaxial:** The stomach folds along its short axis running across from the lesser to the greater curvature. The antrum and pylorus become situated at a level higher than the fundus and the body of the stomach (upside-down stomach) (Fig 23-4). The condition is usually intermittent with chronic symptoms.

Gastric volvulus has also been classified according to the location of the stomach:

- **Primary gastric volvulus (subdiaphragmatic):** One third of cases; occurs below the diaphragm when the stabilizing ligaments are too lax as a result of congenital or acquired causes.
- **Secondary gastric volvulus (intrathoracic):** Two thirds of cases; occurs above the diaphragm and is usually of the organoaxial type. Associated with paraesophageal hernias or other congenital or acquired diaphragmatic hernias. Not associated with sliding hiatal hernias. Multiplanar CT scanning is helpful to determine the type of volvulus.

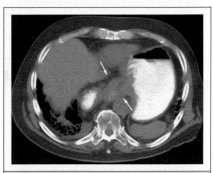

Figure 23-4. Mesenteroaxial gastric volvulus. The stomach is twisted on itself (between *arrows*) with the antrum and duodenum extending cephalad to a higher level than the fundus.

12. **Describe gastric rupture and its CT findings.**

Gastric rupture due to blunt trauma is rare and occurs when the stomach is distended with food. The anterior wall of the stomach is most commonly affected, followed by the greater curvature. CT demonstrates pneumoperitoneum and extravasation of contrast or fluid in the peritoneal cavity. Gastric perforation is more common in neonates and is usually spontaneous or due to necrotizing enterocolitis (NEC). Other causes include instrumentation, such as nasogastric tube placement or endoscopy, perforation of peptic ulcers, and cancer (Fig. 23-5).

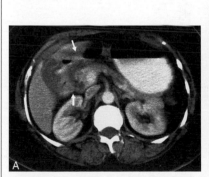
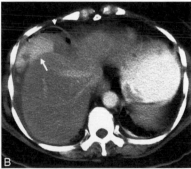

Figure 23-5. Perforated gastric ulcer. *A,* Diffuse edema surrounding the gastric antrum and duodenum *(arrows). B,* Perihepatic accumulation of oral contrast *(arrow)* and free air *(arrowhead).*

13. **What is phlegmonous gastritis?**

It is a purulent streptococcal infection of the stomach that primarily affects the submucosa and may lead to gangrene. Perforation is common with peritonitis and purulent ascites. There is a high mortality rate. Diagnosis is made by endoscopy and bacterial culture. CT demonstrates thick gastric wall with diffuse inflammation and the absence of intramural air.

14. **Describe emphysematous gastritis and its CT findings.**

Emphysematous gastritis is a rare, life-threatening condition characterized by generalized gastric wall infection caused by gas producing organisms, such as *Clostridium, Escherichia coli,* and streptococcal infection. Predisposing factors are ingestion of corrosive substances, alcohol abuse, gastroenteritis, recent abdominal surgery, GI infarction, arterial and venous occlusion, and acute pancreatitis. Patients present with an acute abdomen, fever, chills, and sometimes hematemesis. The major complication is acute perforation. The mortality rate is greater than 60%. CT demonstrates intramural gas and gastric wall thickening.

15. **What is the differential diagnosis of air in the gastric wall?**
In addition to emphysematous gastritis, intramural gas can be encountered in benign gastric emphysema, which can be secondary to the following:
- Severe gastric distention
- Trauma such as following endoscopy
- Pulmonary etiology (chronic obstructive pulmonary disease [COPD], emphysema)
It is a benign condition and can be differentiated from emphysematous gastritis by its benign clinical course and the lesser degree of gastric wall thickening.

KEY POINTS: DIFFERENTIAL DIAGNOSIS OF AIR IN THE GASTRIC WALL

1. Severe gastric distention

2. Trauma such as following endoscopy

3. Pulmonary etiology (COPD, emphysema)

4. Emphysematous gastritis (rare but life-threatening condition)

16. **Describe the multidetector CT enterography protocol.**
- Patients should avoid solid food for 8 hours.
- One hour prior to the scan, administer a single 10-mg dose of metoclopramide orally, together with 450 mL of water. Give 10 mg of Metoclopromide orally, followed by three 450-mL bottles of Volumen (E-Z-EM) over a period of 1 hour; 1200–1500 mL of water can be used instead. (Metoclopramide helps to reduce nausea and gastroesophageal reflux).
- Use 120 mL of IV contrast at a rate of 3 mL/second.
- Acquire a biphasic CT scan at 40 and 70 seconds with 2- to 3-mm slice thickness. View in axial or coronal planes.
- Encourage patients and explain to them the need to drink the required amount of liquid.

CT enterography with negative contrast administered perorally is as accurate as "CT enteroclysis" performed with methyl-cellulose administered through a nasoje-junal tube for the evaluation of Crohn's disease (Fig. 23-6).

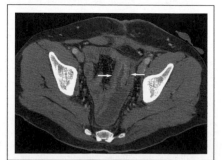

Figure 23-6. CT enterography in a patient with Crohn's disease. Note the thickened wall of an ileal loop with mucosal enhancement *(arrows)* indicating active disease.

17. What is a Meckel diverticulum?

Meckel diverticulum is the most common congenital anomaly of the GI tract and occurs in 2–3% of the population. It results from failure of closure of the omphalomesenteric duct and is located at the antimesenteric side of the ileum within 100 cm of the ileocecal valve. It measures up to 15 cm in length; 60% of patients present before 10 years of age. Heterotopic gastric mucosa and pancreatic mucosa are often found in symptomatic patients. Common complications include hemorrhage, intestinal obstruction, diverticulitis, and intussusception.

18. What is the role of CT in the diagnosis of Meckel diverticulum?

Radiologic evaluation of Meckel diverticulum is usually tailored to the patient's signs and symptoms. CT plays a role in evaluating patients with pain or bowel obstruction (Fig. 23-7). In patients with obstruction, look for an inverted diverticulum within the intestinal lumen, intussusception, volvulus, or the presence of the diverticulum in a hernia (Littre hernia).

In patients with an inflammatory clinical presentation and normal appendix, remember to look for Meckel diverticulitis. The wall of the diverticulum may be thick, with local stranding. It may contain a fluid level, enteroliths, or fecal-like material. If you are proven right, you will be a star!

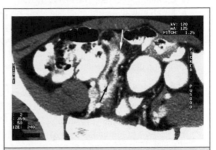

Figure 23-7. Inverted Meckel's diverticulum within an ileal loop *(arrows)* with no signs of obstruction.

19. What is the normal wall thickness of the small intestine?

Less than 3 mm. When the intestine is distended, the wall may not be perceptible. Intestinal wall may appear abnormally thick during peristalsis or if bowel contents are isodense with bowel wall. If in doubt, request a small bowel follow-through examination.

20. Name the benign tumors in the small intestine and their complications.

Benign tumors of the small intestine are rare. They include adenoma, benign stromal tumor, and lipoma. Complications are bleeding, intussusception, and obstruction.

21. What are the small bowel primary malignant tumors? What is their differential distribution?

Small bowel malignant tumors are uncommon and account for less than 3% of GI malignancies. The most common is adenocarcinoma, followed by malignant carcinoid, lymphoma, and sarcomas. Adenocarcinoma is more common in the duodenum (Fig. 23-8). Carcinoid and lymphoma are more common in the terminal ileum. Sarcomas are slightly more common in the jejunum.

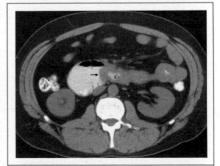

Figure 23-8. Duodenal carcinoma arising from its third portion causing obstruction *(arrow)*.

22. **Describe the GI malignancies in acquired immunodeficiency syndrome (AIDS) and their CT appearance.**
    - **Kaposi's sarcoma:** Most common; related to herpes virus. GI tract is third in frequency after skin and lymph nodes. It is most common in the duodenum and rectum. CT demonstrates large focal masses or nodular wall thickening.
    - **Non-Hodgkin lymphoma:** Related to Epstein-Barr virus; usually more aggressive and less responsive to therapy than non-AIDS lymphoma. It also involves the GI tract more often than in non-AIDS patients. Complications include obstruction, intussusception, and perforation. Distal ileum and rectum are more involved.

    CT findings include the following:
    - **Stomach:** Circumferential or focal mural thickening
    - **Small bowel:** Aneurysmal dilatation, nodular and diffuse wall thickening

23. **What is the CT appearance of carcinoid tumors?**
    Ill-defined mass in right lower quadrant (RLQ). Calcifications occur in 70% of cases. Soft tissue stranding of the mesentery in a stellate pattern, displacing bowel loops (Fig. 23-9) is also seen.

24. **What are the CT features of primary small bowel lymphoma?**
    Non-Hodgkin lymphoma of the small bowel has become more frequent with AIDS. It is more common distally than proximally.
    - The most common form is characterized by multiple nodules (usually larger than lymphoid hyperplasia) of various sizes, giving symmetric bowel wall thickening associated with retroperitoneal lymphadenopathy.
    - A polypoid mass that can be large and may cause intussusception. The junction of the tumor with the normal small bowel is more gradual and difficult to define and extends along a longer segment than adenocarcinoma.
    - It may present as an aneurysmal dilatation of the involved segment of the small bowel (Fig. 23-10).
    - Another form is a large exocentric mass that extends beyond the bowel wall.

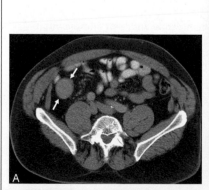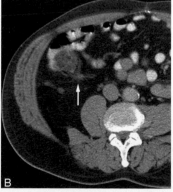

Figure 23-9. Malignant carcinoid tumor of the distal ileum in a 61-year-old man with intermittent right lower quadrant pain. *A,* CT scan of the pelvis shows a well-defined submucosal mass in the distal ileum *(arrows)*. *B,* CT scan at a slightly higher level shows a mild desmoplastic reaction in the adjacent mesentery *(arrow)*.

25. What is the target sign?
It implies the presence of submucosal edema (Fig. 23-11) and can be seen as a two- or three-layer appearance of the bowel wall. The contrast-enhancing inner and outer circles are believed to represent hyperemia of the mucosa and muscularis propria/serosa, respectively. The middle nonenhanced circle represents submucosal edema. Barium in the lumen obscures the mucosal enhancement. It is best seen in the arteriovenous phase of the IV contrast. In severe cases of submucosal edema, it may even be appreciated on the nonenhanced scan.

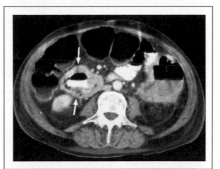

Figure 23-10. Duodenal lymphoma presenting as aneurysmal dilatation with thickened walls *(arrows)*.

KEY POINTS: TUMORS OF THE STOMACH AND SMALL INTESTINE

1. Gastrointestinal stromal tumor (GIST) is the most common nonepithelial neoplasm of the stomach and small bowel. It is rare in the colon and rectum.

2. In recent years, gastric adenocarcinoma has become less common in the body and distal stomach and more prevalent in the gastroesophageal junction.

3. Conventional CT scanning is not sensitive in early gastric cancer (reported sensitivity of about 50%).

4. Small bowel malignant tumors are uncommon and account for less than 3% of GI malignancies. The most common is adenocarcinoma, followed by malignant carcinoid, lymphoma, and sarcomas.

5. GI malignancies in AIDS include Kaposi's sarcoma (most common) and non-Hodgkin lymphoma.

26. What is the differential diagnosis of a target sign?
The target sign is encountered in the small and large intestine. It is associated with Crohn's disease, ischemic bowel, Henoch-Schönlein purpura, radiation damage to the small and large bowel, pseudomembranous colitis, and bowel edema due to portal hypertension.

27. Does the presence of a target sign exclude malignancy?
Yes, because the target sign is associated with inflammatory conditions and not with malignancy. One exception is infiltrating scirrhous carcinoma of the stomach and colon, which is very rare and usually associated with rigidity, narrowing, and regional lymphadenopathy.

28. If you see deposition of fat in the submucosa of the small or large intestine, what does it mean?
Deposition of fat in the submucosa of the bowel is encountered in chronic inflammatory bowel disease, such as Crohn's disease and ulcerative colitis (Fig. 23-12). It could be a response to

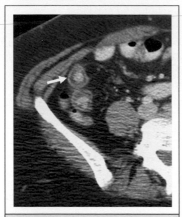

Figure 23-11. Target sign *(arrow)*. CT scan of a patient with Crohn's disease shows mesenteric edema and enhancement of the muscularis propria/serosa. The enhancement of the mucosa is obscured by the presence of barium in the lumen.

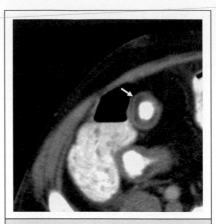

Figure 23-12. Submucosal fat infiltration in the distal ileum of a patient with Crohn's disease *(arrow)*.

chronic inflammation or to steroid therapy. It has also been reported to develop within a few weeks during chemotherapy for leukemia or lymphoma.

29. **What is the Comb sign?**
    Enhancement of engorged vasa recta in the terminal ileum due to hyperemia (Fig. 23-13). It is not present in the jejunum. It is seen mostly in Crohn's disease but can be also encountered in vasculitis, such as lupus, mesenteric thromboembolism, strangulated bowel, and ulcerative colitis.

30. **What are the complications of Crohn's disease?**

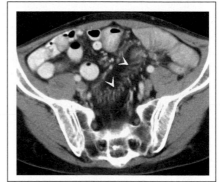

Figure 23-13. Comb sign *(arrowheads)*. CT scan of a patient with Crohn's disease showing enhancement of engorged vasa recta in a distal ileal loop.

    - Bowel perforation, abscess, bowel obstruction, fistula formation (bladder, skin, and vagina), and perianal fissures and fistulas (Fig. 23-14) may be seen.
    - There is an increased risk of colon and small bowel cancer as well as small bowel lymphoma.
    - Malabsorption, cholelithiasis, nephrolithiasis, hepatic abscess, pancreatitis, and toxic megacolon can be found.
    - Primary sclerosing cholangitis (PSC). 1% of Crohn's patients will develop PSC, and 10% of patients with PSC have Crohn's disease.
    - Sacroiliitis can manifest before the enteric form.

31. **Why do patients with Crohn's disease develop gallbladder and kidney stones? What is their frequency?**
    - **Gallstones** are reported in up to 30% in patients with Crohn's disease. Formation of gallstones is due to several factors:
      - Use of total parenteral nutrition (TPN) causes sludge formation.
      - Gallbladder hypomotility found in IBD.
      - Poor absorption of bile salts in the terminal ileum results in diminished bile acid pool size and supersaturation of cholesterol in bile (cholesterol stones).
      - Diseased ileum cannot absorb bile salts that pass in the colon where they combine with unconjugated bilirubin and promotes its absorption. Increased concentration of bilirubin in bile is associated with stone formation.

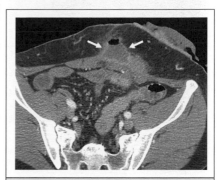

Figure 23-14. Abscess in the anterior abdominal wall complicating Crohn's disease *(arrows).*

    - **Kidney stones** are reported in up to 19% of patients and are more common in those with an ileostomy. Kidney stones are usually calcium oxalate types. They are caused by malabsorption of fatty acids, which combine with calcium and are lost in the stools as calcium soaps. Normally, calcium binds to oxalates and together they are expelled from the colon. Lack of sufficient free calcium in the colon leads to reabsorption of oxalates, resulting in hyperoxaluria and the formation of stones.

32. **Describe the CT findings of Crohn's disease.**
    The most common sites are the distal small bowel and proximal colon (ileocolic). Look for skip lesions. CT findings include bowel wall thickening (1–2 cm), target sign (caused by submucosal edema and found in the acute phase of the disease), Comb sign, fatty infiltration of the submucosa, abscess formation, phlegmon, fibrofatty proliferation in the mesentery (creeping fat), and mesenteric lymphadenopathy (less than 1 cm). If larger lymph nodes are present, suspect lymphoma.

33. **What are the CT findings in *Mycobacterium avium-intracellulare* (MAI) enteritis?**
    MAI affects the GI tract and the hepatobiliary system in patients with AIDS. The condition is diagnosed with blood culture. Clinical, histologic, and radiologic findings are similar to those of Whipple disease, and it is thus often called pseudo-Whipple disease. CT findings include bowel wall thickening especially in the jejunum (Fig. 23-15A) and bulky low-attenuation mesenteric and retroperitoneal lymphadenopathy similar to those found in lymphoma (Fig. 23-15B).

34. **What is Henoch-Schönlein syndrome? How does it affect the GI tract?**
    Also known as anaphylactoid purpura, Henoch-Schönlein syndrome is a systemic allergic vasculitis affecting capillaries, small arterioles, and venules and involving the skin, joints, and kidneys. Immunizations, insect bites, medication, infections, and certain foods are implicated in its etiology. It causes a characteristic skin rash, arthritis involving the large joints, and hematuria. GI findings include colic, nausea, vomiting, diarrhea, and GI bleeding. GI perforation and obstruction are rare. *Important note:* GI symptoms may present as a surgical abdomen and precede the skin rash.

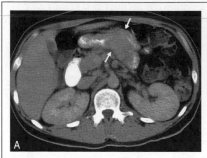
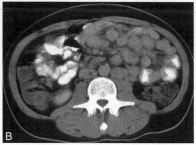

Figure 23-15. Lymph node biopsy-proven MAI infection in a 35-year-old human immunodeficiency virus (HIV)-positive man with AIDS. **A,** CT scan shows thickening of a jejunal loop *(arrows)*. **B,** Scan at a lower lever demonstrates severe mesenteric lymphadenopathy.

35. What are the CT findings of Henoch-Schönlein syndrome?

CT findings are bowel wall thickening with multifocal and skipped segments. The jejunum and ileum are most frequently involved, followed by the duodenum and colon (Fig. 23-16). GI involvement occurs in 29–62% of adult patients. Other findings include regional lymphadenopathy (less than 1.5 cm in diameter), engorgement of mesenteric vessels, edema in mesenteric fat, and free peritoneal fluid.

36. What is graft-versus-host disease (GVHD)?

GVHD is a major complication seen in recipients of allogenic bone marrow transplant. Immunocompetent stem cells introduced in a patient with a destroyed immune system by chemotherapy recognize the body as foreign (reversed rejection). It has various grades of severity

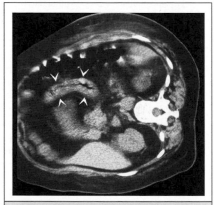

Figure 23-16. Henoch-Schönlein purpura. CT scan of a 72-year-old woman who presented with a 1-week history of watery diarrhea and progressive renal failure. Three days earlier she had developed generalized skin rash following an episode of pharyngitis. CT scan demonstrates a thickened jejunal loop *(arrowheads)*.

(I–IV). The risk of developing GVHD increases with age. The **acute form** occurs in the first 3 months after transplantation (skin rash and peeling, cramps, fever, diarrhea, and liver insufficiency). The **chronic form** occurs later and has similar symptoms. Prognosis depends on early diagnosis and immunosuppressive therapy.

37. What are the CT findings in GVHD?

- Bowel wall thickening (more common in the small than the large bowel)
- Bowel dilatation (may occur proximal to the thickened wall segments)
- Bowel mucosal enhancement
- Engorgement of the vasa recta (common)
- Mesenteric stranding, ascites, and cholecystitis (mesenteric lymphadenopathy is absent). Esophageal thickening in severe forms

38. **What is the pathogenesis of radiation enteritis? What are the CT findings?**
Radiation enteritis occurs 6–24 months following treatment. However, the latent period may be up to 20 years. Doses greater than 45 Gy can predispose to the disease. Radiation causes serositis and adhesions. It also causes narrowing of the arterioles in the submucosa, resulting in bowel ischemia and necrosis. This may lead to perforation and development of a sinus tract to the vagina or bladder. Bowel stricture and adhesions are responsible for bowel obstruction.

CT demonstrates matted bowel loops, thickening of the bowel wall and adjacent mesentery, and a target sign. Increased attenuation of the mesenteric fat may be present (Fig. 23-17).

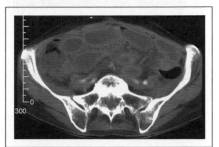

Figure 23-17. Radiation enteritis. CT scan of a patient after radiation therapy for rectal cancer. Note small bowel obstruction with thickened bowel wall.

39. **Describe duodenal hematoma and its CT findings.**
The second and the third portions of the duodenum are vulnerable to blunt trauma due to their retroperitoneal location. The third portion of the duodenum can easily be compressed against the spine during a traumatic event.

Blunt trauma results in either duodenal rupture or duodenal hematoma. It is important to differentiate between these two conditions to determine the clinical management. Perforation requires emergency surgery, whereas duodenal hematoma is treated conservatively.

CT plays an important role in the evaluation of duodenal injury. Extravasation of air and or oral contrast around the duodenum or in the right pararenal space of the peritoneum is an indication of rupture. Duodenal hematoma is shown on CT as circumferential or eccentric wall thickening, having a high attenuation indicating acute bleeding causing narrowing of the lumen. Because of the anatomic proximity of the pancreas, special attention should be give to this organ to evaluate for any signs of traumatic pancreatitis.

40. **What are the causes of periduodenal air?**
Perforation from a duodenal ulcer, foreign body, endoscopic retrograde cholangiopancreatography (ERCP), or trauma. On CT, look for the presence of air, oral contrast, and fat stranding (stranding may not be present at an early stage). Perforation must be differentiated from duodenal diverticula, which are common but not associated with local fat stranding. Perforated peptic ulcer is a common occurrence, and special attention should be given to the duodenum and distal stomach in all cases of abdominal pain (Figs. 23-18 and 23-19).

41. **Regarding the bowel wall, how does intramural hemorrhage look on CT?**
Homogenous, high attenuation of the thickened bowel wall. Intramural hemorrhage does not enhance with IV contrast.

42. **What are the causes of bowel ischemia?**
   - **Arterial compromise:** Thromboembolic occlusion of the superior mesenteric artery (SMA) or its branches, vasculitis (uncommon), and external compression of arteries by volvulus, hernia adhesions, and intussusception
   - **Hypotension:** Hypovolemia, sepsis and congestive heart failure
   - **Vasoconstrictive drugs:** Norepinephrine
   - **Impaired venous drainage:** Thrombosis of mesenteric and portal veins, severe intestinal distention occurring proximal to a stenotic lesion, and compression of mesenteric veins by tumor, adhesion, volvulus, hernia, and intussusception

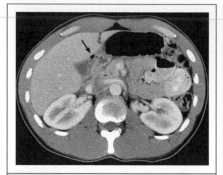

Figure 23-18. Perforated duodenal ulcer. Note the small extraluminal air *(arrow)* with only minimal degree of edema, which is difficult to appreciate due to the paucity of fat.

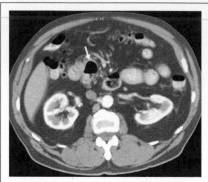

Figure 23-19. Diverticulum arising from the third portion of the duodenum *(arrow)*.

43. **What is shock bowel? How does it look on CT?**

   Shock bowel is defined as diffuse abnormalities in the small bowel caused by prolonged hypoperfusion due to hypovolemic shock. CT findings include diffuse thickening of the small bowel wall associated with strong enhancement after IV contrast. Also seen is dense enhancement of the aorta and inferior vena cava, which is flattened, and increased enhancement of the kidneys (Fig. 23-20).

44. **What are the CT findings of acute bowel ischemia?**

   ■ **Specific CT findings:** Thromboembolism in the mesenteric vessels, intramural gas, portal venous gas, lack of bowel wall enhancement, and ischemia of other organs

   ■ **Nonspecific signs:** Bowel dilatation, submucosal edema (target sign), bowel wall thickening (more severe in venous thrombosis than arterial occlusion), bowel wall enhancement, mesenteric edema, vascular engorgement, and ascites (Figs. 23-21 and 23-22)

   Note: The degree of bowel wall enhancement depends on the pathophysiology of the ischemic process. In complete arterial occlusion, there is no or very little wall enhancement. In transient arterial ischemia, the degree of enhancement increases with the degree of damage affecting the microvascular endothelium and the mucosal epithelium. In extreme ischemia, there is intramural hemorrhage with varying degrees of enhancement. In impaired venous drainage, the degree of enhancement may be mild to severe and is associated with mesenteric venous engorgement and wall thickening.

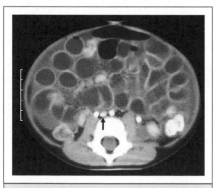

Figure 23-20. Shock bowel. CT scan of a child with hypovolemia following a motor vehicle accident. Note the marked degree of bowel wall enhancement and a small-caliber inferior vena cava (IVC) *(arrow)*.

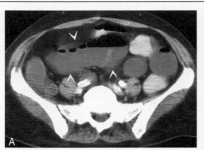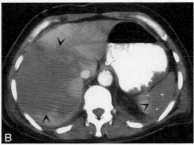

Figure 23-21. Intestinal infarct. **A,** CT scan of an elderly patient showing dilated fluid-filled loops of bowel with no wall enhancement *(arrowheads)*. **B,** CT scan showing extensive liver and spleen infarcts *(arrowheads)*. The SMA (not shown) was calcified and thrombosed.

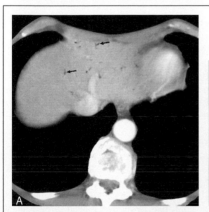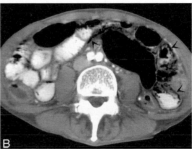

Figure 23-22. **A,** Intestinal infarct with portal venous gas *(arrows)*. **B,** CT scan at the level of the mid abdomen showing pneumatosis intestinalis *(arrowheads)* and lack of bowel wall enhancement.

45. In acute intestinal ischemia, do patients with thick bowel wall have a worse prognosis than those with thin wall?

No. The wall of the infarcted bowel is usually thin compared with transient reversible ischemia, which is usually associated with thick walls. As a result, intestinal ischemia patients with thick bowel wall usually have a better prognosis than those with thin bowel wall.

46. Describe pneumatosis intestinalis.

It is an uncommon condition characterized by the presence of thin-walled, gas-filled cysts located in subserosa or submucosa. It is best diagnosed on CT (Fig. 23-23). There are two forms: primary and secondary.

Primary pneumatosis intestinalis (15%), also known as pneumatosis cystoides intestinalis, is a benign, asymptomatic condition, found in adults older than the fifth decade. On barium studies, it may be mistaken for polyposis. It can be associated with pneumoperitoneum.

Secondary pneumatosis intestinalis (85%) can be associated with a variety of conditions:

- **NEC:** Occurs in infants
- **Mesenteric vascular occlusion:** High mortality rate when pneumatosis is present
- **Trauma:** Colonoscopy, blunt trauma, jejunostomy tube, intestinal anastomosis
- **Infection:** Primary infection, parasites, perforated sigmoid or jejunal diverticulum, appendicitis
- **Inflammatory bowel disease:** Crohn's disease and ulcerative colitis
- **Connective tissue disease, especially scleroderma**
- **Pulmonary disease:** COPD, artificial ventilation
- **Gastric and intestinal obstruction, volvulus**
- **Increased mucosal permeability:** Steroids, chemotherapy
- **Miscellaneous:** Whipple disease, GVHD

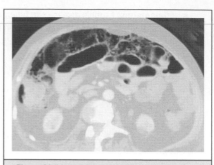

Figure 23-23. Benign pneumatosis cystoides intestinalis in an elderly patient with mild abdominal pain. CT shows diffuse pneumatosis involving the bowel and mesentery and associated with free air.

47. **Why do patients with COPD develop intestinal pneumatosis?**
Pneumatosis of pulmonary origin is caused by ruptured pulmonary bullae and dissection of air along the bronchovascular trunk into the mediastinum and then into the retroperitoneum. It reaches the GI tract as it dissects along the leaves of the mesenteric bed.

48. **What are the causes of pneumoperitoneum?**
- **Perforated hollow viscus:** Peptic ulcer disease, foreign body, necrotic GI tumor, diverticulitis, NEC, and inflammatory bowel disease
- **Ruptured intraabdominal abscess**
- **Iatrogenic:** Laparotomy and laparoscopy (free air seen up to 6 days, but sometimes small amount of air can last up to 24 days), gastrostomy tube placement, leaking surgical anastomosis, enema tip injury, trauma from endoscopy, peritoneal dialysis, paracentesis, dilation and curettage (D&C), placement of chest tube below the diaphragm, hysterosalpingogram, and tubal insufflation
- **Trauma:** Penetrating abdominal injury, rectal injury, ruptured urinary bladder
- **Pneumatosis cystoides intestinalis**
- **Nonsymptomatic causes in females:** Intercourse, squatting, knee-chest movements, and certain sports

49. **List the most common causes of small bowel obstruction.**
- **Adhesions**
- **Internal and external hernias:** (Fig. 23-24)
- **Extrinsic tumors:** Ovarian cancer, mesenteric implant of tumor
- **Intestinal tumors:** (e.g., carcinoma, GIST, lymphoma)

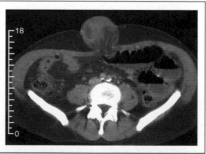

Figure 23-24. Incarcerated umbilical hernia. Patient presenting with small bowel obstruction. Note the umbilical hernia containing an incarcerated small bowel loop together with engorged mesenteric vessels.

- **Inflammation:** Crohn's disease and tuberculosis
- **Vascular etiology:** Radiation enteritis and bowel ischemia
- **Mural hematoma:** (Anticoagulants and trauma)
- **Intussusception**
- **Intraluminal etiology:** Foreign bodies, bezoars, and gallstone ileus

50. What is the most common cause of small bowel obstruction?

Adhesions are responsible for 60% of cases of small bowel obstruction,; 80% of adhesions are postsurgical, and the remainder are due to peritonitis or are congenital in nature. Postsurgical adhesions usually occur near the site of surgical intervention and are most common in the ileum.

51. What is the whirl sign?

It is a mass seen on CT, composed of swirling vessels, twisted loops of bowel, and mesenteric fat. It is found in small and large bowel volvulus and closed loop obstruction (Fig. 23-25).

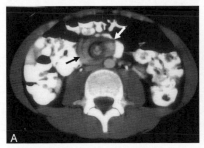
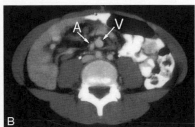

Figure 23-25. **A,** Whirl sign in an infant with mid gut volvulus *(arrows).* **B,** CT scan of the same patient showing reversed position of the superior mesenteric artery/vein. A = superior mesenteric artery, V = superior mesenteric vein.

52. What is the small bowel feces sign?

It is an uncommon CT sign occurring in less than 8% of small bowel obstructions. Characterized by the presence of fecal-like material with air bubbles in the small bowel immediately proximal to the point of obstruction (Fig. 23-26). Usually occurs in subacute or longstanding obstruction. When present, it is a reliable sign in confirming the diagnosis.

53. What is the role of CT in small bowel obstruction?

In complete or high-grade small bowel obstruction, CT has a sensitivity of 90–96% and a specificity of 91–96% and an accuracy of 90–95%. CT is less accurate in partial or low-grade obstruction. In such cases, barium studies are of help.

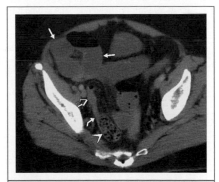

Figure 23-26. Feces sign. Axial CT of pelvis demonstrates "feces sign" *(arrowhead)* demarcating the site of small bowel obstruction *(curved arrow)* with proximal dilated small bowel loops *(arrows)* and normal caliber distal small bowel *(small arrow).*

54. **How do you diagnose small bowel obstruction (SBO) by CT?**

The diagnosis of SBO is made by identifying dilated proximal bowel and collapsed distal bowel. A small bowel with a caliber greater than 2.5 cm is considered dilated. A transition point may not by easily seen especially if there is paucity of intraabdominal fat. Multiplanar images may aid in confirming the diagnosis (Fig. 23-27).

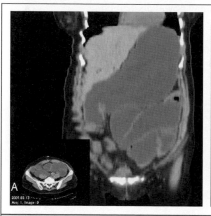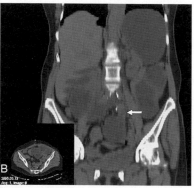

Figure 23-27. Small bowel obstruction due to adhesions in a patient with previous laparotomy. Kidney, ureter, and bladder (KUB, not shown) revealed a gasless abdomen. *A,* CT coronal reformatted images shows diffuse dilatation of the stomach and jejunum. *B,* A coronal image at a more posterior level clearly depicts the point of transition *(arrow)*.

55. **Describe the CT findings in gallstone ileus.**

Dilated loops of small bowel with air in the biliary tree and gallbladder. A stone in the lumen of the small bowel, usually located in the terminal ileum. The stone can be discovered at any location along the small bowel. Note that biliary symptoms are often absent (Fig. 23-28).

56. **What is Bouveret syndrome?**

It is a rare form of gallstone ileus in which the stone is embedded in the duodenum and causes gastric outlet obstruction (Fig. 23-29).

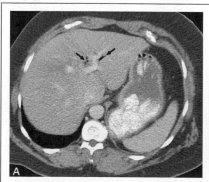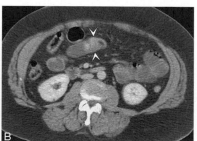

Figure 23-28. Gallstone ileus. *A,* Gas in the biliary tree *(arrows)*. *B,* Large gallstone obstructing the jejunum *(arrowheads)*.

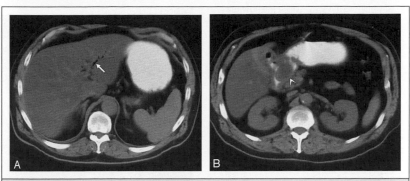

Figure 23-29. Bouveret syndrome. A 65-year-old woman presenting with upper abdominal pain and vomiting. **A,** CT scan of the liver showing pneumobilia *(arrow).* **B,** A scan at a lower level showing a large gallstone obstructing the duodenum *(arrowhead).*

57. Name the types of bezoars and their CT findings.

Bezoars are rare and represent retained masses of animal or vegetable material in the GI tract (Fig. 23-30). Predisposing factors are gastroparesis, gastric surgery, vagotomy, and poor mastication. There are three known kinds of bezoars: Trichobezoars occur in patients suffering of trichophagia and also found in wool-workers and are due to the ingestion of hair that accumulates in the stomach. Lactobezoars occur in neonates and are due to inspissation of feeding formula in the small bowel causing obstruction. Phytobezoars are more common than the other types and are due to the ingestion of large quantities of nonabsorbable fibers or seeds, such as those found in persimmons and oranges, which can accumulate in the stomach or the small bowel. Cactus pear seeds tend to accumulate in the rectum. CT demonstrates fiberlike rings or small organized radiodensities with entrapped air.

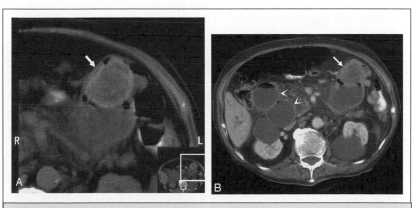

Figure 23-30. Bezoar. **A,** Axial CT demonstrates a bezoar in small bowel *(arrow)* with proximal small bowel obstruction *(arrowheads)* as seen in *B*.

58. Describe pharmacobezoars and their CT findings.

Pharmacobezoars result from the accumulation of compacted large quantities of undigested drugs. Procardia XL has been implicated in bezoar formation in the stomach and the small bowel (Fig. 23-31). The main ingredient, nifedipine (a calcium channel blocker), is contained in an insoluble, cellulose shell. A laser-drilled hole in the shell permits the passage of water from the

GI tract into the shell, which mixes with the medication forming a suspension. Once the volume of this suspension inside the shell reaches a critical amount, it is released into the intestine. The insoluble shell is then evacuated intact. The shells may contain air and barium. The air-filled, undigested shells can mimic pneumatosis intestinalis and may also give focal filling defects on barium enema studies simulating small polyps. Procardia XL should not be taken by patients with any degree of bowel obstruction.

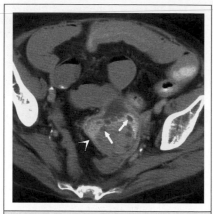

Figure 23-31. Pharmacobezoar. Axial CT demonstrates a pharmacobezoar (Procardia XL) *(arrowhead)*. Multiple hypodensities within this pharmacobezoar represent individual Procardia XL pills *(arrows)*.

59. What is the frequency of intussusception?
In children, it is the most common cause of intestinal obstruction, whereas in adults it is responsible for less than 5% of bowel obstructions. Unlike childhood intussusception, which is usually idiopathic, the adult form is associated with a cause, such as a mass or polyp.

60. What are the types of intussusception?
- **Enteroenteric and enterocolic:** Usually of benign origin, such as lymphoid hyperplasia, adhesions, and Meckel's diverticula; 1% of patients with cystic fibrosis develop an enterocolic intussusception. Malignancy is rare. In the adult, up to 20% of enteroenteric intussusceptions are idiopathic.
- **Colocolic:** This type frequently has a malignant lead point.
- **Other forms are very rare:** Gastrojejunal, jejunogastric.

61. Describe CT features of intussusception.
CT features of intussusception include a target mass with enveloped, eccentrically located areas of low density, frequently associated with a linear structure representing the intussusceptum leading into the area of fat density. This latter area represents the invaginated fat. Other CT features include a stratified pattern caused by differential attenuation of mesenteric fat, luminal air, and layers of bowel wall (Fig. 23-32).

62. How do you differentiate between an idiopathic small bowel intussusception from that caused by a mass in adults?
The idiopathic enteroenteric intussusception is usually shorter in length (less than 3.5 cm) and smaller in diameter (less than 3.5 cm).

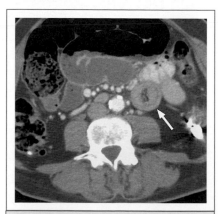

Figure 23-32. Idiopathic transient jejunal intussusception *(arrow)*. A middle-aged man with abdominal pain, treated conservatively. A follow-up barium small bowel examination and a CT scan after a few days showed interval resolution of the intussusception and no intestinal abnormalities.

63. List the types of internal hernias. Which one is the most common?

Internal hernias are rare and represent herniation of bowel through a normal or abnormal aperture within the peritoneal cavity. Symptoms range from intermittent pain to complete obstruction. Paraduodenal hernias represent 50-75% of internal hernias and are usually on the left side. The other types are pericecal, intersigmoid, transmesenteric, and hernias through the foramen of Winslow. Internal hernias can also occur through adhesions and are a radiologic challenge.

64. Describe the left paraduodenal hernia and its CT appearance.

Herniation of the small bowel through a congenital defect in the descending mesocolon situated just to the left of the fourth portion of the duodenum, called the paraduodenal fossa (fossa of Landzert). The lateral margin of this fossa is delineated anteriorly by the inferior mesenteric vein and the ascending left colic artery. The herniated small bowel extends behind the descending mesocolon. On CT, it appears as a cluster of small bowel loops situated between the stomach and pancreatic tail or behind the pancreatic tail. There is usually mass effect on the posterior wall of the stomach and the descending colon. Look for signs of ischemia, such as vascular engorgement, bowel wall thickening, abnormal bowel enhancement, and free fluid (Fig. 23-33).

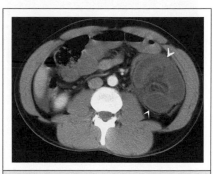

Figure 23-33. Left paraduodenal hernia, surgically proven. Note the clustered small bowel loops in the left side of the abdomen with a hernia sac formed by the descending mesocolon (*arrowheads*).

65. Describe the right paraduodenal hernia and its CT appearance.

Herniation of small bowel through a rare congenital defect called the mesentericoparietal fossa (fossa of Waldeyer) situated just inferior to the third portion of the duodenum and behind the SMA. The herniated bowel is entrapped behind the ascending mesocolon. CT scans demonstrate a cluster of herniated small bowel loops situated lateral and inferior to the second portion of the duodenum in a retroperitoneal location. The SMA can be seen stretched anteriorly to the hernia. Look for any possible signs of ischemia.

66. Describe the transmesenteric hernia and its CT appearance.

Accounts for 5–10% of all internal hernias and is the most common internal hernia in infants. In this age group, it is due to a congenital defect in the mesentery near the ileocecal valve or the ligament of Treitz.

In adults it is due to an acquired defect in the mesentery or omentum and is more common after Roux-en-Y anastomosis. In both the congenital and the acquired types, there is no hernia sac and there is a high incidence of bowel obstruction and ischemia. CT demonstrates signs of closed loop obstruction, with possible vascular engorgement and ischemia. CT may also show clustered small bowel loops positioned at the periphery of the abdomen not covered by omental fat. Causes mass effect on adjacent bowel and mesenteric vessels. Look for signs of obstruction with strangulation including volvulus and the whirl sign.

67. What is closed loop obstruction? What are the CT findings?

Closed loop obstruction is the most common cause of bowel strangulation. The bowel is obstructed at two points along its course. It is caused mostly by an adhesive band or less commonly by an internal hernia or external hernia. When the involved segment of bowel is positioned horizontally a C-shaped, U-shaped, or "coffee bean" configuration can be seen on CT, which is considered a classic sign. The mesenteric vessels appear converging toward the twisted site of obstruction. A beak sign or a whirl sign can be seen at the site of obstruction. The obstructed closed loop is usually filled with fluid. Look for vascular engorgement, mesenteric edema, and fluid as signs of vascular compromise (Fig. 23-34).

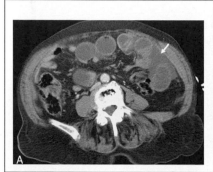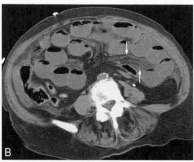

Figure 23-34. Closed loop obstruction. A 75-year-old woman who presented with small bowel obstruction (SBO) associated with leukocytosis and pain. **A,** CT scan shows dilated small bowel with thick walls and mesenteric fluid *(arrow)*. **B,** Unenhanced CT performed 24 hours after A as the patient's conditions worsened. It shows increased intestinal dilatation with increased vascular engorgement and mesenteric edema *(arrows)*. A closed loop obstruction with strangulation caused by adhesions was found during surgery. A necrotic segment of bowel 60 cm long was resected.

68. Define small bowel strangulation and describe its CT findings.

Strangulation is obstructed bowel associated with vascular compromise and resulting in bowel ischemia. Careful analysis of the scan should be made to search for signs of strangulation. The reported prevalence is 5–42% of cases. The CT criteria are as follows:

- Portal or mesenteric venous gas, pneumatosis (late finding)
- Abnormal bowel wall enhancement
- Serrated beak sign
- Unusual mesenteric vascular course
- Diffuse mesenteric vascular engorgement and haziness
- Bowel wall thickening
- Ascites and fluid within the mesentery (highly suspicious finding)

Some of the previous findings can be found in simple obstruction. It is therefore important to discuss the CT results with the clinician.

There are four important clinical signs of strangulation: abdominal tenderness, tachycardia, fever, and leukocytosis. With equivocal CT results, the presence of three or more of these clinical signs is highly suspicious of strangulation.

69. What is the SMA syndrome?

It is characterized by compression of the third, or transverse, portion of the duodenum against the aorta by the SMA, resulting in chronic, intermittent, or acute complete or partial duodenal obstruction. It is seen with marked weight loss, anorexia nervosa, and total body casting. Upper GI series demonstrate a vertical impression on the duodenum caused by the narrow space between the SMA and the aorta. CT reveals dilatation of the duodenum proximal to the SMA. The SMA-aortic distance at the level of the aorta is less than 8 mm. However, this finding alone is not diagnostic and should be correlated with the barium studies and clinical examination (Fig. 23-35).

BIBLIOGRAPHY

1. Ba-Ssallameh A, Prokop M, Uffmann M, et al: Dedicated multidetector CT of the stomach: Spectrum of diseases. Radiographics 23:625–644, 2003.

2. Blachar A, Federle, MP, Dodson SF: Internal hernia: Clinical and imaging findings in 17 patients with emphasis on CT criteria. Radiology 218:68–74, 2001.

3. Buckley JB, Jones B, Fishman EK: Small bowel cancer: Imaging features and staging. Radiol Clin North Am 35:381–402, 1997.

4. Chou CK: CT manifestations of bowel ischemia. AJR 178:87–91, 2002.

5. Fidivi SA, Klein SA: Emphysematous gastritis. Applied Radiology on line. 2002, p 31.

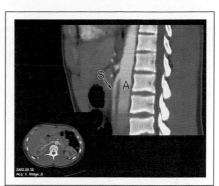

Figure 23-35. SMA syndrome. A 19-year old man with known SMA syndrome who is also hypertensive. CT angiogram is performed to evaluate the renal arteries, which appeared normal (not shown). The SMA-aortic distance is measured on the sagittal images at 5.6 mm. S = superior mesenteric artery, A = aorta.

6. Fuchsjager MH: The small bowel feces sign. Radiology 225:378–379, 2002.

7. Furukawa A, Yamasaki M, Furuichi K, et al: Helical CT in the diagnosis of small bowel obstruction. Radiographics 21:341–355, 2001.

8. Gore RM, Levine MS, Ghahremani GG, et al: Gastric cancer: Clinical and pathologic features. Radiol Clin North Am 35:295–310, 1997.

9. Gore RM, Levine MS, et al: Gastric cancer: Radiologic diagnosis. Radiol Clin North Am 35:311–329, 1997.

10. Horton KM: CT examination of mesenteric vessels and small bowel. Appl Radiol Suppl:45–53, 2004.

11. Horton KM, Fishman EK: Current role of CT in imaging of the stomach. Radiographics 23:75–87, 2003.

12. Joeng YK, et al: Gastrointestinal involvement in Henoch-Schönlein syndrome: CT findings. AJR 168:965–968, 1997.

13. Kalantari BN, Mortele KJ, Cantisani V, et al: CT features with pathologic correlation of acute gastrointestinal graft-versus-host disease after bone marrow transplantation in adults. AJR 181:1621–1625, 2003.

14. Khurana B: The whirl sign. Radiology 226:69–70, 2003.

15. Konen E, Amitai M, Apter S: CT angiography of superior mesenteric artery syndrome. AJR 171:1279–1281, 1998.

16. Levy AD, Hobbs CM: From the archives of the AFIP: Meckel diverticulum: Radiologic features with pathologic correlation. Radiographics 24:565–587, 2004.

17. Macari MM, Balthazar EJ: CT of bowel wall thickening: Significance and pitfalls of interpretation. AJR 176:1105–111, 2001.

18. Madureira AJ: The comb sign. Radiology 230:783–784, 2004.

19. Manganiotis AN, Banner MP, Malkowicz SB: Urologic complications of Crohn's disease. Surg Clin North Am 81:197–215, 2001.

20. Miller FH, Kochman ML, et al: Gastric cancer: Radiologic staging. Radiol Clin North Am 35:331–349, 1997.

21. Mirvis SE, Shanmuganathan K, Erb R: Diffuse small bowel ischemia in hypotensive adults after blunt trauma (shock bowel): CT findings and clinical significance. AJR 163:1375–1379, 1994.

22. Muldowney SM, Balfe DM, et al: Acute fat deposition in bowel wall submucosa CT appearance. J. Comput Assist Tomogr 19:390–393, 1995.

23. Wiesner W, Khurana B, et al: CT of acute bowel ischemia. Radiology 226:635–650, 2003.

24. Wood PB, Fletcher JG, et al: Assessment of small bowel Crohn disease: Noninvasive peroral CT enterography compared with other imaging methods and endoscopy—feasibility study. Radiology 229:275–281, 2003.

CHAPTER 24

COLON AND APPENDIX

Vikram Dogra, MD, and Joseph Crawford, MD

1. **What are the four most common pathologic conditions affecting the colon?**
   - Neoplasm
   - Diverticular disease
   - Inflammatory bowel disease
   - Appendicitis

2. **What are typical technical factors (scan parameters) employed in CT scanning of the abdomen?**
   At our institution, CT abdominal scan parameters include the following:
   - Tube voltage of 120 kV
   - 200–250mAs
   - 750-msec rotation time
   - 5-mm collimation
   - 6.5-mm slice thickness
   - 3.2-mm slice increment

3. **What contrast agents are used in CT scanning of the large bowel?**
   To visualize the large bowel, contrast materials must be given to opacify the bowel lumen. Iodinated contrast agents or dilute mixtures of barium are equally effective. Pre-CT preparation of the bowel by use of clear liquid diet is also helpful. Oral contrast agents are given 30–60 minutes prior to scanning of the abdomen. Earlier administration of these agents, in divided dosages, results in more complete bowel opacification.

   Typically, 500–600 mL of 3% dilute diatrizoate meglumine (or dilute 2% barium solution) is given orally. An enema of water or dilute iodinated contrast material is used at some sites when colonic disease is suspected.

4. **Discuss the use of rectal contrast material in CT examination of the bowel.**
   Rectally administered contrast material is useful in evaluation of mucosal disease in the colon and rectum. Agents that have been used include dilute diatrizoate meglumine, water, room air, carbon dioxide gas, and methylcellulose solution. Air or carbon dioxide are particularly helpful in distending the properly cleansed colon to detect small polyps and small masses. Water or air contrast should be used when performing CT angiography, because positive contrast agents (such as water-soluble iodinated agents) can interfere with data manipulation. Iodinated contrast agents should be used rectally if a colonic fistula or bowel perforation is suspected.

5. **What is the role of intravenous contrast in large bowel evaluation?**
   Intravenous contrast agents are used to opacify blood vessels, to detect solid organ metastases and abscesses, and to evaluate the relative vascularity of the abdominal viscera. Intravenous contrast often does not contribute when evaluating the bowel, especially if positive (dense) oral contrast has been used.

   Low-osmolar iodinated agents are preferable, due to their lower incidence of adverse reactions. The time of scanning with respect to the time of infusion of these intravenous agents is of importance and must be tailored to the organ in question.

6. **What is the third source of contrast that helps evaluate the large bowel?**
The patient's inherent intraperitoneal fat. Intra-abdominal fat sets off wall thickening, adenopathy, and inflammatory changes. Diverticulitis and appendicitis in particular are often revealed by inflammatory changes in the adjacent fat. The diagnosis of extraserosal spread of colon cancer depends on pericolonic fat. Bowel imaging is more difficult in the cachectic, pediatric, or extremely edematous patient.

7. **What is the relative radiation dose to the patient in CT scanning of the abdomen, as compared with the radiation dose from a typical chest radiograph?**
The radiation dose for one abdominal CT scan has been reported to be equivalent to that for 100–250 chest radiographs. Therefore, only CT studies that are medically indicated should be performed.

8. **Describe the anatomic features of the appendix.**
The vermiform appendix is a tubular structure, measuring from 2–20 cm in length, mean length of 8 cm, arising from what was originally the apex of the cecum, and is situated along the medial aspect of the cecum about 2 cm caudal to the ileocecal valve. "Vermiform" means *wormlike*. It may project in any of several directions, including caudally over the pelvic brim, medially and cranially toward the root of the mesentery, or medially anterior to the ileum, but in two thirds of cases it projects into the retrocecal space.

9. **How is the appendix localized on CT?**
The appendix is located between 1 and 4 cm inferior to the ileocecal valve on the medial wall of the cecum. If the cecum is displaced or malrotated, the appendix may be located laterally. In the absence of intraperitoneal fat, the appendix may be difficult to identify.

10. **How is acute appendicitis evaluated on CT scanning?**
The classic CT findings in acute appendicitis include an abnormal appearance of the appendix, measuring greater than 6 mm in diameter, which exhibits a thickened, enhancing wall, associated with periappendiceal inflammation and cecal changes (Fig. 24-1). The latter include regional fat stranding and/or abscess formation. Finding an appendicolith (Fig. 24-2) supports the diagnosis but is not by itself diagnostic. An appendicolith was more important in the pre-CT era, when plain films seldom showed the appendicitis directly.

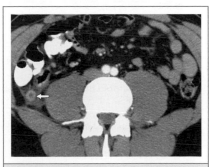

Figure 24-1. Appendicitis. Axial contrast enhanced CT demonstrates an enlarged appendix *(arrow)* with thickened, enhancing walls and periappendiceal inflammatory changes.

11. **How accurate is CT scanning in establishing the diagnosis of acute appendicitis?**
Helical CT scanning is reported to be 98% sensitive, 97% specific, and 97.6% accurate in diagnosing acute appendicitis.

12. **What is mucocele of appendix?**
Mucocele of the appendix is the abnormal accumulation of mucus in the lumen of the appendix, usually due to obstruction of the appendiceal lumen. Causes of such obstruction may include mucosal hyperplasia, cystadenoma, or cystadenocarcinoma. This entity appears as a

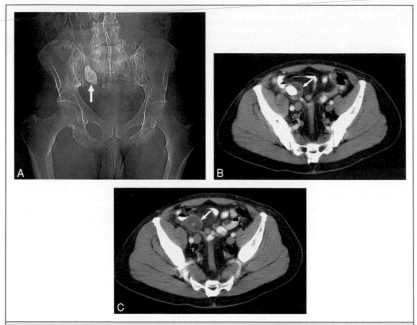

Figure 24-2. Appendicolith. *A*, Plain film demonstrates a large calcific density in the right lower quadrant *(arrow)*. *B* and *C*, Corresponding CT images reveal an enlarged appendix with a large appendicolith within it *(arrows)*.

low-attenuation, encapsulated mass, with smooth, regular walls. It may be distinguished from acute appendicitis by the absence of local inflammatory changes or abscess.

13. **What is carcinoid tumor of the appendix?**
    Carcinoid tumors are rare neuroendocrine tumors that can arise anywhere in the body. Approximately 90% arise in the gastrointestinal (GI) tract. Of all carcinoids, approximately 80% involve the appendix and 20% involve the small bowel, mainly the ileum. Small bowel carcinoids have a tendency to invade the mesentery, which frequently incites an intense desmoplastic reaction, leading to focal deformities of the bowel wall, with kinking and bowel obstruction. Another feature of mesenteric invasion is the formation of a mesenteric mass, causing rigidity of bowel loops. One may also see sharp angulation of a bowel loop or a spoke-wheel arrangement of adjacent loops of small bowel.

14. **Discuss the urine test for carcinoid tumor.**
    Serotonin, elaborated by carcinoid tumors, is metabolized to 5-hydroxy indoleacetic acid (5-HIAA). Urinary 5-HIAA is increased in a number of disease states, including midgut, foregut, and ovarian carcinoid tumors, but also in celiac sprue, tropical sprue, Whipple's disease, and oat cell tumors of the bronchus. The test is useful clinically for the detection of metastatic carcinoid and for the evaluation of flushing attacks.

15. **Describe appendiceal carcinoma.**
    Carcinomas of the appendix are usually well-differentiated adenocarcinomas that tend to produce *pseudomyxoma peritonei* and do not metastasize until late in the disease.

Adenocarcinomas of the appendix are rare (approximately 0.2 cases/100,000/year) and are almost invariably discovered only during pathologic examination of a surgical specimen (Fig. 24-3). Of importance is the high incidence of synchronous colorectal cancer associated with *all* appendiceal tumors, including carcinoids, benign tumors, secondary malignancies, and primary malignancies (89% in the latter).

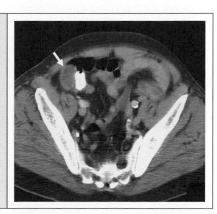

Figure 24-3. Appendiceal carcinoma. Axial CT image demonstrates a dilated appendix *(arrow)* in a patient with right lower quadrant abdominal pain. The appendix was resected, and pathologic examination revealed adenocarcinoma of the appendix.

16. **What is epiploic appendagitis? How is it diagnosed with CT?**

    Epiploic appendices are small peritoneal sacs, filled with vessels and fat, that protrude from the serosal side of the colon. These may become inflamed due to torsion or venous thrombosis and can become clinically painful. The diagnosis of epiploic appendagitis may be made on CT by the findings of discrete, pericolonic collections of fat density, associated with periappendageal fat stranding. Local thickening of adjacent parietal peritoneum and possible mass effect can also be seen.

17. **Give a brief summary of the anatomy of the colon.**

    The ascending and transverse colon are derived from the embryologic midgut and are supplied by branches of the superior mesenteric artery (SMA). The descending colon is derived from the hindgut and is perfused by branches of the inferior mesenteric artery, as are the sigmoid colon and the rectum. The ascending and the descending colon are retroperitoneal in position and are situated in the anterior pararenal spaces. The transverse colon is intraperitoneal and is attached to the mesocolon, which accounts for its relative mobility. The sigmoid colon is intraperitoneal and attaches to the sigmoid mesentery.

18. **What is volvulus of the colon?**

    A volvulus is twisting of a portion of colon on its mesenteric axis, resulting in partial or complete mechanical obstruction of the bowel and frequently resulting in vascular compromise of the affected bowel segment.

19. **What colon segments can be involved in volvulus?**

    Any colon segment that possesses a mesentery can be subject to volvulus. This ordinarily includes the cecum, transverse colon, and the sigmoid colon. In cases of anomalous elongation of the mesentery of the descending colon, volvulus of that colonic segment may occur.

20. **What is the most common type of colonic volvulus?**

    Sigmoid volvulus is the most common form of volvulus of the GI tract and is said to be the cause of 8% of mechanical bowel obstructions. This entity is more common in the aged, and predisposing factors include chronic constipation and megacolon.

21. **What are the radiographic findings in sigmoid volvulus?**
    Barium enema (unless contraindicated by symptoms of peritonitis or the finding of free peritoneal air) reveals obstruction at the rectosigmoid junction. Radiographically, one finds one or two dilated loops of colon, frequently directed upward into the right upper abdomen, with tapering limbs directed into the lower right side of the abdomen. Findings of small bowel obstruction are common.

22. **What are the radiographic findings in cecal volvulus?**
    In cecal volvulus (torsion of the ascending colon), one frequently finds a grossly dilated cecum that extends from the right lower quadrant to the epigastrium or the left upper quadrant (Fig. 24-4). The distal large bowel is relatively empty. Signs of small bowel obstruction are usually present. A single-contrast barium enema is helpful in cases of uncertainty.

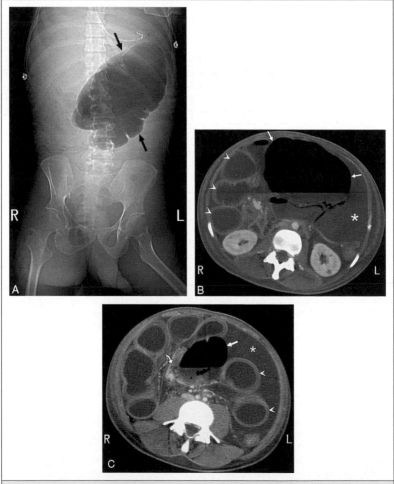

Figure 24-4. Cecal volvulus. **A,** Plain abdominal film demonstrates a large distended cecum occupying the left middle and upper abdomen *(arrows)* secondary to clockwise twisting of cecal mesentery. **B** and **C,** Corresponding CT images reveal CT appearance of cecal volvulus *(arrows)* with evidence of distended proximal small bowel loops *(arrowheads)* and ascites (*). The twist of the cecal mesentery *(curved arrow)* can be seen in C.

Cecal volvulus is of two types: the **axial rotation type** (two thirds of cases) and the **cecal bascule** type. In the latter case, the cecum folds itself anterior and medial to the ascending colon and forms a flap-valve occlusion at the site of folding. This can be associated with marked distension of the cecum, which may be localized in the center of the abdomen.

23. **What is the role of CT in the diagnosis of colonic volvulus?**
CT may clarify the site of obstruction and is helpful in distinguishing mechanical obstruction from adynamic ileus. CT may also find signs of bowel ischemia that may not be apparent with plain radiographs, including bowel wall thickening and infiltration of mesenteric fat. CT is also helpful in finding free peritoneal air, portal venous gas or *pneumatosis intestinalis*.

24. **What is coffee bean sign?**
The coffee bean sign is a plain film sign of sigmoid volvulus. It is also seen on the frontal scout for the CT and on coronal reformats. The air-filled sigmoid looks like a giant coffee bean as it folds back on itself.

25. **What is the whirl sign? How is it helpful in diagnosing volvulus?**
The whirl sign is a sign of intestinal volvulus and consists of a soft tissue mass with an appearance of swirling strands of soft tissue and fat attenuation, simulating the form of a hurricane on a weather map. Originally described as a finding in midgut volvulus, it is now recognized as a non-specific sign of large or small bowel volvulus. It occurs when afferent and efferent loops of bowel rotate about a point of obstruction, resulting in twisted mesentery along the axis of rotation.

26. **What diseases should be considered if a colon mass is found on CT examination?**
   - Polypoid disease
   - Colon neoplasm
   - Mucocele
   - Hematoma
   - Infection

27. **What are typical CT findings in carcinoma of the colon?**
Focal thickening of the bowel wall (Figs. 24-5 and 24-6), irregular luminal surface of the bowel mucosa, polypoid mass in the bowel lumen, circumferential wall thickening with luminal narrowing, soft tissue densities extending from a colonic mass into pericolic fat, regional adenopathy, and metastatic liver or adrenal disease are typical findings.

28. **Other than adenocarcinoma, what neoplastic diseases present as a colon mass on CT examination?**
   - Lymphoma
   - Metastases to the colon
   - Carcinoid
   - Mesenchymal tumor

Colonic lymphoma is uncommon but has an increased prevalence in immunocompromised patients. Non-Hodgkin lymphoma is the most prevalent form of colonic lymphoma, and the cecum and the rectum are the most common sites of involvement. The CT appearance of the bowel may be nonspecific in that entity, but four forms are described: infiltrative, polypoid, cavitary, and diffuse. Associated findings in colon lymphoma may include mesenteric adenopathy, cavitation, and splenomegaly.

Metastases to the colon are frequently serosal implants due to peritoneal seeding, but other routes of involvement include hematogenous spread, direct extension, and lymphatic spread. An important pathway of metastasis to the transverse colon is from pancreatic or gastric carcinoma that extends via the mesenteric reflection.

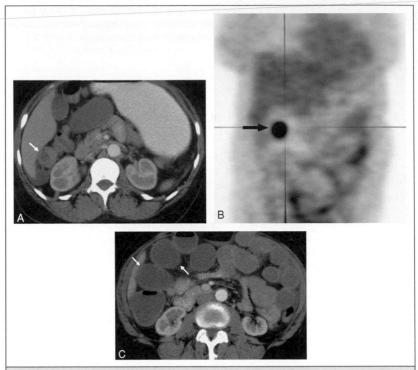

Figure 24-5. Colon carcinoma. **A,** Axial CT reveals thickening of ascending colon *(arrow)*, confirmed by fluro-2-deoxy-D-glucose (FDG) uptake on positron emission tomography (PET) scan *(arrow)* seen in B, resulting in small bowel obstruction *(C, arrows)*. This was confirmed to be an adenocarcinoma of colon.

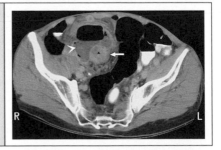

Figure 24-6. Ulcerated colon carcinoma. CT of pelvis reveals a large abscess *(arrowhead)* with an air-fluid level with thickened sigmoid colon *(arrow)*. This appearance is suggestive of ulcerated colonic carcinoma.

29. Describe CT colonography.

CT colonography is under active development and shows promise for the noninvasive detection of intraluminal colon disease. It is a CT air enema designed to see the bowel mucosa for detection of polyps and cancer. Air or carbon dioxide is insufflated into the bowel to get good distension. Acquisition requires thin slices and thus a multidetector scanner. Acquisition is both prone and supine.

Thorough bowel cleansing is the key. Fecal tagging with oral barium (to make residual feces dense) is used at some sites. Bowel-relaxing agents such as glucagon or Buscopan are often used to get better distension and reduce patient discomfort.

The acquired data are initially evaluated for any intraluminal abnormalities. If the initial images are of adequate quality, postprocessing techniques are applied and the images are displayed in any of several workstation formats, including virtual colonoscopy.

30. What is virtual colonoscopy?

Virtual colonoscopy is a display technique that combines endoscopic viewing with cross-sectional imaging and simulating the endoscopist's view of the bowel lumen. Viewing is done in both antegrade and retrograde directions, to view both sides of each haustral fold. The term *virtual* colonoscopy is often used synonymously with *CT colonography,* but in fact it is only one viewing tool.

31. With current techniques, how sensitive is CT colonography in the detection of colonic polyps?

The sensitivity and specificity of this technique vary with the prevalence of polyp disease in the population under study and are related to polyp size. For polyps measuring 10 mm or larger, sensitivities of 82–93% have been reported, with specificities in the range of 90–97%. For polyps measuring 5 mm or smaller, sensitivities in the range of 3–12% are reported. American College of Radiology Imaging Network (ACRIN) is sponsoring a multi-center trial of virtual colonoscopy for colon cancer screening.

32. What pathophysiologic changes are associated with acute diverticulitis of the colon?

Diverticula are small outpouchings of mucosa and submucosa through the muscularis of the colonic wall. These occur primarily in the descending colon and the sigmoid. Whenever the neck of a diverticula becomes occluded, inflammation can set in, causing erosion and perforation of the mucosa and submucosa, resulting in pericolonic inflammation, microabscess, or frank abscess and gross perforation.

33. What are the characteristic CT findings in acute diverticulitis?

Local colonic wall thickening in the presence of diverticula, pericolonic fat stranding (Fig. 24-7), fluid accumulation in the root of the mesentery locally, and dilatation and engorgement of mesenteric vessels, a finding termed the "centipede sign." Acute diverticulitis is mainly a disease of the left colon; fewer than 5% of cases involve the right colon. Diverticulitis of the transverse colon is uncommon.

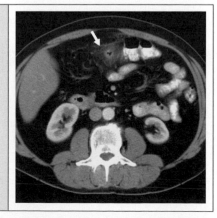

Figure 24-7. Diverticulitis. Axial CT image demonstrates bowel wall thickening with pericolonic stranding *(arrow)* suggestive of acute diverticulitis.

34. **What are the diagnostic implications of the findings of fat stranding associated with thickening of the colonic wall, in the clinical setting of acute abdominal pain?**
These findings indicate a GI etiology of the patient's pain. When the fat stranding is disproportionately prominent relative to the colonic wall thickening, consider an extraluminal or mesenteric-centered etiology of disease, such as appendicitis, omental infarction, epiploic appendagitis, or diverticulitis.

35. **What are the typical CT findings in inflammatory bowel disease?**
Bowel wall thickening, pericolonic stranding, ascites, and bowel wall nodularity. In distinguishing between the various types of inflammatory disease, reliance is placed on the distribution of the pathologic findings within the bowel, the degree of wall thickening, and the clinical setting.

36. **What are the CT findings in *Clostridium difficile* colitis?**
Pseudomembranous colitis is a severe inflammatory disorder related to overgrowth of *C. difficile* following antibiotic use. Typical clinical presentations include watery diarrhea, fever, and leukocytosis. CT findings in this entity are not sensitive (52% sensitivity in one study of 54 patients) but when present are specific: marked bowel wall thickening (Fig. 24-8), usually greater than 10 mm, evidence of mucosal and submucosal edema, ascites, and the "accordion sign." The rectum and sigmoid colon are typically involved.

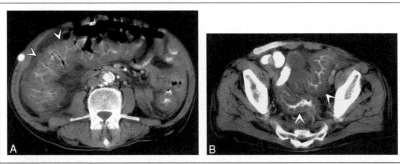

Figure 24-8. Pseudomembranous *(Clostridium difficile)* colitis. *A* and *B*, Axial CT images demonstrate marked bowel wall thickening *(arrowheads)* and the "accordion sign."

37. **What is the accordion sign?**
Alternating edematous, nodular haustral folds, interposed with transverse ridges filled with contrast material, resulting in an appearance suggesting a collapsed accordion *(see* Fig. 24-8).

KEY POINTS: COLON AND APPENDIX

1. If the appendix is not obvious, locate the tip of the cecum and search around it.

2. When you consider bowel ischemia, look at the supplying vessels for occlusion.

3. Perforated colon carcinoma can mimic diverticulitis with thickened bowel and pericolonic stranding. Look for the offending diverticulum itself. Do a follow-up colonoscopy when the patient has recovered if it is not clearly diverticulitis.

4. In bowel obstruction, the distal bowel is seldom totally evacuated.

38. **What are the CT scan findings in Crohn's colitis?**

Bowel wall thickening, skip areas, obstruction, and fistula formation. Abdominal ascites is uncommon in Crohn's colitis, and, if found, raises the possibility of an alternate entity, such as infectious (e.g., *C. difficile* or tuberculous) or ischemic colitis.

39. **Is liver disease associated with colonic wall thickening?**

Approximately one third of patients with severe hepatic cirrhosis exhibit colonic wall thickening In two thirds of these patients, the thickening is limited to the right colon. Colonic wall thickening usually subsides following liver transplantation and is believed to be related to changes in colonic blood flow and hydrostatic pressures due to portal hypertension.

40. **In cases of nonpenetrating abdominal trauma, what are common CT findings of bowel injury?**

Extraluminal oral contrast material, bowel discontinuity, extraluminal air, bowel wall thickening, bowel wall enhancement, mesenteric infiltration ("stranding"), and intraperitoneal or retroperitoneal fluid accumulation. In the setting of blunt abdominal trauma, free fluid in the absence of demonstrated injury to the solid visceral organs suggests bowel injury.

41. **What are common causes of bowel ischemia?**

SMA arterial occlusion due to thrombus or embolism, decreased cardiac output, hypotension, decreased flow states due to arterial or venous disease, mechanical bowel obstruction due to hernia (Fig. 24-9) or adhesions, neoplasm with mesenteric invasion, vasculitis, inflammatory bowel or mesenteric disease, trauma, chemotherapy, and radiation therapy can all result in bowel ischemia.

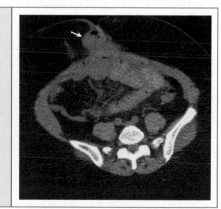

Figure 24-9. Incarcerated hernia of the colon *(arrow).*

42. **What are common CT findings in bowel ischemia?**

In the case of arterial insufficiency without reperfusion, CT shows thinning of the bowel wall with poor enhancement. With infarction of the mucosa and submucosa, bacteria proliferate and gas can enter the bowel wall and ultimately the portal venous system and the liver.

In the case of transient arterial insufficiency with reperfusion of the bowel, various degrees of mucosal and submucosal enhancement may be present. There is frequently wall thickening due to passage of water and/or red blood cells into the intramural space, which can result in a thumbprinting appearance. Fluid may accumulate in the bowel lumen (Fig. 24-10).

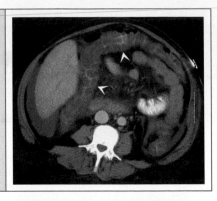

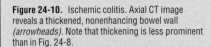

Figure 24-10. Ischemic colitis. Axial CT image reveals a thickened, nonenhancing bowel wall *(arrowheads)*. Note that thickening is less prominent than in Fig. 24-8.

43.   What is graft-versus-host disease? What are the colon CT scan findings?

This disease may occur after organ transplantation, when lymphoid cells of the donor attack certain cells of the host. This process may be seen anywhere from 1 day and up to 2 months after transplantation. The frequent initial clinical manifestation is that of a skin rash, but subsequent sites of involvement include the liver and the gut, including both the small bowel and the colon.

In cases of small bowel involvement, one finds multiple fluid-filled loops of bowel, with enhancing layer of bowel wall mucosa, which may later be replaced with granulation tissue.

CT findings in the colon include luminal narrowing, wall thickening, and stasis of contrast coating in the bowel wall. The scan findings are not distinguishable from those of viral enteritis.

Additional CT findings in this entity include small bowel wall thickening, engorgement of the vasa recta adjacent to affected bowel segments, fat stranding of the mesentery, bowel dilatation proximal to thickened bowel wall segments, abdominal ascites, periportal edema, and, occasionally, serosal enhancement.

BIBLIOGRAPHY

1. Dodd GD, Dodds WJ, Mahieu PG, et al: Colon. In Margulis AR, Burhenne HJ (eds): Practical Alimentary Tract Radiology, 5th ed. St. Louis, Mosby, 1993, pp 221–291.

2. Feldman D: The coffee bean sign. Radiology 216:178–179, 2000.

3. Ha HK, Kim JK: The gastrointestinal tract. In Haaga JR, Lanzieri CF, Gilkeson RC (eds): CT and MR Imaging of the Whole Body, Vol 2, 4th ed. St. Louis, Mosby, 2003, pp 1154–1269.

4. Johnson CD: The National CT Colonography Trial. ACRIN Protocol 6664.

5. Raman SS, Lu DS, Kadell BM, et al: Accuracy of nonfocused helical CT for the diagnosis of acute appendicitis: A 5-year review. Am J Roentgenol 78:1319–1325, 2002.

CHAPTER 25

CT IMAGING OF THE LIVER

Srinivasa R. Prasad, MD, and Kedar Chintapalli, MD

1. How does the liver develop embryologically?

The liver develops as an endodermal diverticulum of the primitive foregut that forms the duodenum. While the cranial portion of the diverticulum forms the liver, the caudal portion develops into the gallbladder and biliary system. The liver capsule is derived from the surrounding mesoderm.

2. Explain the segmental anatomy of the liver.

According to the Couinaud classification system, the liver is divided into eight segments, each supplied by a central vasculobiliary sheath (Fig. 25-1). Segment I is the caudate lobe. The right liver segments (V, VI, VII, VIII) are separated from the left liver segments (II, III, IV) by the middle hepatic vein. The anterior (V, VIII) and the posterior (VI, VII) right liver segments are separated by a plane containing the right hepatic vein. Superior (VII, VIII) and inferior (V, VI) right liver segments are separated by an axial plane containing the horizontal portion of the right portal vein. Segment III is separated from the segment IV by the falciform ligament.

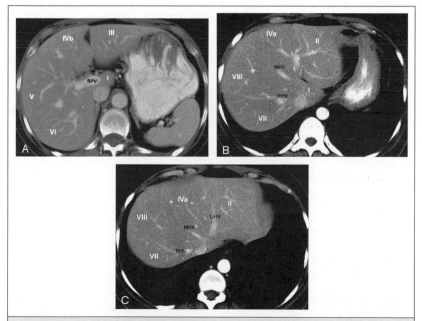

Figure 25-1. A–C, CT segmental anatomy of the liver: Couinaud classification system. Hepatic veins and portal vein branches divide the liver into eight segments, each supplied by a central vasculobiliary sheath. RHV = right hepatic vein, MHV = middle hepatic vein, LHV= left hepatic vein, RPV = right portal vein, horizontal portion.

3. **What is the clinical relevance of the Couinaud classification system?**
The knowledge of segmental anatomy is crucial in planning hepatic surgeries, including tumor resection and transplantation.

4. **What is the "bare area" of the liver?**
The bare area of the liver the portion of the liver that is not covered by the peritoneum. The bare area lies between the anterior-superior and the posterior-inferior layers of the coronary ligament.

5. **How is the liver perfused?**
The liver derives 70–80% of its blood supply from the portal vein; the hepatic artery contributes 20–30% of hepatic blood flow.

6. **What are the advantages of multidetector CT in the evaluation of the liver?**
Due to faster z-axis speed, better anatomic coverage, and improved longitudinal resolution, multidetector CT permits multiphase imaging in a single breath-hold. While allowing faster injection rates, it is ideally for imaging the liver during different vascular phases.

7. **What are the advantages and disadvantages of fast rates (>3 mL/sec) of contrast injection?**
Faster injection shortens the injection duration and shortens the time to peak liver enhancement, thereby permitting faster scanning. Also, it is possible to reduce contrast volume injected. Disadvantages include increased potential for contrast extravasation and physiologic complications.

8. **What determines how bright the liver looks on contrast-enhanced CT?**
The iodine load mainly determines peak liver enhancement. The other factors impacting liver enhancement include patient size, blood volume, cardiovascular physiology, and hepatic conditions.

9. **What are the phases of hepatic enhancement at helical CT?**
   - Arterial phase (18–35 seconds after contrast injection)
   - Portal venous phase (60-second delay)
   - Equilibrium phase (100-second delay)

10. **What is the portal-inflow phase?**
Also referred to as late arterial phase (approximately 35-second delay), the portal-inflow phase is the optimal phase for detecting hypervascular tumors that are fed by hepatic artery branches (e.g., hepatoma, neuroendocrine metastases). The early arterial phase (approximately 20-second delay) provides exquisite CT angiographic data.

11. **What tumors are best seen during portal venous phase?**
Most hepatic metastases (metastases from breast, lung, colon) and lymphomas are hypovascular and are best depicted during portal venous phase (Fig. 25-2).

12. **What is THAD? How do THADs appear on CT?**
THAD is an acronym for **t**ransient **h**epatic **a**ttenuation **d**ifference. THAD refers to sectoral or lobar parenchymal enhancement during arterial phase imaging. They are typically peripheral and wedge-shaped with a straight border (Fig. 25-3).

13. **What causes THAD?**
THAD can result from a variety of causes:
   - Increase in arterial inflow (hypervascular focal lesions, inflammation of adjacent organs, aberrant arterial supply)
   - Portal hypoperfusion
   - Hepatic venous thrombosis

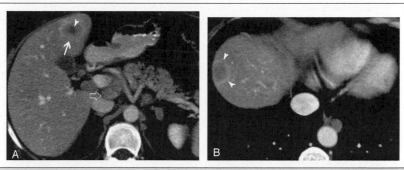

Figure 25-2. *A,* Liver metastasis. Metastatic breast adenocarcinoma to the liver showing low-density center *(arrowhead)* and peripheral rim enhancement *(arrow).* Note the metastatic lymphadenopathy *(open arrow).* *B,* Colon cancer metastasis. Peripheral rim enhancement during portal venous phase imaging *(arrowheads).*

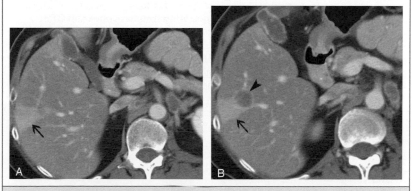

Figure 25-3. *A* and *B,* Transient hepatic attenuation difference (THAD). Contrast-enhanced computed tomography (CECT) shows a peripheral, wedge-shaped hyperattenuation focus *(arrow)* distal to a metastasis *(arrowhead).*

14. **What are the causes of portal venous gas?**

    Causes of portal venous system gas include bowel ischemia/infarction, abdominal sepsis, bowel obstruction, necrotizing pancreatitis, perforated stomach, diverticulitis, inflammatory bowel disease, trauma, and colonoscopy.

15. **What are the causes of air in the biliary system?**

    Causes of pneumobilia (biliary air) include biliary-enteric anastomosis, biliary procedures, endoscopic retrograde cholangiopancreatography (ERCP), biliary-enteric fistulae, infection, trauma, and gallstone ileus.

16. **How do you differentiate portal venous gas from pneumobilia?**

    Air in the biliary tree (pneumobilia) tends to collect in the large bile ducts at the hilum, owing to the centripetal flow of bile. It typically does not extend to within 2 cm of the liver capsule (Fig. 25-4A). Portal venous gas appears as peripheral, subcapsular branching hypodensities in the liver, predominantly in the left lobe because of its ventral location (Fig. 25-4B).

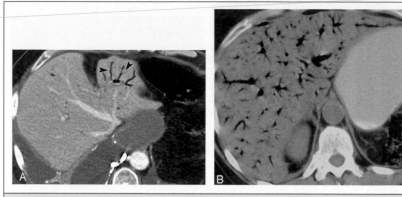

Figure 25-4. *A,* Pneumobilia. Contrast-enhanced computed tomography (CECT) shows biliary air secondary to a surgical anastomosis. *B,* Portal venous air. CECT demonstrates diffuse portal venous gas secondary to bowel infarction.

17. **How does an "injured" liver (blunt/penetrating trauma) appear on CT?**
    Typical lacerations are parallel to hepatic veins or portal vein branches (Fig. 25-5). Contusion appears as a hypodense area with irregular margins (Fig. 25-6). Hematomas are hyperattenuating. Periportal tracking may either be due to blood in periportal tissues or lymphatic congestion likely due to overhydration.

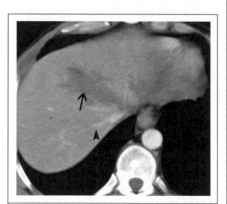

Figure 25-5. Liver laceration. Contrast-enhanced computed tomography (CECT) illustrates a typical traumatic laceration *(arrow)* that parallels the course of the hepatic vein *(arrowhead).*

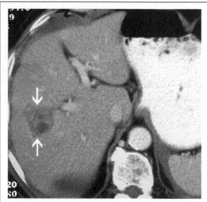

Figure 25-6. Liver contusion. Contrast-enhanced computed tomography (CECT) shows a heterogenous, hypoattenuating contusion *(arrows)* secondary to blunt trauma.

18. **How is liver injury graded by CT?**
    The CT-based grading of hepatic injury is as follows:
    - **Grade 1:** Capsular avulsion, superficial laceration(s) less than 1 cm deep, subcapsular hematoma less than 1 cm in thickness, and periportal blood tracking
    - **Grade 2:** Laceration(s) 1–3 cm deep and central-subcapsular hematoma(s) 1–3 cm in diameter

- **Grade 3:** Laceration greater than 3 cm deep and central-subcapsular hematoma(s) greater than 3 cm in diameter
- **Grade 4:** Massive central subcapsular hematoma greater than 10 cm and lobar tissue destruction (maceration) or devascularization
- **Grade 5:** Bilobar tissue destruction (maceration) or devascularization

19. **What are the types of choledochal cysts?**
    - **Type I:** Diffuse dilation of the extrahepatic bile ducts
    - **Type II:** Saccular diverticulum of the common duct
    - **Type III:** Choledochocele within the wall of the duodenum
    - **Type IVA:** Similar to type I, but in addition intrahepatic ducts are involved
    - **Type IVB:** Multiple dilatations of the extrahepatic ducts and normal intrahepatic ducts
    - **Type V:** Dilatation confined to intrahepatic bile ducts, Caroli's disease

20. **What are the complications of choledochal cysts?**
    Patients with choledochal cysts are predisposed to biliary obstruction, stone formation, cholangitis, and (rarely) development of cholangiocarcinoma.

21. **How do you differentiate Caroli's disease from polycystic liver disease (PLD)?**
    Patients with PLD often present with both hepatic and renal cysts. The liver cysts in PLD are noncommunicating and the intrahepatic biliary ducts are normal (Fig. 25-7).

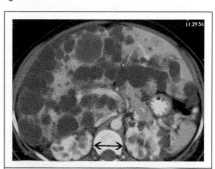

22. **What is central-dot sign?**
    The central-dot sign refers to small enhancing vessels in relation to cystic dilatation of the intrahepatic bile ducts and is suggestive of Caroli's disease.

Figure 25-7. Polycystic liver disease. Contrast-enhanced computed tomography (CECT) demonstrates numerous hepatic cysts in a patient with autosomal dominant polycystic kidney disease *(arrows)*.

23. **What are the CT signs associated with biliary stones?**
    The stone may appear as a central density surrounded by hypoattenuating bile (target sign) (Fig. 25-8). With the rim sign, one can see a faint rim of increased density along the margin of the bile duct. A hyperattenuating calculus that is surrounded by a crescent of low-attenuation bile constitutes the crescent sign. Indirect signs of obstruction, such as ductal narrowing or ductal dilatation, are helpful for the diagnosis of stones.

24. **What percentage of common duct stones are not seen with CT?**
    Fifteen to 25% of stones are isoattenuating with bile and are not detectable on CT.

25. **What are the indications for CT cholangiography?**
    CT cholangiography is useful in patients who require noninvasive evaluation of the biliary

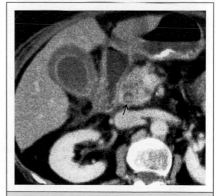

Figure 25-8. Choledocholithiasis. Contrast-enhanced computed tomography (CECT) shows a high-density calculus *(arrow)* within the distal common bile duct.

system in the following scenarios: failed/difficult ERCP, contraindications to magnetic resonance imaging (MRI) exam (e.g., claustrophobia, aneurysm clips, pacemaker), and contraindications to percutaneous transhepatic cholangiography.

26. **How do you perform CT cholangiography?**
   CT cholangiography can be performed in several ways: obtaining CT following oral (iopanoate) or intravenous (IV) (iotroxic acid) administration of cholecystographic agents or without use of cholecystographic agents.

27. **What are the disadvantages of CT cholangiography?**
   Oral absorption and hepatic excretion of the oral cholecystographic agents are variable leading to suboptimal opacification of gall bladder and biliary system. Also, adverse reactions (mainly allergic) are seen predominantly with IV cholecystographic agents.

28. **What is primary sclerosing cholangitis?**
   Primary sclerosing cholangitis is an idiopathic, chronic fibrosing inflammation of the biliary system characterized clinically by a cholestatic syndrome and radiologically by segmental biliary stenoses or occlusion alternating with saccular ductal dilatation. It mainly occurs in young adult males and is associated with ulcerative colitis. Complications include cholangiocarcinoma and cirrhosis.

29. **How do you diagnose focal fat in the liver?**
   Hepatic focal fat is typically peripheral and located in periligamentous areas (likely related to anomalous perfusion) (Fig. 25-9). The blood vessels may traverse through focal fat.

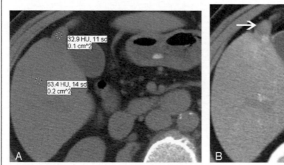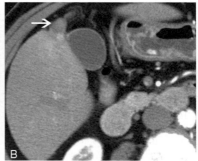

Figure 25-9. *A* and *B*, Focal hepatic steatosis. Typical location of focal hepatic steatosis adjacent to the gallbladder *(arrow)*.

30. **What is the typical distribution of focal hepatic steatosis? Why?**
   Focal hepatic steatosis typically occur near the falciform ligament, medial segment of the left hepatic lobe, and around the hepatic hilum. It is postulated that focal hepatic steatosis is related to either aberrant systemic venous supply or nonportal splanchnic venous supply that is rich in insulin.

31. **Describe the distribution, mechanism, and importance of focal fatty sparing.**
   Regions of focal fatty sparing within diffuse hepatic steatosis occur typically along the liver hilum, pericholecystic area, and peritumoral regions. Likely hypotheses for such changes include absence of portal venous inflow that is rich in dietary triglycerides and fatty acids and

"nonportal" splanchnic venous supply with low levels of dietary fat and insulin. At imaging, focal fatty sparing may simulate a neoplasm.

32. How is diffuse hepatic steatosis diagnosed?

Normally, the liver attenuation on unenhanced CT averages 8 HU greater than the spleen. Hepatic steatosis is diagnosed when the liver attenuation is less than that of the spleen on noncontrast CT (Fig. 25-10).

33. How is hepatic steatosis quantified?

Hepatic steatosis may be quantified at dual-energy CT. When scanned with 80 and 140 kVp, hepatic steatosis shows greater change in attenuation than does normal liver. Attenuation changes of 6 HU, 11 HU, and 20 HU are associated with < 25%, 50%, and 75% steatosis, respectively. Dual-energy CT is not done routinely.

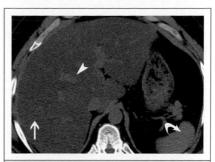

Figure 25-10. Diffuse hepatic steatosis. Noncontrast CT shows diffuse low attenuation of the liver *(arrow)* compared with the internal reference organ, the spleen *(curved arrow)*. Also, note the "bright"-appearing hepatic vessels *(arrowhead)*.

34. How is hepatic iron deposition diagnosed?

Hepatic iron deposition results in increased attenuation of the liver (CT attenuation values in hepatic hemochromatosis varies from 75–130 HU.)

35. What are the causes of a "bright liver" on noncontrast CT?

Primary or secondary hemochromatosis, glycogen storage disease, amiodarone toxicity, and Wilson's disease all cause increased attenuation of the liver (bright liver appearance).

36. What are the causes of portal vein thrombosis?

The most common risk factor for portal vein thrombosis is cirrhosis. Other predisposing conditions include infections (e.g., sepsis, pancreatitis, cholangitis), tumors, hypercoagulable states, and surgery.

37. How does portal vein thrombus appear on CT?

Acute thrombus may have high attenuation on noncontrast CT. Contrast-enhanced CT shows either partial or complete luminal filling defect (Fig. 25-11). Rim enhancement of the vessel wall may be seen. Indirect signs of portal vein thrombosis include cavernous transformation of the portal vein and the presence of portosystemic collateral vessels. Calcification may be seen in a chronic thrombus.

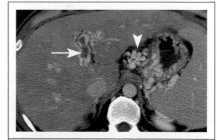

Figure 25-11. Portal vein thrombosis (bland thrombus). Contrast-enhanced computed tomography (CECT) shows a filling defect in the left portal vein *(arrow)*. Note the perigastric collateral vessels *(arrowhead)*.

38. **What is the mechanism of flow-related filling defect within the portal vein?**
   During the hepatic arterial scanning phase, mixing of enhanced splenic venous return and the nonenhanced superior mesenteric venous return in the main portal vein simulates a thrombus. However, in these cases of "portal vein pseudothrombus," the portal vein shows uniform contrast enhancement during the portal venous phase.

39. **What are the characteristics of tumor thrombosis of the portal vein?**
   The tumor thrombus demonstrates three key features: venous expansion, enhancement characteristics similar to the primary tumor, and neovascularity (Fig. 25-12).

40. **What is Budd-Chiari syndrome?**
   Budd-Chiari syndrome refers to a disorder characterized by portal hypertension due to occlusion and/or stenosis of the hepatic veins or hepatic segment of the inferior vena cava (IVC).

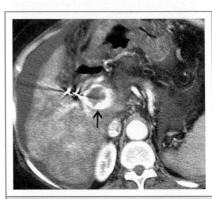

Figure 25-12. Malignant tumor thrombus. The main portal vein *(arrow)* is expanded and shows complete thrombosis in a patient with hepatocellular carcinoma.

41. **What are the causes of Budd-Chiari syndrome?**
   About half the cases are due to thrombotic disorders: polycythemia vera, pregnancy, paroxysmal nocturnal hemoglobinuria, contraceptive pills, and hepatocellular carcinoma (HCC). Other causes include myeloproliferative disorders, infections, membranous webs, and trauma. About 30% of cases are idiopathic.

42. **What are the CT findings of Budd-Chiari syndrome?**
   CT findings of Budd-Chiari syndrome include hepatomegaly, hepatic venous/IVC thrombosis, diffuse, heterogenous parenchymal enhancement ("nutmeg liver"), caudate hypertrophy, and ascites (Fig. 25-13). Large, hypervascular regenerative nodules can also occur.

43. **What is hepatic thorotrastosis?**
   Thorotrastosis refers to visceral deposition of thorotrast, a radiologic contrast medium used in the early 20th century. Thorotrast appears as high-density deposits within the liver, spleen, and lymph nodes. Hepatic thorotrastosis predispose to development of HCC, cholangiocarcinoma, and angiosarcoma.

44. **What are the CT findings of hepatic cirrhosis?**
   CT findings of cirrhosis include small, nodular liver, compensatory hypertrophy of caudate and left hepatic lobe, and features of portal hypertension (Fig. 25-14).

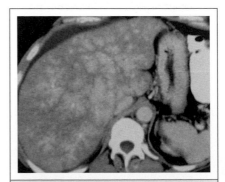

Figure 25-13. Budd-Chiari Syndrome. Contrast-enhanced computed tomography (CECT) shows typical "nutmeg" appearance of the liver.

The most dreaded complication is development of HCC.

45. What conditions cause pseudocirrhosis?

Pseudocirrhosis simulates cirrhosis and is characterized by a lobular hepatic contour and segmental atrophy and/or compensatory hypertrophy (Fig. 25-15). Pseudocirrhosis is described in several conditions, including systemic chemotherapy (typically breast cancer patients with liver metastases), chemoembolization for liver tumors, hereditary hemorrhagic telangiectasia, congenital hepatic fibrosis, and cardiac pseudocirrhosis (chronic right heart failure).

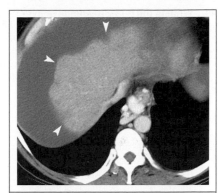

Figure 25-14. Hepatic cirrhosis. Note the irregular, nodular surface of the liver *(arrowheads)*.

46. What are the CT manifestations of portal hypertension?

Ascites, splenomegaly, and portosystemic shunts constitute the triad of portal hypertension. The portosystemic shunts include esophageal, perigastric, paraumbilical, perisplenic, and retroperitoneal collateral vessels (Fig. 25-16).

47. What is confluent hepatic fibrosis? How does it appear on CT? Why?

Confluent hepatic fibrosis is seen in patients with advanced cirrhosis. They appear as peripheral bandlike, wedge-shaped lesions in a segmental or lobar distribution with associated capsular retraction (Fig. 25-17). They show variable enhancement on early phases (due to variable proportion of fibrous tissue, tissue edema, and vessels) and uniform enhancement on delayed phases (because of increased interstitial space and slow venous drainage).

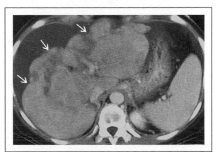

Figure 25-15. Pseudocirrhosis secondary to systemic chemotherapy. Nodular contour of the liver *(arrows)* in a patient with hepatic metastases from a breast adenocarcinoma following chemotherapy.

48. What are the causes of liver abscesses?

The liver abscesses may be pyogenic, fungal, mycobacterial, or parasitic in origin. Pyogenic abscesses can be due to hematogenous spread, superinfection of necrotic tissue, spread from contiguous organ, or secondary to biliary obstruction (cholangitic abscesses).

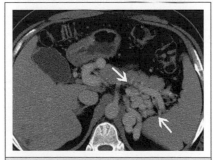

Figure 25-16. Portal hypertension. Contrast-enhanced computed tomography (CECT) in a patient with cirrhosis demonstrates dilated, tortuous retroperitoneal collateral vessels *(arrows)*.

49. What is the CT appearance of liver abscesses?

Liver abscesses appear as unilocular or multiseptate hypoattenuating lesions with a low-attenuation halo of edema (Fig. 25-18). Peripheral rim enhancement and presence of gas are unusual.

50. How do hydatid cysts appear on CT?

Hydatid cysts can be single or multiple and appear unilocular or multilocular (Fig. 25-19). The cyst wall is usually thin and well-defined. Separation of the laminated membrane from the pericyst results in a "split wall" appearance. Complete collapse of the laminated membrane results in "water lily sign." Calcification occurs in up to 50% of cases. Daughter cysts seen in 75% of cases are initially solid then become cystic. A fluid level may be due to hydatid sand or infection. A fat-fluid level indicates rupture into biliary system.

51. What is the cluster sign?

The cluster sign is considered a characteristic CT sign of hepatic pyogenic abscesses. The pyogenic abscesses appear to "cluster" in a pattern that suggests coalescence into a single, larger abscess cavity (Fig. 25-20).

52. How do fungal microabscesses appear on CT?

Fungal microabscesses usually appear as multiple round targetoid lesions with central, punctate contrast enhancement.

53. What is amebiasis? How is amebic liver abscess caused?

Amebiasis refers to infection by a protozoan parasite, *Entamoeba histolytica*. Ingestion of protozoan cysts in fecally contaminated food and water leads to colonic colonization and subsequent colitis. Following invasion of the colonic mucosa by trophozoites, the protozoa infects the liver through portal vein branches.

54. What are the CT findings of amebic liver abscess?

Amebic abscess typically appears as a unilocular, low-attenuation lesion

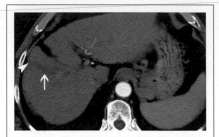

Figure 25-17. Confluent hepatic fibrosis. Hypoattenuating, fibrotic bands causing capsular retraction in a patient with cirrhosis *(arrows).*

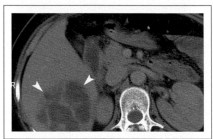

Figure 25-18. Pyogenic liver abscess. Contrast-enhanced computed tomography (CECT) shows multiple, low-attenuation coalescent abscesses in the left lobe of the liver *(arrowheads).*

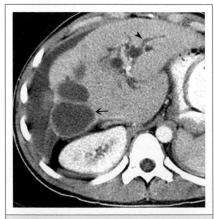

Figure 25-19. Hydatid cyst. Multifocal hepatic hydatid disease *(arrow)* with associated biliary dilatation *(arrowhead).*

(10–20 HU) with an enhancing wall of variable thickness and a peripheral zone of edema (Fig. 25-21). Septations, fluid-debris levels, and air are uncommon.

55. **What are the complications of amebic liver abscess?**
Complications of amebic liver abscess result from rupture of the abscess with extension into the peritoneum, pleural cavity, or pericardium. Extrahepatic amebic abscesses may occur in the lung and brain presumably from hematogenous spread.

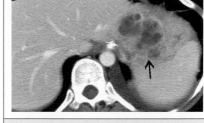

Figure 25-20. Cluster sign of abscess. Multiple, coalescing pyogenic abscesses *(arrow)*.

56. **What is hepatic peliosis?**
Peliosis hepatis refers to a benign hepatic condition characterized by disseminated blood-filled cavities of variable size and shape. It may be associated with malignancy, acquired immune deficiency syndrome (AIDS), and anabolic steroids usage.

57. **What is bacillary angiomatosis? What are CT findings of bacillary angiomatosis?**
Bacillary angiomatosis refers to liver infection by *Rochalimaea henselae*. This condition occurs almost exclusively in patients with AIDS. Contrast-enhanced CT scan reveals multiple, punctate hypervascular nodules scattered throughout the liver.

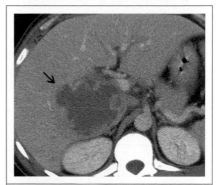

Figure 25-21. Amebic liver abscess. Large, hypodense lesion in the liver with an enhancing, thick wall and nodularity *(arrow)*.

58. **What are the manifestations of AIDS-related cholangiopathy?**
Radiologic manifestations of AIDS-related cholangiopathy are protean and include papillary stenosis, sclerosing cholangitis involving extrahepatic and intrahepatic biliary system, and long-segment extrahepatic biliary strictures.

59. **What are the causes of hepatic calcifications?**
Punctate calcifications are usually secondary to healed granulomatous conditions, such as tuberculosis, histoplasmosis, toxoplasmosis, *Pneumocystis carinii* infection, and sarcoidosis. Vascular calcifications including hepatic arterial aneurysmal and venous calcifications are segmental, curvilinear, or ovoid in configuration. Hepatic echinococcosis and schistosomiasis may show capsular calcification. Metastatic and primary liver tumors may show punctuate or coarse calcification. Old hematomas and abscesses may calcify.

60. **What is sarcoidosis? What are the CT findings of hepatic sarcoidosis?**
Sarcoidosis is an idiopathic, multisystem disorder characterized by noncaseating granulomas commonly affecting younger adult patients. Usually hepatic sarcoidosis manifests as hepatomegaly. In 5–15% of patients, coalescing granulomas appear as hypoattenuating nodules and may be mistaken for lymphoma or metastases (Fig. 25-22).

61. How does a typical liver hemangioma appear on dynamic CT?
A typical hemangioma exhibits peripheral globular/nodular enhancement and a centripetal fill-in pattern with the attenuation of enhancing areas identical to that of the blood pool (Fig. 25-23).

62. What is the bright-dot sign?
The bright-dot sign is suggestive of a liver hemangioma. The sign refers to tiny enhancing dots in the hemangioma that do not progress to the classic globular enhancement because of the small size of the lesion and the propensity for very slow contrast fill-in (Fig. 25-24).

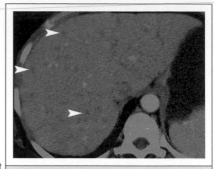

Figure 25-22. Hepatic sarcoidosis. Multiple, small hypoattenuation lesions scattered in the liver parenchyma *(arrowheads)*.

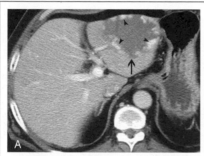
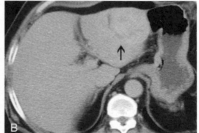

Figure 25-23. *A,* Liver hemangioma. Arterial phase images demonstrate peripheral nodular enhancement pattern *(arrowheads* and *arrow)* that is pathognomonic of a hemangioma. *B,* Liver hemangioma. Five-minute delay contrast-enhanced computed tomography (CECT) demonstrates progressive, centripetal contrast fill-in, the classic sign of liver hemangioma.

63. How does focal nodular hyperplasia (FNH) appear on dynamic CT?
FNH is a benign tumor that shows intense, uniform arterial phase enhancement and uniform portal venous phase contrast washout (Fig. 25-25). The scar demonstrates delayed contrast enhancement.

64. What is the pathologic basis for CT findings of FNH?
The rich network of capillaries, which provides arterial blood to the lesion is responsible for the intense, arterial phase enhancement of the FNH. The central scar comprised of fibrous connective tissue and malformed vessels shows delayed contrast enhancement.

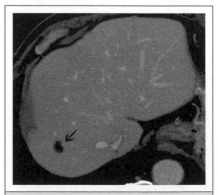

Figure 25-24. Bright-dot sign: Liver hemangioma. Contrast-enhanced computed tomography (CECT) showing an enhancing focus in a small hemangioma *(arrow)*.

65. **What are the risk factors for development of hepatic adenomas?**
    Use of high-estrogen oral contraceptive pills, anabolic steroids, and type 1 glycogen storage disease are risk factors.

66. **How does hepatic adenoma appear on CT?**
    Hepatic adenoma appears as a well-encapsulated, heterogeneous tumor with frequent areas of hemorrhage and infrequent foci of macroscopic fat (Fig. 25-26).

67. **What are the complications of liver adenomas?**
    The complications of liver adenomas include hemorrhage, rupture (typically subcapsular adenomas in pregnant women), and malignant change to a HCC.

68. **Why are hepatic adenomas more prone for bleeding?**
    The presence of dilated sinusoids (with scanty connective tissue support) that are fed by prominent arteries predispose hepatic adenomas to hemorrhage.

69. **What are the risk factors for HCC?**
    Cirrhosis (secondary to chronic hepatitis, alcohol abuse) is by far the commonest risk factor for HCC. Other less common risk factors include type I glycogen storage disease, tyrosinemia, hemochromatosis, Wilson's disease, and α1-antitrypsin deficiency.

70. **What are CT findings of HCC?**
    HCC has a variable appearance on CT, depending on size, histologic differentiation, and degree of neovascularity. Typical HCC shows arterial phase hypervascularity and may show contrast-washout on delayed phases. Although small tumors show uniform enhancement, larger tumors tend to be of heterogeneous attenuation (Fig. 25-27). Well-differentiated HCC may be hypoattenuating to liver. HCC may show mosaic appearance or capsular rim enhancement (Fig. 25-28). Multicentric and diffusely infiltrating forms of HCC also exist. Foci of calcification and macroscopic fat may occur. Findings of portal vein and hepatic venous thrombosis may be associated with HCC.

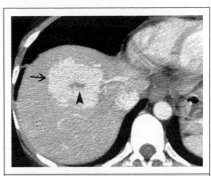

Figure 25-25. Focal nodular hyperplasia (FNH). Typical features of a hepatic FNH: Homogenous, intense contrast enhancement *(arrow)* with a central scar *(arrowhead)*.

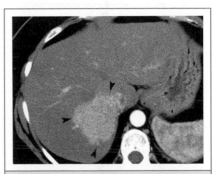

Figure 25-26. Hepatic adenoma. Uniform, hypervascular tumor *(arrowheads)* in an asymptomatic young woman.

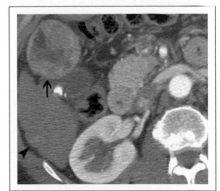

Figure 25-27. Hepatocellular carcinoma. Heterogeneously enhancing tumor *(arrow)* in a patient with cirrhosis *(arrowhead)*.

71. **What is lipiodol? How do lipiodol deposits appear on CT? How is lipiodol-enhanced CT performed?**
Lipiodol is iodized poppy seed oil that is known to concentrate semiselectively in liver tumors, specifically HCC. Lipiodol deposits appear as hyperattenuating foci on CT (Fig. 25-29). Liver CT is performed 10–14 days after lipiodol administration to allow for hepatic lipiodol clearance and selective tumor staining. Lipiodol is commonly mixed with chemotherapy agents as part of an intra-arterial chemoembolization protocol.

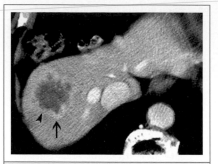

Figure 25-28. Hepatocellular carcinoma. Contrast-enhanced computed tomography (CECT) shows a hepatoma with thick, irregular rim-enhancement *(arrowhead* and *arrow)*.

72. **Why are small HCCs seen predominantly on the arterial phase?**
HCC derives its blood supply from hepatic artery branches. It shows arterial phase hypervascularity and hence is best seen on the late arterial phase (35-second delay).

73. **What lesions can mimic HCC?**
HCC can be radiologically confused with other tumors such as hemangioma, FNH, adenoma, and hypervascular metastases. Regenerative nodules (especially in Budd-Chiari syndrome), dysplastic nodules, and arterioportal shunts may show arterial phase hypervascularity and can mimic HCC.

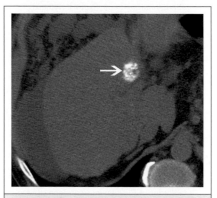

Figure 25-29. Lipiodol deposition. High-density lipiodol deposition *(arrow)* within a small hepatoma.

74. **What are the characteristics of fibrolamellar HCC?**
Fibrolamellar HCC is characterized by young patients with no history of cirrhosis or chronic liver disease, absence of serum tumor markers, characteristic histomorphology, increased chance of resectability, and better prognosis when compared with patients with conventional HCC. At CT, they appear as large, lobulated, heterogeneous tumors with a characteristic central, stellate, fibrous scar (70% of cases) that frequently calcifies (Fig. 25-30).

75. **What is a Klatskin tumor?**
Adenocarcinomas that originate from the confluence of the right and left hepatic ducts are called Klatskin tumors.

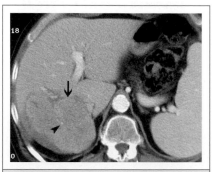

Figure 25-30. Fibrolamellar hepatocellular carcinoma. Contrast-enhanced computed tomography (CECT) shows a large, lobulated tumor *(arrow)* with a central speck of calcification *(arrowhead)*. Note the smooth contour of the liver.

76. **What are the CT findings of an intrahepatic cholangiocarcinoma?**
Intrahepatic cholangiocarcinoma appears as a well-defined, homogeneous mass with irregular borders and frequent satellite nodules. Peripheral rim enhancement is commonly seen as well as gradual centripetal enhancement on delayed phase images (Fig. 25-31). Associated segmental biliary dilatation, lobar atrophy, capsular retraction, and angio-invasion are relatively frequent.

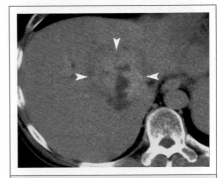

Figure 25-31. Intrahepatic cholangiocarcinoma. Thirty-minute delayed contrast-enhanced computed tomography (CECT) shows gradual enhancement of a cholangiocarcinoma *(arrowheads)*.

77. **Why do cholangiocarcinomas show delayed enhancement?**
Most cholangiocarcinomas are well-differentiated sclerosing adenocarcinomas that produce florid desmoplastic reaction (synthesis of collagenous tissue). The fibrous tissue accounts for delayed contrast enhancement.

78. **What liver tumors are associated with capsular retraction?**
Desmoplastic liver tumors, such as cholangiocarcinoma, atypical hemangioma, epithelioid hemangioendothelioma, and sclerosing metastases, cause capsular retraction.

79. **What liver tumors are associated with central scar?**
Liver tumors associated with a central scar include FNH, scirrhous HCC, fibrolamellar HCC, and large hemangioma. Rarely, scar can occur in cholangiocarcinoma and metastases.

80. **Name some calcifying liver metastases.**
Calcifications are seen most commonly with hepatic metastases from mucinous colon carcinoma; other tumors include primary tumors from ovary, breast, lung, kidney, and thyroid.

81. **What liver metastases demonstrate hypervascularity?**
Hypervascular hepatic metastases are seen in patients with renal cell carcinoma, pheochromocytoma, islet cell tumors, melanoma, and sarcoma (Fig. 25-32).

82. **What tumors give rise to cystic hepatic metastases?**
Cystic hepatic metastases occur in patients with ovarian adenocarcinoma and pancreatic cystic malignancies. Treated hepatic metastases from gastrointestinal stromal tumors may undergo cystic degeneration.

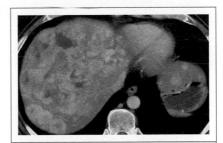

Figure 25-32. Hypervascular carcinoid metastases. Contrast-enhanced computed tomography (CECT) shows numerous heterogeneously enhancing, hypervascular liver metastases.

83. **What are the types of liver lymphoma?**
Liver lymphoma may be primary (rare) or secondary (most common), Hodgkin or non-Hodgkin variety (more common).

84. **What are the CT findings of hepatic lymphoma?**
CT findings of liver lymphoma can be varied; they can present as hepatomegaly without focal lesions or as solitary/multiple lesion(s) or as a diffusely infiltrating process (Fig. 25-33). Focal lesions may exhibit "targetoid" appearance.

85. **What is a hepatic angiosarcoma?**
Liver angiosarcoma is a highly aggressive mesenchymal neoplasm (with disseminated metastases) that is typically associated with exposure to vinyl chloride or thorotrast.

86. **What is a hepatoblastoma?**
Hepatoblastoma is an infantile, embryonal, malignant hepatic tumor that typically affects children younger than 3 years. It is characterized by elevated alpha fetoprotein levels, angio-invasion, and metastases.

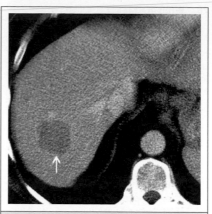

Figure 25-33. Biopsy-proven primary liver lymphoma. Contrast-enhanced computed tomography (CECT) demonstrates a solitary, low-attenuation tumor in the right hepatic lobe.

KEY POINTS: CT IMAGING OF THE LIVER

1. Central dot sign is characteristic of Caroli's disease.

2. Cluster sign suggests a liver abscess.

3. Peripheral nodular, globular enhancement and progressive, centripetal contrast fill-in are pathognomic of a hepatic hemangioma.

4. Hepatocellular carcinoma should be strongly considered when an arterially enhancing lesion is seen in a cirrhotic liver.

5. If cholangiocarcinoma is suspected, a 10-minute delayed CT should be obtained.

---

87. **What are the CT findings of a hepatoblastoma?**
Hepatoblastoma typically occurs as a large, well-circumscribed heterogeneously enhancing mass lesion within the liver. Diffuse infiltrating and multifocal forms also occur. Calcifications occur in up to 50% of cases. Angio-invasion and metastases chiefly to lymph nodes and lungs can occur.

88. **What is an infantile hemangioendothelioma?**
Infantile hemangioendothelioma is the most common benign infantile vascular hepatic tumor. Patients may present with abdominal symptoms, rupture, congestive heart failure, and consumptive coagulopathy (Kasabach-Merritt syndrome).

89. **What is a hepatic epithelioid hemangioendothelioma? How does it appear on CT?**
Hepatic epithelioid hemangioendothelioma is a rare, malignant tumor of vascular origin. It may present as multiple, peripheral nodules with calcification, capsular retraction, and peripheral contrast enhancement or as a diffusely infiltrating tumor with marked angio-invasion.

90. What is the role of CT in patients treated by radiofrequency ablation of HCC?

CT is the most widely used modality in evaluating patients with HCC treated by radiofrequency ablation. CT is invaluable in showing completeness of ablation, presence of residual tumor, differentiation of tumor from pseudolesions, and detection of complications.

91. Can CT demonstrate patency of transjugular intrahepatic portosystemic shunt (TIPS)?

Yes. CT angiography (50-second delay) has been successfully used to document patency of TIPS. In addition, stenosis and thrombosis of the stent or draining hepatic vein can be detected.

92. What is the role of multidetector CT in liver transplantation?

Multidetector CT provides comprehensive hepatic vascular and parenchymal evaluation in both transplant donors and recipients. Preoperative mapping of hepatic arterial, portal, and hepatic venous anatomy provides a roadmap to the surgeons. In addition, important parenchymal information including the presence of diffuse disorders, such as steatosis and liver tumors determines the criteria for liver transplantation.

93. What are the complications of liver transplantation?

The complications of liver transplantation include hemorrhage, infection, hepatic necrosis, rejection, biliary (strictures, biliary necrosis, bile leaks), vascular complications, and development of post-transplantation lymphoproliferative disorders (Fig. 25-34). Vascular complications include arterial (stenosis, thrombosis, pseudoaneurysm), portal, and hepatic venous (stenosis, thrombosis) complications.

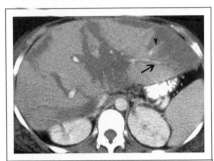

Figure 25-34. Multifocal infarction in a liver transplant recipient. Contrast-enhanced computed tomography (CECT) shows scattered areas of hepatic infarction *(arrow* and *arrowhead).*

BIBLIOGRAPHY

1. Baron RL: Common bile duct stones: Reassessment of criteria for CT diagnosis. Radiology 162:419–424, 1987.

2. Choi BI, Yeon KM, Kim SH, Han MC: Caroli disease: central dot sign in CT. Radiology 174:161–163, 1990.

3. Chopra S, Chintapalli KN, Dodd GD III: Helical CT angiography of transjugular intrahepatic portosystemic shunts. Semin Ultrasound CT MR 20:25–35, 1999.

4. Dodd GD III Baron RL, Oliver JH III, et al: Spectrum of imaging findings of the liver in end-stage cirrhosis. Part I: Gross morphology and diffuse abnormalities. AJR 173:1031–1036, 1999.

5. Dodd GD III, Baron RL, Oliver JH III, et al: Spectrum of imaging findings of the liver in end-stage cirrhosis. Part II: Focal abnormalities. AJR 173:1185–1192, 1999.

6. Foley WD, Kerimoglu U: Abdominal MDCT: Liver, pancreas, and biliary tract. Semin Ultrasound CT MR 25:122–144, 2004.

7. Horton KM, Bluemke DA, Hruban RH, et al: CT and MR imaging of benign hepatic and biliary tumors. Radiographics 19:431–451, 1999.

8. Itai Y, Saida Y: Pitfalls in liver imaging. Eur Radiol 12:1162–1174, 2002.

9. Jang HJ, Choi BI, Kim TK, et al: Atypical small hemangiomas of the liver: "Bright dot" sign at two-phase spiral CT. Radiology 208:543–548, 1998.

10. Kawamoto S, Soyer PA, Fishman EK, et al: Nonneoplastic liver disease: Evaluation with CT and MR imaging. Radiographics 18:827–848, 1998.

11. Lim JH, Park CK: Hepatocellular carcinoma in advanced liver cirrhosis: CT detection in transplant patients. Abdom Imag 29:203–207, 2004.

12. Mirvis SE, Whitley NO, Vainwright JR, Gens DR: Blunt hepatic trauma in adults: CT-based classification and correlation with prognosis and treatment. Radiology 171:27–32, 1989.

13. Mortelé KJ, Segatto E, Ros PR: The infected liver: Radiologic-pathologic correlation. Radiographics 24: 937–955, 2004.

14. Paulson EK, McDermott VG, Keogan MT, et al: Carcinoid metastases to the liver: Role of triple-phase helical CT. Radiology 206:143–150, 1998.

15. Poletti PA, Mirvis SE, Shanmuganathan K, et al: CT criteria for management of blunt liver trauma: Correlation with angiographic and surgical findings. Radiology 216:418–427, 2000.

16. Redvanly RD, Nelson RC, Stieber AC, Dodd GD III: Imaging in the preoperative evaluation of adult liver-transplant candidates: Goals, merits of various procedures, and recommendations. AJR 164:611–617, 1995.

17. Sahani D, Mehta A, Blake M, et al: Preoperative hepatic vascular evaluation with CT and MR angiography: Implications for surgery. Radiographics 24:1367–1380, 2004.

18. Sahani D, Saini S, Pena C, et al: Using multidetector CT for preoperative vascular evaluation of liver neoplasms: Technique and results. AJR 179:53–59, 2002.

19. Soyer P, Bluemke DA, Bliss DF, et al: Surgical segmental anatomy of the liver: Demonstration with spiral CT during arterial portography and multiplanar reconstruction. AJR 163:99–103, 1994.

20. Wong K, Paulson EK, Nelson RC: Breath-hold three-dimensional CT of the liver with multi-detector row helical CT. Radiology 219:75–79, 2001.

CHAPTER 26

GALLBLADDER AND BILIARY TRACT

Raj Mohan Paspulati, MD

1. **What are the indications for CT imaging of the gallbladder (GB) and biliary tract?**
   - GB carcinoma
   - Emphysematous cholecystitis
   - Porcelain GB
   - Obstructive jaundice
   - Right upper quadrant pain unexplained by ultrasonography
   - Postcholecystectomy complications

2. **What are the risk factors for GB carcinoma?**
   - 3–4 times more common in females
   - Native Americans, Spanish Americans, and Eskimos are at high risk
   - Gallstones and chronic cholecystitis
   - Porcelain GB

KEY POINTS: CT IMAGING OF THE GALLBLADER

1. CT is not the primary imaging modality of the gallbladder.

2. CT is indicated for evaluation of complications of acute cholecystitis and gallbladder mass.

3. Emphysematous cholecystitis and porcelain gallbladder suspected on ultrasound should be evaluated with CT.

---

3. **What are the various morphologic forms of GB carcinoma?**
   There are three morphologic forms of presentation:
   - Focal or diffuse thickening of the GB wall is present.
   - An intraluminal polypoidal mass arises from the GB wall (Fig. 26-1).
   - Mass in the GB fossa, replacing the GB and often infiltrating the hepatic parenchyma. Unfortunately, this is the most common form of presentation.

4. **What is the most common type of GB carcinoma?**
   Adenocarcinoma is the most common type of carcinoma. Anaplastic and squamous cell carcinomas are other less common forms of carcinoma.

5. **What are the reasons for dismal prognosis of GB carcinoma?**
   The clinical presentation of GB carcinoma is nonspecific and can mimic various other causes of right upper quadrant pain. This presentation is most often confused with cholelithiasis and cholecystitis. Radiologic imaging with ultrasound and CT is also insensitive in differentiating early carcinoma from inflammation. When a definitive diagnosis is made, the cancer has already infiltrated into the hepatic parenchyma and other adjacent organs. The 5-year survival rate is less than 5%.

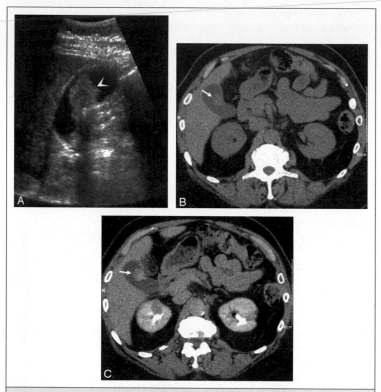

Figure 26-1. Gallbladder carcinoma. *A,* Ultrasonography of the gallbladder demonstrates a polypoidal intraluminal mass *(arrowhead). B* and *C,* Corresponding pre- and postenhanced CT of the abdomen reveals an enhancing gallbladder mass *(arrow).*

6. **What is the differential diagnosis of an infiltrating mass in the GB fossa?**
   - Complicated cholecystitis with perforation and pericholecystic inflammatory mass
   - Hepatocellular carcinoma invading the GB fossa, usually with underlying chronic hepatitis and cirrhosis of the liver
   - Metastases to the GB fossa

7. **What are the causes for biliary dilatation in GB carcinoma?**
   Biliary dilatation is seen in 50% of patients with GB carcinoma at the time of initial presentation. It is due to the following:
   - Metastatic lymphadenopathy compressing the common bile duct (CBD)
   - Tumor invasion of the hepatoduodenal ligament
   - Intraductal tumor invasion
   - Associated choledocholithiasis
   Metastatic lymphadenopathy and hepatoduodenal ligament invasion are the most common causes of bile duct obstruction.

8. **What are other malignant neoplasms of GB?**
   Other less common malignant neoplasms of GB include the following:

- Metastases (most commonly malignant melanoma, although may originate from any primary malignancy)
- Carcinoid tumor
- Lymphomas
- Sarcomas

KEY POINTS: BILIARY DILATATION

1. Normal intrahepatic bile ducts can be visualized with multichannel thin-slice CT and should not be mistaken for bile duct dilatation.

2. Mirizzi's syndrome should be suspected when acute cholecystitis is associated with intrahepatic biliary dilatation.

9. **What is porcelain GB?**
It is a form of chronic cholecystitis with mural calcification of the GB. The term *porcelain* derives from the bluish discoloration and brittle consistency of the GB. It is five times more frequent in men. The mural calcification is either a continuous calcification of muscularis (Fig. 26-2) or an interrupted calcification of the mucosa and submucosa. There is high incidence (11–33%) of GB carcinoma. Whenever porcelain GB is suspected on ultrasound, CT has to be performed to confirm the diagnosis and to evaluate for malignancy.

10. **What are the causes for high attenuation contents of the GB?**
    - Milk of calcium or limey bile
    - Sludge
    - Vicarious excretion of intravenous (IV) contrast medium
    - Hemobilia
    - Hemorrhagic cholecystitis
    - Prior endoscopic retrograde cholangiopancreatography (ERCP)

11. **What is milk of calcium or limey bile?**
Milk of calcium bile is puttylike material composed of calcium carbonate and less commonly calcium phosphate or calcium bilirubinate. It is secondary to cystic duct obstruction and chronic cholecystitis.

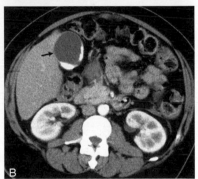

Figure 26-2. Porcelain gallbladder. Contrast-enhanced axial CT images (*A* and *B*) show diffuse mural calcification of the gallbladder.

12. **What is the role of CT in evaluation of acute cholecystitis?**
Ultrasonography is the primary imaging modality for diagnosis of acute cholecystitis. Cholescintigraphy is complementary, when ultrasonography is inconclusive. CT should not

be used as a primary modality for the diagnosis of acute cholecystitis. However, acute cholecystitis is frequent and symptoms can be nonspecific, so it is a relatively common CT diagnosis.

13. **What are the CT findings of acute cholecystitis?**
    Although CT is not a primary imaging modality for acute cholecystitis, it will be seen frequently. The CT features (Fig. 26-3) include the following:
    - GB distention (>5 cm in transverse or anteroposterior [AP] dimension)
    - Gallstone or stone impacted in the cystic duct
    - Mural thickening (>3 mm), nodularity
    - Pericholecystic fluid
    - Poor definition of GB wall at the interface with the liver
    - Pericholecystic fat stranding
    - Focal areas of pericholecystic transient hepatic parenchymal enhancement

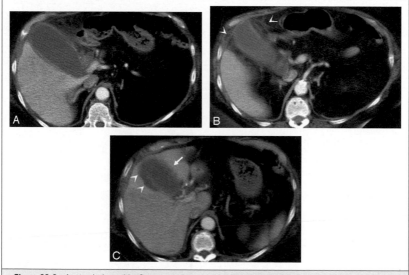

Figure 26-3. Acute cholecystitis. Contrast-enhanced axial CT images show diffuse mural thickening of the gallbladder *(A)* with pericholecystic inflammatory fat stranding *(arrowheads, B)* and pericholecystic fluid *(arrowheads, C)*.

14. **What are the complications of acute cholecystitis?**
    - Empyema
    - Perforation and pericholecystic abscess
    - Biliary-enteric fistula
    - Mirizzi's syndrome

15. **What are the characteristics of gangrenous cholecystitis?**
    This is a severe form of GB inflammation with intramural hemorrhage, necrosis, and microabscesses. This is a surgical emergency due to high incidence of GB perforation. CT may show intraluminal hemorrhage, intraluminal membranes, asymmetric GB wall thickening due to intramural hemorrhage and microabscesses, diminished mural enhancement, and pericholecystic abscess.

16. **What is emphysematous cholecystitis?**

It is a severe form of acute cholecystitis seen more commonly in elderly patients with diabetes and splanchnic ischemia. It is characterized by intramural and intraluminal gas due to infection by the gas-forming bacteria, *Clostridium welchii, Clostridium perfringens, Escherichia coli,* and *Klebsiella* spp. There is fivefold increased risk of GB perforation. CT demonstrates changes of acute cholecystitis and intramural, intraluminal, and pericholecystic gas (Fig. 26-4). CT confirmation should be obtained, when sonographic findings are suspicious for emphysematous cholecystitis.

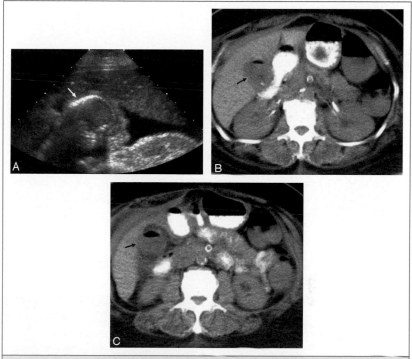

Figure 26-4. Emphysematous cholecystitis. *A,* Ultrasonography demonstrates nondependent linear hyperechoic focus *(arrow)* within the GB suggestive of gas. *B* and *C,* Corresponding contrast enhanced axial CT images show changes of acute cholecystitis and confirms intraluminal gas in the GB *(arrow)*.

17. **How common is GB perforation? What are the risk factors?**

GB perforation occurs in 5–10% of patients with acute cholecystitis and is more common a sequela of gangrenous, emphysematous, and acute acalculous cholecystitis.

18. **When are the CT findings of GB perforation?**

The fundus is the most common site of perforation because of its poor blood supply. A complex pericholecystic fluid collection is seen and may be associated with focal disruption of the GB wall. The GB may become decompressed following perforation. Gallstones may be seen outside the GB.

19. **What is the incidence of acute acalculous cholecystitis? What are its predisposing factors?**

GB inflammation in the absence of gallstones is seen in 2–15% of patients undergoing cholecystectomy. In children, it constitutes 50% of cases of acute cholecystitis.

It is common in the following clinical situations:

- Nonbiliary trauma
- Burns
- Postoperative
- Hyperalimentation
- Mechanical ventilation
- Diabetes
- Vascular insufficiency due to atherosclerosis or cardiac arrest
- Sepsis
- Acquired immunodeficiency syndrome (AIDS)
- Hepatic arterial chemotherapy

20. What is xanthogranulomatous cholecystitis?
It is an uncommon chronic inflammation of the GB. The GB wall is markedly thickened due to infiltration with round cells, lipid-laden histiocytes, multinucleate giant cells, and fibroblastic proliferation of the muscularis propria.

CT scan shows marked mural thickening of the GB or a mass in the GB fossa. The chronic inflammatory process may infiltrate the adjacent hepatic parenchyma or bowel. It is indistinguishable from GB carcinoma on all imaging modalities and is thus a pathologic diagnosis.

21. What are the characteristics of GB torsion?
GB torsion is a rare cause of acute abdomen due to twisting of an unusually mobile GB. The presence of a long mesentery (mesocyst) predisposes to torsion. The incidence of gangrene is much higher than in acute cholecystitis. The clinical features and imaging findings closely mimic those of acute cholecystitis. When changes of acute cholecystitis are associated with an abnormal location of GB on cross-sectional imaging, GB torsion may be suspected.

22. Can CT demonstrate normal intrahepatic bile ducts?
With multichannel thin-slice CT, it is possible to see normal central intrahepatic bile ducts. This should not be mistaken for biliary dilatation.

23. What are the CT criteria for intrahepatic biliary dilatation?
- When intrahepatic bile ducts measure more than 2 mm in diameter
- When intrahepatic bile duct diameter is >40% of the diameter of the adjacent intrahepatic portal vein
- When duct visualization is confluent without discontinuity (Fig. 26-5)

24. What are normal dimensions of extrahepatic bile ducts on CT scan?
Unlike in ultrasound, there is no standardized location for measurement of extrahepatic bile duct in CT scan. Moreover, measurement of the bile duct in CT includes the duct wall. Hence, 8–10 mm is considered upper limits of a normal extrahepatic duct in CT and 6–7 mm in ultrasonography. The extrahepatic bile duct may increase in diameter following cholecystectomy and with aging.

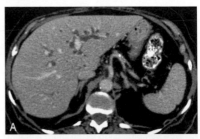

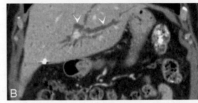

Figure 26-5. Dilated intrahepatic bile ducts. Axial *(A)* and coronal *(B)* contrast-enhanced CT images demonstrate dilated intrahepatic bile ducts *(arrowheads)*.

25. **Does absence of biliary dilatation on CT scan exclude the presence of obstruction?**
There is a time lag between the onset of acute obstruction and the biliary dilatation. The extra-hepatic bile ducts are the first to dilate, usually about 2–3 days after the onset of obstruction. The intrahepatic bile ducts dilate about 1 week after the onset of obstruction. Hence, absence of biliary dilation does not preclude the presence of biliary obstruction.

26. **What are different causes of biliary obstruction?**
See Table 26-1.

TABLE 26-1. CAUSES OF BILIARY OBSTRUCTION

Intrahepatic	Porta Hepatis	Suprapancreatic	Intrapancreatic
Recurrent pyogenic cholangitis	Primary sclerosing cholangitis	Pancreatitis	Choledocholithiasis
Primary sclerosing cholangitis	Mirizzi's syndrome	Pancreatic carcinoma	Pancreatitis
Space-occupying lesions	Cholangiocarcinoma	Cholangiocarcinoma	Pancreatic carcinoma
	Gallbladder carcinoma	Iatrogenic	Ampullary stenosis
	Metastatic disease		Periampullary carcinoma

27. **What are various types of choledocholithiasis?**
CBD calculi are either primary or secondary. Secondary calculi are formed in the GB and passed into the CBD and are the most common type. These are predominantly cholesterol calculi. The primary bile duct calculi are pigment stones secondary to stasis and bacterial or parasitic infection. *E. coli, Klebsiella,* and gram-negative enteric bacteria are common bacterial infections. *Clonorchis sinensis* and *Ascaris* sp. are major parasitic infections in Southeast Asia, which cause primary bile duct calculi.

28. **What are the CT appearances of biliary calculi?**
The CT appearance of biliary calculi varies with their chemical composition. Only 20% of the CBD calculi are of high attenuation and can be detected even without biliary dilatation. Other calculi are of either soft tissue or very low attenuation due to pure cholesterol composition. These noncalcified calculi are identified by crescent or target sign due to the surrounding low-attenuation bile (Fig. 26-6). The crescent sign is also seen with a papillary soft tissue tumor. Concentric focal thickening of the CBD wall on an enhanced CT is a nonspecific sign due to inflammation of the duct wall at the site of calculus.

29. **What is Mirizzi's syndrome?**
An impacted stone in the cystic duct and surrounding inflammation causes obstruction of the adjacent common hepatic duct. This is more common when cystic duct has a low insertion, has a long parallel course with the common hepatic duct, and sometimes is enclosed within a common sheath. Mirizzi's syndrome should be suspected when acute cholecystitis is associated with biliary obstruction. The diagnosis can be made with both ultrasound and CT. The diagnosis can be confirmed with a preoperative ERCP or intraoperative cholangiography.

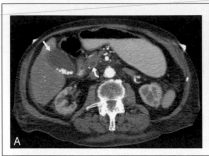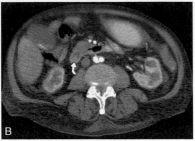

Figure 26-6. Choledocholithiasis. **A,** Contrast-enhanced CT image of the abdomen shows multiple calcified gallstones in the gallbladder *(straight arrow)* and dilated CBD *(curved arrow)*. **B,** Hyperdensity in the distal CBD *(arrow)*, representing a calculus.

30. What is gallstone ileus?

Erosion of a gallstone into the gastrointestinal tract, usually the duodenum, with passage of the gallstone until it obstructs the bowel. Gallstone ileus is usually a sequela of chronic cholecystitis. The eroded gallstone should be >2 cm to cause obstruction. The common sites of obstruction are at the ligament of Treitz, ileocecal valve, sigmoid colon, or a preexisting stricture.

KEY POINTS: CT SIGNS OF GALLSTONE ILEUS

1. Pneumobilia

2. Bowel obstruction

3. Gallstone in the bowel

31. What are the CT features of gallstone ileus?

The classic triad of gallstone ileus is pneumobilia, bowel obstruction, and demonstration of a gallstone in the bowel lumen (Fig. 26-7). All the three features may not be seen. The gallstone may not be sufficiently calcified and pneumobilia may not be consistently seen. However, these findings should be sought in all patients with small bowel obstruction.

32. What is Bouveret syndrome?

Gastric outlet obstruction due to a large gallstone impacted in the duodenum is referred to as Bouveret syndrome. It is a rare form of gallstone ileus, which is more common in the elderly.

33. What are the predisposing factors for acute cholangitis?

Biliary obstruction and bile stasis predisposes to bacterial infection. The biliary obstruction is either due to a benign cause such as choledocholithiasis, anastomotic stricture, or papillary stenosis or malignant causes such as cholangiocarcinoma, pancreatic carcinoma, and hilar lymphadenopathy. Biliary intervention, such as ERCP and stent placement also predispose to cholangitis.

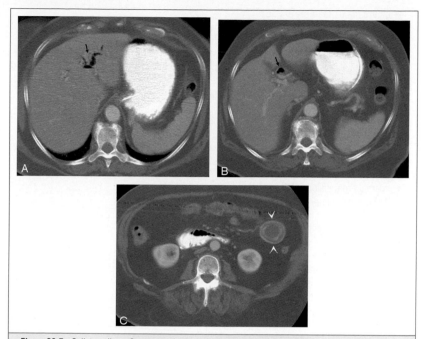

Figure 26-7. Gallstone ileus. Contrast-enhanced CT images show pneumobilia *(arrows)* in the intrahepatic bile ducts *(A)* and extrahepatic bile duct *(B)*. *C,* Well-defined calcified intraluminal filling defect *(arrowheads)* in the proximal jejunum representing a gallstone.

34. **What are the CT features of acute cholangitis?**
    - Biliary dilatation with identification of the level and cause of obstruction
    - Diffuse thickening and enhancement of the bile duct wall
    - Increased attenuation of the purulent bile
    - Hepatic abscesses in close relation to the dilated bile ducts is a usual complication of cholangitis

35. **What is sclerosing cholangitis?**
    Sclerosing cholangitis is characterized by chronic fibrosing inflammation of the bile ducts. This can be primary (idiopathic) or secondary to prior biliary infection. Primary sclerosing cholangitis (PSC) is more common in males and is associated with ulcerative colitis in 70%. Multiple strictures of the intrahepatic and extrahepatic bile ducts due to inflammatory fibrosis is the hallmark of PSC.

36. **What is best imaging modality for diagnosis of PSC?**
    Conventional cholangiography is the gold standard for diagnosis of PSC. Magnetic resonance cholangiography (MRCP) is slowly replacing the invasive cholangiography. MRCP is the imaging modality of choice for follow-up of patients with known PSC.

37. **What is the role of CT in PSC?**
    CT is not the primary imaging modality for diagnosis of PSC. The key role of CT is in screening for cholangiocarcinoma. It is less sensitive than magnetic resonance imaging (MRI) in screening for cholangiocarcinoma.

38. **What are the CT features of PSC?**
CT demonstrates mural thickening and enhancement of the bile ducts, multiple segmental strictures with intervening normal or dilated bile ducts. The mural thickening is less than 5 mm in thickness. Segmental or lobar atrophy of the liver due to chronic biliary obstruction and compensatory hypertrophy of the unaffected liver. The major advantage of cross-sectional imaging is the ability to visualize the peripheral bile ducts, when a distal stricture has prevented peripheral filling of the bile ducts on conventional cholangiography.

39. **What is the incidence of cholangiocarcinoma in PSC? When do you suspect cholangiocarcinoma?**
About 15% of patients with PSC develop cholangiocarcinoma. Cholangiocarcinoma should be suspected under the following circumstances:
- Mural thickening of the bile duct is >5 mm
- Interval progression of biliary dilatation proximal to a stricture
- Periductal or periportal soft tissue mass

40. **What are the risk factors for cholangiocarcinoma?**
- PSC
- Choledochal cyst
- Familial polyposis
- Congenital hepatic fibrosis
- *C. sinensis* (Chinese liver fluke) infection
- Prior exposure to thorium dioxide (Thorotrast; Thorotrast was used instead of iodine for IV injections between 1930 and 1955 but is an alpha-emitter, which is retained in the reticuloendothelial system and causes carcinomas)

41. **How do you classify cholangiocarcinomas?**
Cholangiocarcinomas are classified based on tumor location:
- Intrahepatic or peripheral
- Central or hilar near the confluence of the right and left hepatic ducts (Klatskin tumors)
- Distal duct type involving the distal CHD and CBD

42. **What are the morphologic types of cholangiocarcinoma?**
- Scirrhous infiltrating type causing stricture of the larger ducts
- Exophytic mass lesions, commonly involving the peripheral intrahepatic ducts
- Polypoid intraluminal mass lesions of the distal extrahepatic duct

43. **Which is the most common location of cholangiocarcinoma?**
The most common location for cholangiocarcinoma is from the extrahepatic bile duct. They constitute 65% of all cholangiocarcinomas.

44. **What percentage of cholangiocarcinomas is intrahepatic or peripheral?**
Ten percent of cholangiocarcinomas are peripheral or intrahepatic. These tumors arise from bile ducts peripheral to the second-order branches of the right and left hepatic ducts.

45. **What are Klatskin tumors?**
Hilar cholangiocarcinomas, arising from the confluence of the right and left hepatic ducts and proximal common hepatic duct are called Klatskin tumors. They constitute about 25% of all cholangiocarcinomas (Fig. 26-8).

46. **What is the CT technique for diagnosis of cholangiocarcinoma?**
A standard liver protocol with pre and post IV contrast scans in arterial, portal venous, and delayed phase. A 10- to 15-minute delayed phase scan is important for diagnosis of cholangiocarcinoma and to differentiate it from other benign or malignant mass lesions.

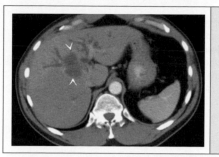

Figure 26-8. Cholangiocarcinoma (Klatskin tumor). Axial contrast-enhanced CT of the liver demonstrates a hypodense mass *(arrowheads)* at the confluence of the right and left hepatic ducts causing intrahepatic biliary dilatation.

KEY POINTS: CHOLANGIOCARCINOMA

1. Delayed CT after IV contrast medium is crucial for diagnosis.

2. Fifteen percent of patients with primary sclerosing cholangitis develop cholangiocarcinoma.

3. Extrahepatic bile duct is the most common site (65%).

47. **What is the significance of a post-IV contrast delayed scan?**
Cholangiocarcinomas have a predominant desmoplastic composition and show characteristic delayed enhancement between 8 and 15 minutes following IV contrast administration.

48. **What CT imaging features differentiate intrahepatic cholangiocarcinoma from hepatocellular carcinoma?**
Intrahepatic cholangiocarcinomas show delayed enhancement and persistent retention of contrast medium up to 15–20 minutes. Hepatocellular carcinomas enhance predominantly in the arterial phase and demonstrate washout in the delayed phase.

49. **Which type of bile duct tumors enhance in the arterial phase of a CT scan?**
The carcinoid or neuroendocrine tumors of the bile duct enhance in the arterial phase. They are rare.

50. **What are cystic bile duct neoplasms?**
Biliary cystadenoma and cystadenocarcinoma are rare cystic neoplasms lined by mucin-secreting columnar epithelium. They manifest as uniloculated or multiloculated intrahepatic cystic mass lesions. Mural nodules are more common in cystadenocarcinoma. Benign cystadenomas tend to undergo malignant transformation. They have to be differentiated from benign hepatic cysts, hydatid cysts, liver abscesses, cystic metastases, and choledochal cysts.

51. **What are choledochal cysts?**
Choledochal cysts are congenital cystic dilatations of the extra- or intrahepatic bile ducts.

52. **Which is the most common type of choledochal cyst?**
Type 1 choledochal cyst is the most common type. It is due to segmental fusiform dilatation of the extrahepatic bile duct.

53. **What is choledochocele?**
Choledochocele is a type 3 choledochal cyst, which is due to focal dilatation of the intraduodenal portion of the CBD.

54. **What is Caroli's disease?**

Caroli's disease is due to cavernous ectasia of the intrahepatic bile ducts. It is characterized by multifocal, segmental, and saccular dilatation of the intrahepatic biliary ducts. It may be segmental, lobar, or diffuse. It is classified as a type 5 choledochal cyst.

55. **What are the complications of Caroli's disease?**
   - Choledocholithiasis
   - Recurrent cholangitis
   - Increased incidence of cholangiocarcinoma

56. **What are the CT features of Caroli's disease?**

Contrast-enhanced CT in the portal venous phase reveals the following:
   - Multiple small cystic foci represent ectatic ducts.
   - Central enhancing dots within these cystic foci due to portal veins encased by the ectatic ducts is called the "central dot sign."

57. **How do you confirm the diagnosis of Caroli's disease?**

Although ERCP is the gold standard for diagnosis of Caroli's disease, contrast-enhanced MRI with MRCP is also an accurate method for diagnosis of Caroli's disease.

BIBLIOGRAPHY

1. Baron RL, Tublin ME, Peterson MS: Imaging the spectrum of biliary tract disease. Radiol Clin North Am 40:1325–1354, 2002.

2. Bortoff GA, Chen MY, Ott DJ, et al: Gallbladder stones: Imaging and intervention. Radiographics 20:751–766, 2000.

3. Campbell WL, Peterson MS, Federle MP, et al: Using CT and cholangiography to diagnose biliary tract carcinoma complicating primary sclerosing cholangitis. Am J Roentgenol 177:1095–1100, 2001.

4. Grand D, Horton KM, Fishman EK, Fishman E: CT of the gallbladder: Spectrum of disease. Am J Roentgenol 183:163–170, 2004.

5. History of thorium compounds as contrast agents: www.orau.org/ptp/collection/Radiology/thorotrast.htm

6. Urban BA, Fishman EK: Tailored helical CT evaluation of acute abdomen. Radiographics 20:725–749, 2000.

CHAPTER 27

PANCREAS

Raj Mohan Paspulati, MD

1. **What is the technique for optimal CT imaging of the pancreas?**

   The optimal technique for evaluation of the pancreas is a triphasic CT: pre-intravenous (IV) contrast and post-IV contrast in the pancreatic and in the portal venous phase. Oral water is preferable to dense contrast medium for identification of terminal common bile duct (CBD) calculi and better evaluation of the periampullary region. In general, slice thickness should be 5 mm or less with a slice interval of 2 mm. With multidetector CT, 1.25-mm thick, overlapping images are reconstructed for detection of small pancreatic tumors and for proper staging of pancreatic cancer. Multiple-row detector CT (MDCT) protocol for unenhanced and enhanced CT is outlined in the following. The acquisition parameters are outlined in Table 27-1.

   Unenhanced scan
   - **IV contrast:** 1000 cc of oral water 20 minutes prior to study and 250 cc before the scan
   - **Scan range:** From diaphragm to mid-pelvis
   - **Slice collimation:** 5 mm
   - **Increment:** 5 mm

   Enhanced scan
   - **IV contrast:** 125–175 cc (300 mg of iodine/ml) injected at 4 cc/sec

TABLE 27-1. MULTIPLE-ROW DETECTOR DCT PROTOCOL ACQUISITION PARAMETERS FOR PANCREAS

Phase	Delay	Collimation	Table Speed	Rotation Speed	MPR
Pancreatic	40 sec	4 or 8 × 1.25 16 × 0.75	7.5–15/Rev	0.5 sec	1.25 RI
Portal venous	65 sec	4 or 8 × 1.25 16 × 0.75	7.5–15/Rev	0.5 sec	1.25 RI

2. **What are the benefits of a preliminary unenhanced CT of the pancreas?**
   - Detection of distal CBD calculi
   - Detection of pancreatic parenchymal and ductal calcifications
   - Detection of hemorrhage in post-trauma patients and in acute hemorrhagic pancreatitis

3. **What are normal CT dimensions of the pancreas?**

   Absolute numbers should not be used to diagnose pancreatic enlargement. The proportion of the various parts of the pancreas, with head of the pancreas being slightly larger in anterior-posterior dimension than the body and tail is important. The anterior-posterior dimension of the pancreas should be less than transverse diameter of the adjacent vertebral body. The pancreatic tail can be bulbous in some normal patients and measure larger than the head.

4. **What is the normal appearance of pancreas on CT scan?**

The morphologic appearance of pancreas varies with age of the patient. In younger patients, the pancreas has a smooth contour with homogeneous attenuation similar to the spleen and muscle and less than that of liver on an unenhanced scan. It enhances homogeneously after IV contrast (Fig. 27-1). In the elderly, there is progressive deposition of fat, and the pancreas has a lobulated contour with inhomogeneous attenuation.

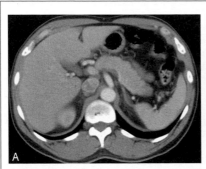

Figure 27-1. Normal pancreas. Axial contrast-enhanced CT image in a young man shows homogeneous enhancement of the body and tail of the pancreas *(A)* and head of the pancreas *(B)* with distal CBD *(arrow)* and pancreatic duct *(arrowhead)*.

5. **Can you see a normal pancreatic duct on CT?**

Yes. The normal pancreatic duct is seen in 70% of normal patients as a thin, linear, low-attenuation region coursing along the center of the pancreas (Fig. 27-2). In young adults, it measures < 3 mm in width. In the elderly, the normal pancreatic duct may be larger than 3 mm in width due to parenchymal atrophy. The normal fat plane between the splenic vein and pancreas should not be mistaken for pancreatic duct. Of course, the better your scanner, the more often you will see it.

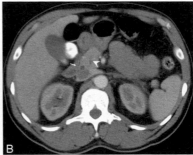

Figure 27-2. Normal pancreatic duct. Axial contrast-enhanced CT image in a young man demonstrates a normal pancreatic duct *(arrowheads)*.

6. **What is pancreas divisum?**

This is the most common anatomic variation of the pancreatic duct due to failure of fusion of the ventral and dorsal anlage of the pancreas. The dorsal and ventral pancreatic ducts drain separately into the duodenum without any communication between the two ducts. The major dorsal pancreatic duct, which drains the body, tail, and superior portion of the head, courses anterior to the CBD and opens into the duodenum at the minor papilla, proximal to the major papilla. The minor ventral pancreatic duct, which drains the inferior head and uncinate process, opens along with the CBD at the major papilla.

7. **What is the significance of pancreas divisum?**
   Although pancreas divisum may be an incidental finding on cross-sectional imaging, it has been associated with acute pancreatitis due to obstruction of the main dorsal pancreatic duct at the minor papilla.

8. **What are CT imaging features of acute pancreatitis?**
   In early and mild pancreatitis, the pancreas will be normal in appearance. Later findings (Fig. 27-3) may include the following:
   - Focal or diffuse enlargement of pancreas
   - Heterogeneous enhancement of pancreas
   - Diminished enhancement of parenchyma due to edema or necrosis
   - Shaggy pancreatic contour with peripancreatic fat stranding
   - Peripancreatic thickening of facial planes
   - Peripancreatic fluid collections in the anterior pararenal space
   - Free intraperitoneal fluid

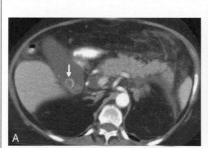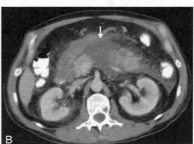

Figure 27-3. Acute pancreatitis. **A,** Axial contrast-enhanced CT image of the abdomen shows peripancreatic inflammatory fat stranding, thickened left Gerota's fascia, and gallbladder calculi *(arrow)*. **B,** Peripancreatic fluid collections *(arrow)*.

9. **What is CT grading of acute pancreatitis?**
   Based on the CT appearance, acute pancreatitis can be graded into five types:
   - **Grade A:** Normal pancreas
   - **Grade B:** Focal or diffuse enlargement of gland
   - **Grade C:** Pancreatic and peripancreatic inflammation
   - **Grade D:** Single peripancreatic fluid collection
   - **Grade E:** Two or more fluid collections or gas in the pancreas or retroperitoneum

   Patients with grades D and E have higher incidence of morbidity and mortality than patients with grades A, B, and C.

10. **What are the advantages of IV contrast medium in CT imaging of acute pancreatitis?**
    The normal pancreas enhances homogeneously in the arterial phase of IV contrast medium. Focal or diffuse areas of diminished enhancement of the parenchyma indicate pancreatic necrosis (Fig. 27-4). Mild inflammation and interstitial edema do not interfere with pancreatic enhancement. Peripancreatic planes are well delineated following IV contrast medium. Contrast-enhanced CT also helps in evaluation of peripancreatic vasculature for complications.

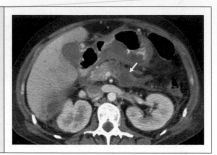

Figure 27-4. Acute necrotizing pancreatitis. Axial contrast-enhanced CT of the abdomen demonstrates changes of acute pancreatitis with a nonenhancing area *(arrow)* in the body of the pancreas, representing pancreatic necrosis.

11. **Which is the single most CT imaging feature that correlates with prognosis?**
    Demonstration of presence and extent of pancreatic necrosis in acute pancreatitis correlates with morbidity and mortality. CT has an overall sensitivity of 85% in detection of necrosis. The degree of necrosis is an important factor. Patients with <30% necrosis have no mortality and 40% morbidity. With 50% or more necrosis, there is 75–100% morbidity and 11–25% mortality.

12. **What local complications of acute pancreatitis can be identified with CT imaging?**
    The abdominal complications develop usually between 2 and 5 weeks after the onset of acute pancreatitis. CT imaging can identify both nonvascular and vascular complications.
    Nonvascular complications
    - Pseudocyst
    - Pancreatic abscess
    - Distal CBD obstruction
    - Duodenal or colonic obstruction
    Vascular complications
    - Splenic vein thrombosis
    - Pseudoaneurysm
    - Mesenteric vascular compromise
    - Splenic infarcts

13. **What are pseudocysts?**
    Pseudocysts are encapsulated fluid collections in or adjacent to the pancreas that evolve 4 or more weeks following acute pancreatitis. Most fluid collections associated with acute pancreatitis are absorbed in 2–3 weeks. Unabsorbed fluid collections develop a nonepithelialized capsule, composed of inflammatory, granulation, and fibrotic tissue to form a pseudocyst.

14. **What are the CT features of a pseudocyst?**
    - Well-defined fluid collection with a uniformly thin (1–2 mm) capsule (Fig. 27-5)
    - Variable in size
    - Usually peripancreatic in location but can dissect along fascial planes to distant locations such as mediastinum or pelvis
    - Uncomplicated pseudocysts have fluid attenuation of <15 HU

15. **What is spontaneous resolution of a pseudocyst?**
    Pseudocysts can resolve spontaneously by the following mechanisms:
    - Rupture of the cyst wall
    - Drainage into a communicating pancreatic ductal system
    - Spontaneous drainage into an adjacent hollow viscous, such as stomach or colon

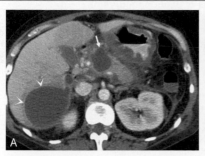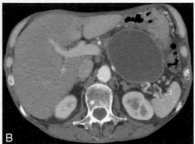

Figure 27-5. Acute pancreatitis with pseudocysts. **A,** Axial, contrast-enhanced CT image of the abdomen demonstrates acute pancreatitis with two well-defined, thin-walled pseudocysts in the body of the pancreas *(arrow)* and in the Morison's space *(arrowheads)*. **B,** A large pseudocyst in the lesser sac displacing the stomach anteriorly.

16. **What are the indications for surgical or percutaneous drainage of a pseudocyst?**
    - Enlarging cysts or cysts larger than 5 cm
    - Symptomatic cysts: Abdominal mass, pain, and gastric outlet and biliary obstruction
    - Complications, such as hemorrhage or infection

17. **Which is the ideal time for drainage of a pseudocyst?**
    A pseudocyst should have a mature capsule for placement of a drainage catheter or surgical drainage. This is usually seen in pseudocysts that are older than 6 weeks.

18. **What are the CT features of pancreatic abscess?**
    Pancreatic abscess develops in 3–21% of cases of acute pancreatitis as peripancreatic fluid collections with gas. In the absence of gas, they are indistinguishable from noninfected fluid collections (Fig. 27-6). In the proper clinical setting, abscess should be suspected in all persistent peripancreatic fluid collections, and CT-guided aspiration is necessary to establish the diagnosis.

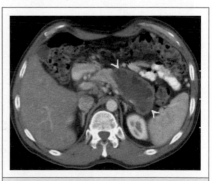

Figure 27-6. Pancreatic abscess. Axial contrast-enhanced CT in a patient with known acute pancreatitis, presenting with fever and elevated white cell count, demonstrates a well-defined, thick-walled fluid collection *(arrowheads)* at the tail of the pancreas. Subsequent CT-guided drainage of this collection revealed frank pus.

19. **Can CT demonstrate infected pancreatic necrosis?**
    The demonstration of gas within the necrotic pancreas is indicative of infection but is seen in only about 12–18% of cases. When there are clinical manifestations of sepsis (fever, elevated white cell count, and hypotension), imaging-guided aspiration is necessary to exclude infection.

20. Which are the most common locations of pseudoaneurysms?

The most common locations of pseudoaneurysms are splenic, gastroduodenal, and pancreaticoduodenal arteries. The less commonly affected are the left gastric, middle colic, hepatic, and small peripancreatic arteries. The pseudoaneurysms can be free or located within a pseudocyst.

21. What is groove pancreatitis?

Rare segmental form of chronic pancreatitis affecting the groove between the head of the pancreas, duodenum, and CBD. Symptoms may be due to duodenal or CBD stenosis. CT demonstrates a poorly enhancing mass between the head of pancreas and duodenal wall (Fig. 27-7). Cysts may be seen in the duodenal wall or the groove. Groove pancreatitis can not be differentiated from pancreatic carcinoma and needs tissue diagnosis.

22. What are the causes of chronic pancreatitis?

- Alcohol (most common cause)
- Chronic biliary tract disease
- Hereditary pancreatitis
- Cystic fibrosis
- Pancreas divisum
- Hyperlipidemia
- Hyperparathyroidism

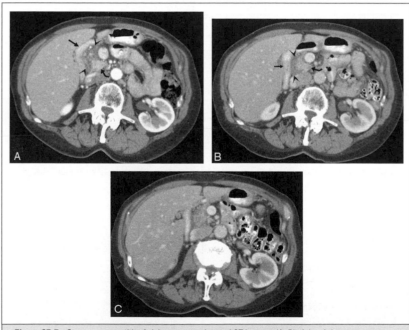

Figure 27-7. Groove pancreatitis. Axial contrast-enhanced CT images *(A, B)* of the abdomen demonstrate a hypodense mass *(arrowheads)* in the groove between the head of the pancreas *(curved arrow)* and second stage of duodenum *(straight arrow)*. A follow-up CT *(C)* after 3 months demonstrates interval partial resolution of the inflammatory mass.

23. **What are the characteristic CT features of chronic pancreatitis?**
    - Pancreatic parenchymal atrophy
    - Main pancreatic duct dilatation (Fig. 27-8)
    - Pancreatic calcifications (see Fig. 27-8)

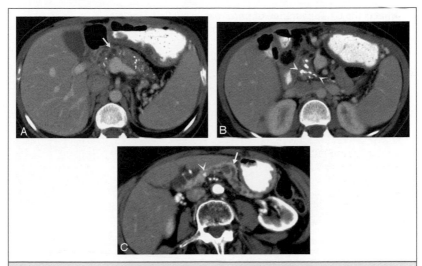

Figure 27-8. Chronic pancreatitis. Axial contrast-enhanced CT images (A, B, C) show diffuse pancreatic parenchymal calcification (arrowheads) and pancreatic duct dilatation (arrow).

24. **Which is the most reliable CT finding in chronic pancreatitis?**
    Pancreatic intraductal calcification is the most reliable CT finding in chronic pancreatitis.

25. **Can CT differentiate changes of focal chronic pancreatitis from carcinoma?**
    Although chronic pancreatitis manifests as diffuse parenchymal atrophy, it may occasionally present as focal areas of enlargement indistinguishable from pancreatic carcinoma. Both of them appear hypodense and show progressive gradual enhancement following IV contrast medium administration. This distinction has to be made by biopsy as risk of carcinoma is increased in chronic pancreatitis.

KEY POINTS: PANCREATITIS

1. The extent of pancreatic necrosis correlates with the morbidity and mortality in acute pancreatitis.

2. Pancreatic intraductal calcification is the most reliable CT feature of chronic pancreatitis.

3. Groove pancreatitis is a segmental form of chronic pancreatitis.

4. Groove pancreatitis cannot be differentiated by imaging from pancreatic carcinoma.

26. What are the complications of chronic pancreatitis?
- Pseudocyst
- CBD obstruction
- Pseudoaneurysms
- Chronic splenic vein thrombosis

27. What is the CT appearance of pancreas in cystic fibrosis?
- Fatty replacement is the most common feature (Fig. 27-9)
- Pancreatic calcifications
- Single or multiple parenchymal cysts of variable size

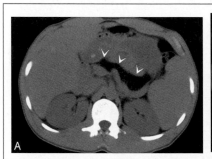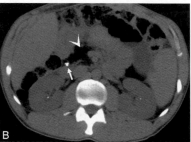

Figure 27-9. Cystic fibrosis. Axial unenhanced CT images *(A, B)* of the abdomen in a patient with known cystic fibrosis show diffuse fatty replacement *(arrowheads)* of the pancreas and calcification *(arrowhead)* in the head of pancreas.

28. Which is the most common type of malignant neoplasm of the pancreas?
Adenocarcinoma arising from the ductal epithelium is the most common malignant neoplasm of the pancreas. It accounts for more than 75% pancreatic tumors.

29. Name the hereditary syndromes associated with pancreatic adenocarcinoma.
- Hereditary pancreatitis
- Ataxia telangiectasis
- Gardner's syndrome
- Familial pancreatic and colon cancer
- Familial aggregates of pancreatic cancer

30. Which is the most common site of ductal adenocarcinoma of pancreas?
Head of the pancreas is the most common site of pancreatic carcinoma. The distribution of pancreatic carcinoma is as follows:
- **Head of the pancreas:** 60%
- **Body of the pancreas:** 13%
- **Tail of the pancreas:** 5%
- **Diffuse involvement:** 22%

31. What are the reasons for the dismal prognosis of pancreatic carcinoma?
Pancreatic adenocarcinoma has an extremely poor prognosis with an overall 5-year survival rate of about 4%. This dismal outcome is due to the advanced stage in which the patients initially present for evaluation. This is due to the nonspecific symptoms and signs in the early stages and no reliable tumor marker for screening. Surgical resection is the only treatment that offers long-term survival rate; however, 10–20% of the tumors are surgically resectable at the time of initial diagnosis.

32. **What is the role of CT in imaging of pancreatic carcinoma?**
CT is the primary imaging modality of pancreas. It plays a crucial role in diagnosis and staging of pancreatic carcinoma and to determine resectability of the tumor.

33. **What are the key objectives of CT scan parameters in the imaging of pancreatic carcinoma?**
The aim is to attain maximal enhancement of the pancreatic parenchyma and peripancreatic vasculature. Multidetector CT with thin collimation and good IV bolus provides high-resolution scans in various phases of contrast enhancement and provides multiplanar reconstruction images. This improves the accuracy of diagnosis and staging of pancreatic carcinoma.

34. **What are the CT findings in pancreatic carcinoma?**
Primary signs are as follows and depend on the size and extent of the tumor:
   - Focal low-attenuation lesion (pancreatic tumor enhances less than normal parenchyma)
   - Focal contour abnormality
   - Enlarged head or uncinate process without discrete mass
   - Peripancreatic fat infiltration
   - Peripancreatic vascular encasement

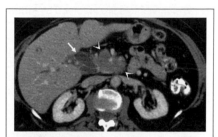

Figure 27-10. Pancreatic adenocarcinoma. Axial contrast-enhanced CT of the abdomen demonstrates a hypodense mass *(arrowheads)* in the head and uncinate process of the pancreas causing CBD *(arrow)* obstruction.

Secondary signs may include the following:
   - Pancreatic and /or CBD dilatation proximal to the mass (Fig. 27-10)
   - Abrupt termination of a dilated pancreatic and/or CBD without a discrete mass
   - Pancreatic parenchymal atrophy proximal to the mass

35. **What are the CT criteria of an unresectable tumor?**
Multidetector CT with multiplanar imaging provides an accuracy of 90–100% in determining resectability. The CT signs of unresectable tumors include the following:
   - Peripancreatic invasion of adjacent organs with the exception of duodenum
   - Vascular invasion of peripancreatic vessels
   - Hepatic metastases, peritoneal implants, and other distant metastases

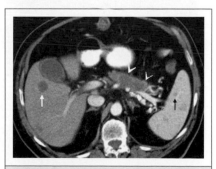

Figure 27-11. Pancreatic adenocarcinoma with liver metastases. Axial contrast-enhanced CT of the abdomen demonstrates a hypodense mass *(arrowheads)* in the body of the pancreas representing primary pancreatic carcinoma with hypodense metastases *(arrows)* in liver and spleen.

36. **Which is the most common site of metastases from pancreatic carcinoma?**
The liver is the most common site of metastases from a pancreatic adenocarcinoma. They appear as hypodense lesions in the portal venous phase of IV contrast enhancement (Fig. 27-11).

KEY POINTS: PANCREATIC CARCINOMA

1. Head is the most common site (60%).

2. It appears as a hypodense mass relative to the enhancing normal parenchyma.

3. Multidetector CT with MPR is the best imaging modality for accurate staging.

4. Liver is the most common site of metastases.

37. **Which vessels are involved by infiltrating pancreatic carcinoma? What are the CT criteria for vascular invasion?**

    The celiac trunk and its branches, superior mesenteric artery (SMA), superior mesenteric vein (SMV), splenic vein, and portal vein are the peripancreatic vessels that are involved by infiltrating pancreatic cancer. Of these, the SMA and SMV are more commonly involved. The CT signs of vascular invasion are occlusion and stenosis and when more than 50% of the vessel circumference is in contact with the tumor (*see* Fig. 27-12).

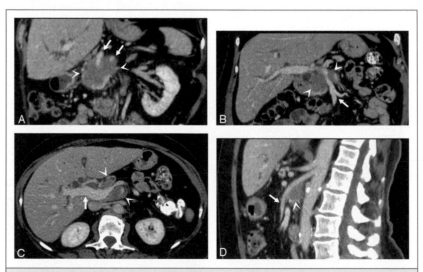

Figure 27-12. Infiltrating pancreatic carcinoma with perivascular invasion. Contrast-enhanced coronal *(A, B)* and sagittal *(D)* reconstructed CT images demonstrate infiltrating pancreatic head mass *(arrowheads)* encasing the superior mesenteric vessels *(arrows)*. Axial CT image *(C)* shows tumor encasing *(arrowheads)* the splenoportal confluence. The portal vein *(arrow)* at the porta hepatis is patent.

38. **What are the different types of cystic pancreatic neoplasms?**

    The cystic neoplasms of the pancreas constitute 10–15% of all the cystic lesions of the pancreas. They are broadly classified into four categories:

    - Serous cystadenomas (microcystic adenomas)
    - Mucinous cystic tumors (cystadenomas and cystadenocarcinomas)
    - Intraductal papillary mucinous tumors (IPMTs)
    - Unusual cystic neoplasms (lymphangioma, papillary cystic tumor, cystic teratoma)

39. **What are CT characteristics of a serous (microcystic) cystadenoma?**
   - Predilection for pancreatic head
   - Increased frequency in von Hippel-Lindau disease
   - Large well-circumscribed mass with a thin fibrous pseudocapsule
   - Multiple small cysts separated by thin septa radiating from the center of the mass
   - Multiple cysts (six or more)
   - Individual cyst less than 2 cm in size
   - Central stellate scar with possible calcifications
   - Septations and central scar with enhancement on contrast-enhanced CT scan (Fig. 27-13)

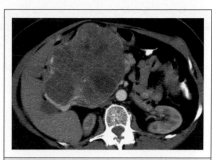

Figure 27-13. Serous (microcystic) cystadenoma. Axial contrast-enhanced CT of the abdomen demonstrates an incidental large, well encapsulated, multilocular cystic mass arising from the head of the pancreas. The loculations are predominantly <2 cm with thin septations.

40. **What are the CT characteristics of mucinous (macrocystic) cystadenoma of pancreas?**
   - Seventy to 90% in the distal body and tail of pancreas
   - Large, lobulated well-encapsulated mass
   - Unilocular or multilocular with cystic spaces separated by septations
   - Relatively few cysts (<6) as compared with serous cystadenoma
   - Individual cyst >2 cm
   - Capsule and septal calcifications in 10% of lesions
   - Capsule and septations with enhancement on contrast-enhanced CT scan
   - Thick septations and enhancing mural nodules—features of malignancy

41. **What are the CT features of a malignant mucinous cystadenoma?**
   Mucinous cystic tumors can be benign or malignant. Differentiation of benign from malignant tumors by imaging is difficult in the absence of metastases. Thick septations and enhancing mural nodules are features of malignancy (*see* Fig. 27-14).

42. **What are IPMTs?**
   IPMT is characterized by cystic dilatation of the pancreatic duct due to proliferation of the ductal epithelium and excess production of mucin. It is classified into main duct, branch duct, and mixed types. The main duct and mixed types have malignant potential. Their clinical presentation is similar to that of chronic pancreatitis. Small branch duct type is asymptomatic and detected incidentally.

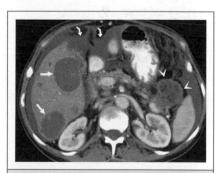

Figure 27-14. Mucinous cystadenocarcinoma. Axial contrast-enhanced CT of the abdomen demonstrates a complex cystic mass (*arrowheads*) with thick septations, arising from the tail of the pancreas. Note multiple cystic hepatic metastases (*straight arrows*) and ascites (*curved arrows*).

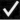
43. **What are the CT characteristics of main duct type IPMT?**
    The CT appearance is often indistinguishable from chronic pancreatitis (Fig. 27-15):
    - Diffuse or segmental dilatation of the main pancreatic duct
    - May be associated with branch duct dilatation preferentially in the uncinate process
    - Intraductal filling defects or amorphous calcification due to mucin
    - Parenchymal atrophy
    - Prominent papilla bulging into the duodenum

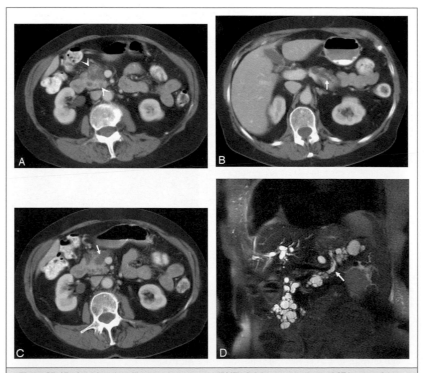

Figure 27-15. Intraductal papillary mucinous tumor (IPMT). Axial contrast-enhanced CT images of the abdomen *(A, B, C)* show diffuse dilatation of the main pancreatic duct and side branches *(arrows)*. The CT features are indistinguishable from chronic pancreatitis. *D,* A corresponding MRCP shows dilated main pancreatic duct *(arrow)* and cystic dilatation of side branches. A diagnosis of IPMT was later established with an ERCP.

44. **What are the CT characteristics of branch duct type of IPMT?**
 - Head and uncinate process are more frequently involved.
 - Cluster of cysts (1–2 cm) are separated by thin septations.
 - Unilocular cyst is found, if only one side branch is involved.
 - Main pancreatic duct may be dilated.

45. **What is the differential diagnosis of IPMT?**
 The main duct type has to be distinguished from chronic pancreatitis and branch duct type from other cystic neoplasms and pseudocyst of the pancreas.

46. **How do you confirm the diagnosis of IPMT?**
 Magnetic resonance cholangiopancreatography (MRCP) and endoscopic retrograde cholangiopancreatography (ERCP) are both useful in confirmation of IPMT. However, ERCP can demonstrate communication between the cystic lesions and pancreatic duct. It will also demonstrate the bulging duodenal papilla with mucin protruding from the patulous orifice into the duodenum, which is characteristic of IPMT.

47. **What are islet cell tumors?**
 These are rare neoplasms arising from neuroendocrine cells of pancreas and the periampullary region. They can be functional or nonfunctional.

48. **Name the various functioning islet cell tumors and describe their clinical presentations.**
 See Table 27-2.

TABLE 27-2. CLINICAL FEATURES OF FUNCTIONING ISLET CELL TUMORS

Islet Cell Tumor	Clinical Presentation	Laboratory Findings
Insulinoma	Hypoglycemic attacks	Hypoglycemia Hyperinsulinemia
Gastrinoma	Multiple peptic ulcers Diarrhea Malabsorption	Elevated serum gastrin
Glucagonoma	Necrolytic migratory erythema	Hyperglycemia
Vipoma	Watery diarrhea	Hypokalemia Hypochlorhydria Acidosis

49. **Which is the most common functioning islet cell tumor?**
 Insulinoma is the most common functioning islet cell tumor.

50. **What is an ideal CT protocol to detect a functioning islet cell tumor?**
 The functioning islet cell tumors are very small and hypervascular as compared with other pancreatic neoplasms, particularly adenocarcinomas. Hence the two most important parameters of the CT protocol are as follows:
 - Thin collimation with 1.25-mm thin reconstructions at 1-mm intervals
 - Good IV bolus (3–4 mL/sec) with arterial and venous phase scans

51. **What are the imaging characteristics of an insulinoma?**
    - Hyperattenuating lesion in the arterial and venous phase
    - Ninety percent of them are solitary (those associated with multiple endocrine neoplasia [MEN] 1 are multiple)
    - Small, usually less than 2 cm

52. **What is the gastrinoma triangle? What are the characteristics of gastrinomas?**
    Unlike insulinomas, gastrinomas are frequently (60%) multiple and malignant. They are predominantly located in the gastrinoma triangle, which is formed by the junction of the CBD and cystic duct superiorly, the second and third portions of the duodenum inferiorly, and the junction between the head and neck of pancreas medially. They are small, hypervascular, and appear as enhancing lesions in the arterial phase.

53. **Which is the common site of metastases from a malignant islet cell tumor?**
    Liver and regional lymph nodes are the common site of metastases. Similar to the primary islet cell tumor, metastases are hypervascular and appear as enhancing lesions in the arterial phase.

54. **What are the characteristics of nonfunctioning islet cell tumors?**
    The nonfunctioning islet cell tumors are often large with metastases at the time of initial diagnosis (Fig. 27-16). They demonstrate heterogeneous enhancement with areas of necrosis, cystic degeneration, and calcification.

55. **What are the characteristics of solid and papillary epithelial neoplasm of pancreas?**
    - Low grade malignant pancreatic tumor
    - Most common in young black females
    - Tail of the pancreas is the most common location (although it can arise from any portion of the pancreas)
    - Large mass lesions with an average size of 10 cm
    - On CT, large well-defined heterogeneous mass lesions with variable internal attenuation due to hemorrhage, necrosis, cystic degeneration, and calcification
    - **Differential considerations:** Other neoplasms arising from the tail of pancreas such as nonfunctioning islet cell tumors and mucinous cystic neoplasm

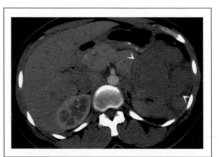

Figure 27-16. Nonfunctioning islet cell tumor. Axial contrast-enhanced CT demonstrates a large hypodense mass *(arrowheads)* arising from the tail of pancreas. Histopathology following distal pancreatectomy demonstrated nonfunctioning islet cell tumor.

KEY POINTS: ISLET CELL TUMORS

1. Insulinoma is the most common functioning islet cell tumor.

2. Gastrinomas are more often multiple, extrapancreatic, and malignant.

3. Gastrinomas and insulinomas may be associated with MEN type I.

4. Enhancement in the arterial phase is the characteristic CT feature.

56. **What are secondary pancreatic neoplasms?**
Secondary pancreatic neoplasms are either due to contiguous spread from an adjacent primary malignancy or due to hematogenous metastases from a distant primary. Primary cancers of the stomach, colon, and duodenum directly invade the pancreas. Primary malignancies of the lung, breast, kidney, ovary, thyroid, liver, gastrointestinal (GI) tract, and melanoma metastasize to the pancreas.

57. **What are periampullary carcinomas?**
Carcinomas arising within 2 cm of the duodenal papilla are termed periampullary carcinomas. They comprise the following:
- Carcinoma of the ampulla of Vater
- Carcinoma of the distal intrapancreatic CBD
- Carcinoma of the head of pancreas
- Carcinoma of the of duodenum

58. **What are the characteristics of periampullary carcinomas?**
They all have common clinical presentation, anatomic location, and therapeutic approach. However, the long-term survival rates are different for each of these tumors. The survival rate is highest for ampullary and duodenal carcinomas, intermediate for CBD carcinoma, and lowest for pancreatic carcinoma.

59. **What are the CT imaging features of periampullary carcinoma?**
The CT appearance depends on the location, extent, and obstruction of the CBD and pancreatic duct.
- Mass at the duodenal papilla with variable involvement of the duodenum and pancreas
- Dilated CBD and pancreatic duct ("double duct sign")
- Isolated dilatation of CBD or pancreatic duct

BIBLIOGRAPHY

1. Balthazar EJ: Complications of acute pancreatitis: Clinical and CT evaluation Radiol Clin North Am 40:1211–1227, 2002.
2. Demos TC, Posniak HV, Harmath C, et al: Cystic lesions of the pancreas. Am J Roentgenol 179:1375–1388, 2002.
3. Lim JH, Lee G, Oh YL: Radiologic spectrum of intraductal papillary mucinous tumor of the pancreas. Radiographics 21:323–337, 2001.
4. Prokesch RW, Chow LC, Beaulieu CF, et al: Local staging of pancreatic carcinoma with multidetector row CT: Use of curved planar reformations initial experience. Radiology 225:759–765, 2002.
5. Vargas R, Nino-Murcia M, Trueblood W, et al: MDCT in Pancreatic adenocarcinoma: Prediction of vascular invasion and respectability using a multiphasic technique with curved planar reformations. Am J Roentgenol 182:419–425, 2004.

CHAPTER 28

SPLEEN

Dean Nakamoto, MD

1. **Name the two types of tissues that make up the spleen.**
   The spleen is made of red pulp and white pulp. The **red pulp** is made of the splenic sinuses, which are thin-walled venous vessels; splenic cords, which are plates of cells that lie between the sinusoids; and terminal branches of the central arteries and pulp veins. The **white pulp** is composed of lymphatic tissue. The marginal zone is the transition between the red and white pulp.

2. **What is the normal size of the spleen?**
   The average spleen weighs 150 gm, with a range of 100–250 gm.

3. **How do you determine spleen size?**
   There are various methods to measure spleen size. One method is as follows:

$$\text{Splenic volume} = 30 + 0.58 \, (W \times L \times Th)$$

   where W = maximum width, Th = maximum thickness, and L = length. With this formula, splenic volume averages 214 cc, with a range of 107–314 cc. From a practical point of view, the normal spleen is less than 13 cm in maximal length. Measurements of 12 cm in length, 7 cm in anteroposterior (AP) diameter, and 5 cm in transverse diameter are borderline.

4. **Describe the normal attenuation of the spleen on CT.**
   The spleen is usually completely within the peritoneum. On unenhanced CT scans, it ranges from 40–60 Hounsfield units, typically 5–10 Hounsfield units less than normal liver. Following intravenous (IV) contrast enhancement, the spleen can have a mottled heterogeneous or arciform and cordlike appearance during the arterial phase and early portal venous phase, believed to be due to differential enhancement of the cords and sinuses of the red pulp. On the middle to late portal venous phase, the spleen becomes uniform in appearance.

5. **Why is it important to recognize the mottled appearance of the normal spleen on the arterial and early portal venous phase images?**
   Typically, the spleen has a mottled, arciform appearance during this phase, with bands of enhancing tissue between bands of nonenhancing tissue. This appearance can be exaggerated in patients with heart failure, decreased cardiac output, or delayed splenic flow due to splenic vein thrombosis. Splenic lacerations may be missed during this phase. In addition, this enhancement pattern can simulate a mass (Fig. 28-1). Therefore, it is important to obtain delayed images in patients in whom a splenic process is suspected (e.g., trauma or suspected masses).

6. **What are some normal variants of the spleen?**
   - **Splenic clefts** are common. These are usually easily recognized due to their sharp smooth borders. Typically, they are located superiorly and medially but can occur anywhere.
   - **Accessory spleens** are also common. Typically, they are located near the splenic hilum but can occur anywhere in the peritoneal cavity. They are important to differentiate from peritoneal metastases.

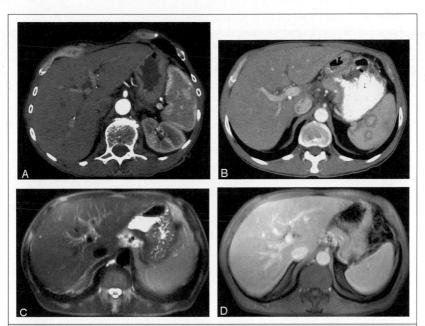

Figure 28-1. Normal splenic enhancement—unusual appearances. Typically, the spleen has an arciform or mottled appearance during the arterial phase of contrast enhancement. However, other patterns of enhancement can occur. It is important to recognize these other patterns as normal. Delayed scans or MRI can be helpful in some instances. ***A,*** Predominantly peripheral enhancement. ***B,*** The CT scan demonstrates nodular enhancement. However, the T2-weighted MRI *(C)* and the T1-weighted 3-minute post-gadolinium MRI *(D)* demonstrate no focal splenic lesions.

- **Wandering spleens** are mobile due to lack of fusion or abnormal development of the splenic suspensory ligaments (gastrosplenic and splenorenal ligaments).

7. **What are some unusual locations for accessory spleens?**
   Accessory spleens have been described in paratesticular, diaphragmatic, gastric, and pararenal sites. They are usually solitary but can be multiple. If multiple, they may be clustered. The diagnosis is confirmed by technetium-labeled heat-damaged red blood cells.

8. **Name the common causes of splenomegaly.**
   - **Mild-to-moderate splenomegaly:** Portal hypertension, infection, acquired immunodeficiency syndrome (AIDS)
   - **Marked splenomegaly:** Leukemia, lymphoma, myelofibrosis

9. **What are the primary neoplasms of the spleen?**
   The **benign** neoplasms are hemangioma, hamartoma, and lymphangioma. The **malignant neoplasms** are lymphoma and angiosarcoma. **Metastases** may occur but are rare.

10. **What is the most common benign neoplasm of the spleen?**
    Although rare, hemangioma is the most common primary neoplasm of the spleen. The incidence ranges from 0.3–14%. Typically the patient is asymptomatic; however, 25% of splenic hemangiomas may rupture or cause symptoms of hypersplenism.

11. **What are the different types of splenic hemangiomas?**
   Splenic hemangiomas arise from sinusoidal epithelium and range from capillary to cavernous. Most are cavernous and can be solitary or multiple. The smaller hemangiomas, both capillary and cavernous, tend to be solid; the larger cavernous hemangiomas can be mixed solid and cystic.

12. **Describe the typical CT appearances of hemangiomas.**
   Splenic hemangiomas can have variable appearances, from solid to mixed solid and cystic. Capillary hemangiomas are typically well-defined solid masses, which are hypoattenuating or isoattenuating to the spleen on unenhanced scans and demonstrate marked homogeneous contrast enhancement (Fig. 28-2).

   Cavernous hemangiomas can have solid and cystic components. The early-phase postcontrast images shows marked enhancement of the solid components. The late- or delayed-phase contrast enhancement pattern may be discrete mottled areas of heterogeneous enhancement rather than peripheral nodules with centripetal enhancement typical of liver hemangiomas. The lesions are usually small but can be as large as 17 cm. Curvilinear or eggshell calcifications can occur in cystic hemangiomas, and central calcifications can occur in solid hemangiomas.

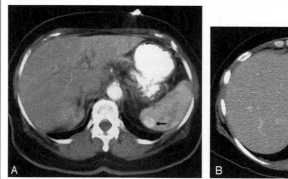

Figure 28-2. Splenic hemangioma. *A,* Typical hemangioma in the posterior upper pole. It demonstrates peripheral early enhancement *(arrow).* *B,* Multiple small low-attenuation hemangiomas *(arrows).*

13. **Are any syndromes associated with splenic hemangioma?**
   Kasabach-Merritt syndrome (anemia, thrombocytopenia, and coagulopathy) has been reported with large hemangiomas. When splenic hemangiomas are multiple, the patient may have generalized angiomatosis (**Klippel-Trenaunay-Weber syndrome**). If the entire organ is replaced by hemangiomas, it is called **hemangiomatosis.**

14. **How does one confirm the diagnosis of splenic hemangioma?**
   The typical splenic hemangiomas appear similar to liver hemangiomas. On CT, they are low in attenuation and demonstrate peripheral enhancement. On magnetic resonance imaging (MRI), they are typically low in signal on T1-weighted images and increased in signal relative to normal spleen on T2-weighted images. They demonstrate progressive enhancement following IV gadolinium and retain contrast on the delayed images. However, atypical splenic hemangiomas may be difficult to differentiate from malignant lesions. On technetium-99m-tagged red cell study, they usually take up pharmaceutical.

15. **What are other benign tumors of the spleen?**
   Other benign splenic neoplasms are rare but include splenic hamartoma and lymphangioma.

16. **What is a splenic hamartoma?**
Splenic hamartoma is a rare benign tumor; approximately 120 cases have been reported in the English literature. They consist of a mixture of normal splenic red pulp elements, likely congenital in origin. They are usually solitary and may be solid or cystic. They may be associated with hamartomas elsewhere in the body and have been reported in tuberous sclerosis and Wiskott-Aldrich-like syndrome. On CT scans, they can be similar to the normal spleen on pre- and postcontrast images and therefore difficult to visualize.

17. **What is splenic lymphangioma?**
Splenic lymphangiomas are rare slow-growing benign tumors composed of lymphatic vessels. They are typically cystic and can be solitary or multiple. They tend to occur in the periphery and trabeculae of the spleen, where lymphatics are located. A subcapsular cystic lesion with septations and small mural nodules incidentally noted in a child should raise the possibility of lymphangioma.

18. **What is lymphangiomatosis?**
Lymphangiomatosis is a syndrome in which multiple organs are involved with lymphangiomas. With lymphangiomatosis, the spleen may be completely replaced by lymphangiomas, but it can also be relatively spared.

19. **What is littoral cell angioma?**
Littoral cell angioma is a rare vascular neoplasm of the spleen that arises from littoral cells (from red pulp sinuses). Typically, there is splenomegaly and multiple focal tumors. The patients may present with anemia or thrombocytopenia. They were originally described as benign but may have malignant features. On early-phase contrast-enhanced CT, they appear as multiple low-attenuation lesions, which is nonspecific. However, on delayed images they become isointense to normal spleen. On MRI, these lesions typically appear hypointense on both T1- and T2-weighted images due to hemosiderin in the lesions resulting from hemophagocytosis by the neoplastic cells.

20. **What is splenic peliosis?**
Peliosis is a rare disease in which multiple blood-filled spaces involve the spleen and liver. Most cases occur with wasting diseases, such as AIDS, anabolic steroid use, and hematologic disorders, such as aplastic anemia. Surface lesions may rupture. On contrast-enhanced CT, they have been described as both enhancing lesions and as low-attenuation nodules, sometimes with fluid-fluid levels.

21. **What are the nonneoplastic cystic lesions of the spleen?**
There are three main types of nonneoplastic cystic lesions of the spleen: congenital epithelial cysts, post-traumatic pseudocysts, and hydatid cysts. Splenic abscesses and infarcts may appear cystic. Pancreatic pseudocysts may also extend into the spleen.

KEY POINTS: SPLENIC MASSES

1. Most are malignant.

2. Lymphoma is the most common malignancy.

3. Hemangioma is the most common benign neoplasm.

22. **What are epithelial cysts?**
Epithelial (also called epidermoid, mesothelial, or primary) cysts are congenital in origin and are true cysts with an epithelial lining. They are usually unilocular and solitary but may be multiple.

23. What are post-traumatic pseudocysts?

Post-traumatic pseudocysts are thought to represent the end stage of splenic hematomas. They do not have an epithelial lining and are therefore called pseudocysts. Although they are presumed to be post-traumatic, a history of previous trauma is present in only one fourth to one half of the cases; however, the trauma may have been in the distant past and not recalled. Post-traumatic pseudocysts are more likely to have peripheral curvilinear calcification than epithelial cysts. Post-traumatic pseudocysts are the most common splenic cystic lesions in the United States.

24. What are hydatid cysts?

Hydatid disease of the spleen is uncommon and occurs in less than 2% of all patients with echinococcus. The appearance varies depending on the age of the cyst and the associated complications. They can range from homogeneous fluid content to complex cysts with debris, hydatid sand, peripheral daughter cysts, and peripheral calcifications.

25. What is the most common malignant neoplasm of the spleen?

Lymphoma is the most common malignancy of the spleen. Splenic lymphoma can be primary, which accounts for up to 2% of all lymphomas, or secondary as part of diffuse systemic involvement. The spleen is involved in 25–33% of patients with Hodgkin or non-Hodgkin lymphoma.

26. Describe the appearance of splenic lymphoma on CT.

There are four gross pathologic patterns of splenic lymphoma:
- Homogeneous enlargement without discrete mass
- Miliary nodules less than 5 mm in size
- Multifocal masses of various sizes from 1–10 cm
- Solitary mass

Focal lesions are more common in non-Hodgkin lymphoma than in Hodgkin lymphoma. Lymphomatous lesions usually do not enhance; however, they occasionally can enhance and become isoattenuating with the spleen. The most common imaging finding is splenomegaly, but splenomegaly may be absent in one third of the patients (*see* Fig. 28-3).

27. Does splenomegaly in a patient with lymphoma always indicate splenic lymphoma?

No. Up to 30% of enlarged spleens in lymphoma patients are benign in origin.

28. What is an angiosarcoma of the spleen?

Angiosarcoma of the spleen as a primary tumor is rare. Hepatic angiosarcomas may be associated with toxic exposure (vinyl chloride, arsenic); primary splenic angiosarcoma may not have this association.

29. Which primary neoplasms metastasize to the spleen?

Splenic metastases are relatively uncommon and occur in approximately 7% of patients with malignancy at autopsy. The common sites of primary tumor are breast, lung, ovary, stomach, melanoma, and prostate. Most of these are due to hematogenous spread. Although melanoma is not the most common source of splenic metastases, it has the highest frequency of metastases to the spleen. Up to 36% of melanomas will metastasize to the spleen. The most common metastasis to the spleen is from lung carcinoma.

30. Which primary neoplasms can cause cystic splenic metastases?

Cystic metastases can be seen with melanoma and ovary, breast, and endometrial carcinoma.

31. What are the different mechanisms of infection of the spleen?

The causes of splenic infection can be divided into five groups:

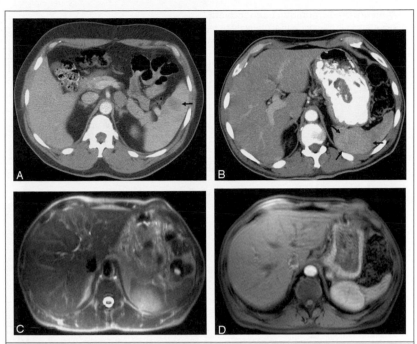

Figure 28-3. Splenic lymphoma. *A,* Non-Hodgkin lymphoma presents as a focal lesion in the midpole anteriorly *(arrow).* *B,* Enhancing, poorly defined focal B-cell lymphoma in the midpole posteriorly in a different patient *(arrows).* However, it is seen on the T2-weighted MRI *(C)* as a high signal intensity mass and demonstrates early enhancement on the T1-weighted 20-second post-gadolinium image *(D).* Typically, lymphomas do not enhance relative to the spleen.

- Metastatic or embolic infection (i.e., subacute bacterial endocarditis, sepsis)
- Contiguous infection (i.e., perinephric abscess, infected pancreas)
- Immunodeficiency states
- Trauma
- Embolic noninfectious events causing ischemia and subsequent infection

The abscesses may be bacterial, fungal, or mycobacterial in origin. Although splenic abscesses are uncommon, they have become more frequent due to an increasing number of immunosuppressed patients, including patients with leukemia who receive aggressive chemotherapy and bone marrow transplants and patients with human immunodeficiency virus (HIV) and AIDS.

32. **Describe the CT appearances of bacterial splenic abscesses.**
Pyogenic splenic abscesses are usually solitary but may be multiple. Initially, an abscess may appear as a low-attenuation mass. They may subsequently form septations, debris, and thick walls. The presence of gas is diagnostic; however, the majority of splenic abscesses do not contain gas (Fig. 28-4).

33. **In a patient with fever, left upper quadrant pain, malaise, and cystic lesions in the spleen, how can one distinguish between a splenic abscess and a necrotic or cystic splenic lymphoma?**
In general, splenic abscess rarely presents with lymphadenopathy, unlike lymphoma. Necrosis in lymphoma is rare; however, large lymphoma lesions can have cystic components. Splenic infarcts may occur in conjunction with lymphoma.

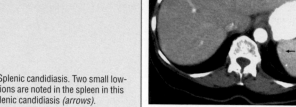

Figure 28-4. Splenic candidiasis. Two small low-attenuation lesions are noted in the spleen in this patient with splenic candidiasis *(arrows)*.

34. **What are the features of fungal abscesses?**

    Fungal microabscesses are usually 5–10 mm in size, although they can be up to 2 cm. The liver and spleen are usually both involved. They can be very difficult to visualize by CT. When visualized, fungal microabscesses may appear as small low-attenuation lesions, although there can be a central focus of higher attenuation, giving a "wheel-within-a-wheel" appearance. Magnetic resonance imaging (MRI) is probably the best way to detect and characterize fungal microabscesses (Fig. 28-5).

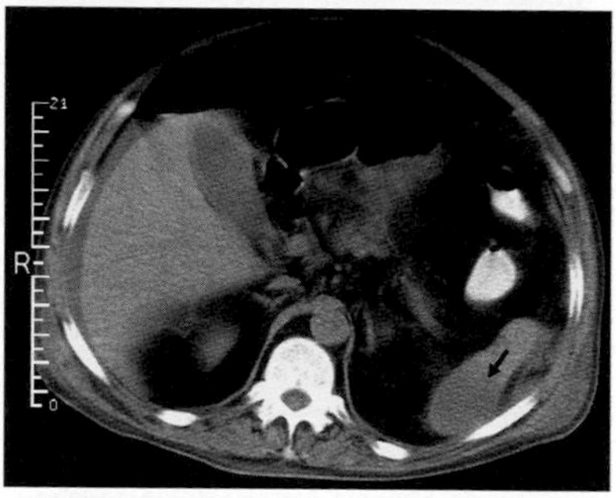

Figure 28-5. Splenic abscess. Pyogenic splenic abscess *(arrow)* in a patient with a history of alcohol abuse.

35. **What types of splenic abnormalities can be seen in AIDS patients?**

    The most common finding is splenomegaly, usually moderate. Focal lesions may be due to opportunistic infections, such as *Candida, Pneumocystis,* or *Mycobacterium.* These can present as foci of low attenuation, "wheel-within-a-wheel" lesions, or small calcifications. Peliosis due to bacillary angiomatosis can occur. Neoplastic lesions, such as Kaposi's sarcoma or lymphoma, can also be seen.

36. **What is the appearance of splenic infarcts?**

    Splenic infarcts are a common cause of a focal splenic lesion. The typical CT appearance is a peripheral, wedge-shaped, and low-attenuation lesion (Fig. 28-6). They can be irregular in contour. Contrast-enhanced CT best delineates the areas of splenic infarct. Over time, they decrease in size. Occasionally, infarct can be difficult to differentiate from abscess or tumor. The lack of mass effect can help differentiate an infarct from splenic abscess or neoplasm, such as lymphoma. However, in leukemia and lymphoma, splenic infarcts may be round and central and thus may mimic neoplasm or abscess.

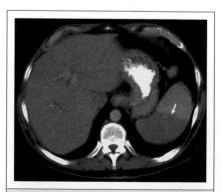

Figure 28-6. Splenic infarct. A patient with a large splenic infarct *(arrow)* involving the posterior aspect of the spleen.

37. **What are the common causes of splenic infarct?**
    In younger patients, splenic infarcts may occur from local thrombosis due to hematologic diseases, such as the various sickle hemoglobinopathies. In elderly patients, splenic infarcts are most commonly due to embolic events from cardiovascular diseases. Other causes include myeloproliferative disorders, splenic artery aneurysm, pancreatitis, splenic torsion, and portal hypertension.

38. **What are the potential complications of splenic infarct?**
    Complications may be seen in up to 20% of splenic infarcts. These include abscess, pseudocyst formation, and hemorrhage.

39. **What are the typical splenic manifestations of sickle cell disease?**
    - **Homozygous form:** Splenomegaly in the first year of life with progressive loss of function due to microinfarcts. These microinfarcts lead to gradual decrease in size, which progresses to fibrosis and calcification.
    - **Heterozygous form:** Splenomegaly may persist into adulthood because there is partial splenic function.

40. **What is splenic sequestration?**
    Splenic sequestration is a complication of sickle cell disease and is due to a sudden trapping of a large amount of blood in the spleen, resulting in rapid enlargement of the spleen and fall in hematocrit. Areas of infarction, hemorrhage, and necrosis are present. Infants and children are most susceptible, because their spleens are still distensible.

41. **What is the role of CT in blunt splenic trauma?**
    The spleen is the most frequently injured solid abdominal organ. In general, contrast-enhanced CT is the modality of choice to image stable patients with trauma. The spleen is the most frequently injured solid parenchymal organ in the abdomen. Contrast-enhanced CT allows for grading of splenic injuries (Table 28-1) and allows for evaluation of active extravasation. Although CT grading scales are important, the need for surgical intervention is determined by a combination of multiple factors, including clinical, laboratory, and radiologic findings (Fig. 28-7).

TABLE 28 1. AMERICAN ASSOCIATION FOR THE SURGERY OF TRAUMA SPLENIC INJURY SCALE		
Grade*	Type of Injury	Description
I	Hematoma	Subcapsular, <10% surface area
	Laceration	Capsular tear, ≤1-cm parenchymal depth
II	Hematoma	Subcapsular, 10–50% surface area; intraparenchymal, <5 cm in diameter
	Laceration	1- to 3-cm parenchymal depth that does not involve a trabecular vessel
III	Hematoma	Subcapsular, >50% surface area or expanding; ruptured subcapsular or parenchymal hematoma; intraparenchymal, >5 cm or expanding
	Laceration	>3-cm parenchymal depth or involving trabecular vessels
IV	Laceration	Laceration involving segmental or hilar vessels producing major devascularization (>25% of spleen)
V	Laceration	Completely shattered spleen
	Vascular	Hilar vascular injury that devascularizes spleen

*Advance one grade for multiple injuries, up to grade III.
Adapted from Moore EE, Cogbill TH, Jurkovich GJ, et al: Organ injury scaling: spleen and liver (1994 revision). J Trauma 38:323–324, 1995.

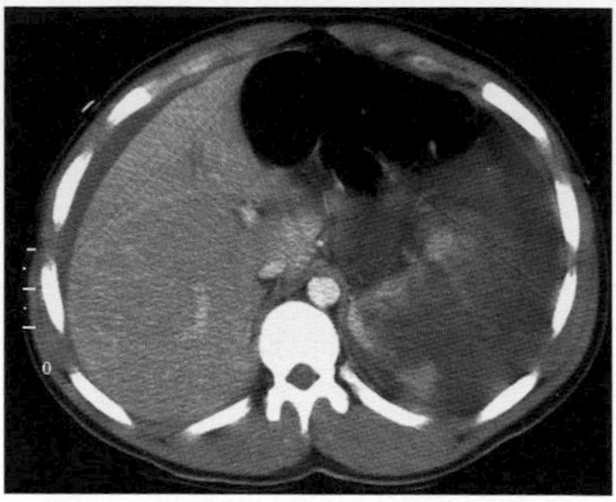

Figure 28-7. Splenic rupture. A patient after a fall from a ladder with a ruptured spleen (grade V). This injury required splenectomy.

42. What important findings from blunt trauma can be identified by CT?
Subcapsular hematomas, perisplenic hematomas, lacerations, fractures, vascular injuries, and active extravasation can be identified by CT.

43. What are potential CT pitfalls in the interpretation of blunt splenic trauma?
False-positive results
- Normal lobulation or clefts may mimic laceration. However, here the margins are smooth, with no evidence of adjacent hematoma.
- Adjacent unopacified loop of bowel may cause a false-positive result.
- Differential enhancement of red pulp of the spleen during early arterial enhancement can mimic laceration.
- Previous splenic infarct can mimic laceration.
- Perisplenic fluid from ascites can mimic trauma.

False-negative results: Poor or delayed contrast infusion may cause an isoattenuating splenic hematoma to be missed.

KEY POINTS: SPLENIC EMERGENCIES

1. Splenic rupture (trauma, pathologic splenomegaly)

2. Infection and abscess

3. Infarct (splenic sequestration, wandering spleen, and torsion)

44. What is the role of CT to monitor healing of blunt splenic injury?
CT can demonstrate interval decrease in size of hematomas and lacerations. Progressive increase in spleen size can be seen, because the spleen may contract acutely following the trauma due to decreased intravascular volume and adrenergic stimulation. CT can also detect pseudoaneurysms of the spleen that may result from nonoperative management of splenic lacerations or with spleen-salvaging surgery.

45. What is the significance of a splenic pseudoaneurysm?
These may expand and cause delayed splenic rupture with a risk from 6–10% (Fig. 28-8).

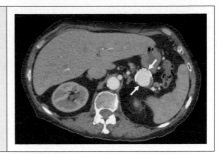

Figure 28-8. Splenic artery pseudoaneurysm. Incidentally noted 3-cm pseudoaneurysm of the splenic artery *(arrows)*.

46. **How are splenic pseudoaneurysms treated?**
    Rarely, these resolve spontaneously. Usually, catheter embolization is performed, with a reported 77% success rate. If embolization fails, open repair is an option.

47. **What is the differential diagnosis of multiple spleens?**
    The main differential considerations are polysplenia, post-traumatic splenosis, and multiple accessory spleens.

48. **What is the difference between polysplenia and asplenia?**
    Polysplenia and asplenia are two of the major congenital splenic anomalies. These conditions are part of the spectrum of visceral heterotaxy. Patients with polysplenia may have bilateral left-sidedness or a dominance of left-sided over right-sided body structures. Polysplenia patients may have two morphologic left lungs, left-sided azygous continuation of an interrupted inferior vena cava, biliary atresia, absence of the gallbladder, gastrointestinal malrotation, and cardiovascular abnormalities.
    Asplenic patients may have bilateral right-sidedness. They may have two morphologic right lungs, reversed position of the abdominal aorta and inferior vena cava, anomalous pulmonary venous return, and horseshoe kidneys.

49. **What are the indications for splenic biopsy?**
    ■ Diagnosis of infections, especially in the immunocompromised population, including tuberculosis (TB), *Candida* spp., *Pneumocystis carinii*
    ■ Biopsy of a focal solid mass, usually lymphoma or metastasis
    ■ Aspiration of a fluid collection for diagnosis of infection

50. **What complications are encountered?**
    The major complication risk is bleeding, which occurs in up to 10% of patients. As many as 8% of patients have major bleeding requiring splenectomy. Bleeding may be a delayed complication, occurring hours to days following the biopsy. Risk factors for bleeding include coagulopathy, low platelet count, and peripherally located lesions. If trying to diagnose metastatic disease, it is still deemed safer to biopsy sites other that the spleen, because the splenic risk of bleeding complications exceeds that of most other sites.

51. **Does the needle size relate to biopsy success or bleeding risk?**
    No. Commonly used needles include 20–23 gauge for fine needle aspiration and 18–20 gauge core needles, with biopsy accuracy of 85–90% for most series, independent of needle. Similarly, the bleeding risk seems to be equivalent, independent of needle size.

52. What are important features of splenic artery aneurysms?

Splenic artery aneurysms and pseudoaneurysms are not uncommon. Surgical repair may be indicated if they become 3 cm or larger. Splenic artery aneurysms may be mistaken for a pancreatic or peripancreatic fluid collection or mass; thus it is important to obtain images during a good bolus of IV contrast prior to performing an interventional procedure.

BIBLIOGRAPHY

1. Dachman AH, Friedman AC: Radiology of the Spleen. St. Louis, Mosby, 1993.

2. Moore EE, Cogbill TH, Jurkovich GJ, et al: Organ injury scaling: Spleen and liver (1994 revision). J Trauma 38:323–324, 1995.

3. Nakamoto DA, Onders RP: The spleen. In Haaga JR, Lanzieri CF, Gilkeson RC (eds): CT and MRI of the Whole Body (ed 4). Mosby, St. Louis, 2002.

4. Prassopoulos P, Daskalogiannaki M, Raissaki M, et al: Determination of normal splenic volume on computed tomography in relation to age, gender and body habitus. Eur Radiol 7:246–248, 1997.

CHAPTER 29

RETROPERITONEUM

Shweta Bhatt, MD, and Kedar Chintapalli, MD

1. **Define the retroperitoneum and describe its boundaries.**
   The retroperitoneum is a large potential space bounded anteriorly by the posterior parietal peritoneum, posteriorly by the transversalis fascia, superiorly by the diaphragm, inferiorly by the levators, and laterally by the flank muscles at the level of the anterior superior spine of the iliac crest to the tip of the twelfth rib.

2. **Describe the subdivisions of the retroperitoneal space.**
   The retroperitoneum is divided into three spaces by the lateral conal fascia, which is formed by the fusion of the anterior (Gerota's) and posterior (Zuckerkandl's) renal fascia (Fig. 29-1). The three retroperitoneal spaces are as follows:
   - Anterior pararenal space
   - Perinephric space
   - Posterior pararenal space

3. **Describe the contents of the retroperitoneal spaces.**
   - The **anterior pararenal space** lies between the parietal peritoneum and the anterior renal fascia and continues in the midline to join the lateral conal fascia laterally. It contains the pancreas, duodenum, and ascending and descending colon.
   - The **perinephric space** is the space limited by the anterior and posterior renal fascia and contains the kidneys, adrenal glands, inferior vena cava (IVC), aorta, renal vessels, ureters, and fat.
   - The **posterior pararenal space** is contiguous with the peritoneal fat and lies within the posterior renal fascia and the transversalis fascia. It contains the psoas muscle and fat.

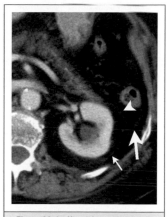

Figure 29-1. Normal renal fasciae. Contrast-enhanced computed tomography (CECT) of the left kidney shows the anterior Gerota's fascia *(arrowhead)* and posterior Zuckerkandl's fascia *(small arrow)*, which fuse laterally to form the lateral conal fascia *(large arrow)*.

4. **What is the modality of choice for the imaging of the retroperitoneum?**
   CT scan with use of intravenous contrast is considered the gold standard for the imaging of the retroperitoneum. CT angiography (CTA) can be used to depict the retroperitoneal vasculature.

5. **What is the most common cause of presence of fluid in the anterior pararenal space?**
   Pancreatitis (Fig. 29-2). Other causes include pathologies involving the duodenum, such as duodenal hematoma (Fig. 29-3) and the ascending and descending colon.

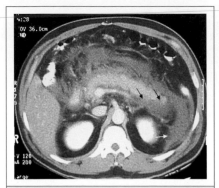

Figure 29-2. Pancreatitis. Fluid from pancreatitis is seen around the pancreas and extends lateral to the kidney in the anterior pararenal space *(arrows).*

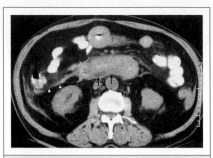

Figure 29-3. Duodenal hematoma. Note thickening of the duodenal wall from duodenal hematoma *(arrows).* Note also the thickening of renal fascia *(arrowheads).*

6. **What is the cause of presence of air in the perinephric spaces?**
   Extension of emphysematous pyelonephritis of either kidney can show presence of air in either or both the perinephric spaces due to the communication between the two perinephric spaces through the midline (Fig. 29-4). Other causes include renal intervention procedures or postoperative status and perinephric abscess.

7. **Describe the etiology of retroperitoneal abscesses.**
   Retroperitoneal abscesses can be primary resulting from hematogenous spread or secondary due to contiguous spread from an adjacent organ. Various causes of retroperitoneal abscesses are listed in descending order of frequency:

   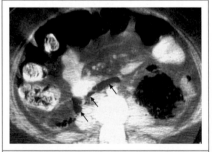

   Figure 29-4. Emphysematous pyelonephritis. In this patient with left emphysematous pyelonephritis, air is also seen in right perirenal space *(arrows)* as the two spaces communicate with each other.

   - Renal infections
   - Gastrointestinal diseases such as diverticulitis, Crohn's disease, and appendicitis
   - Hematogenous spread from remote infections
   - Postoperative complications
   - Bone infections, such as tuberculosis of spine
   - Trauma
   - Malignancies involving the retroperitoneum

8. **Describe the CT appearance of a retroperitoneal abscess.**
   CT demonstrates a low-attenuation mass in the retroperitoneum with peripheral enhancing walls and surrounding inflammatory changes (Fig. 29-5). Gas may be seen in about one third of retroperitoneal abscesses. CT can also depict the relationship of the abscess with adjacent organs, indicating the possible source of infection.

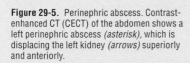

Figure 29-5. Perinephric abscess. Contrast-enhanced CT (CECT) of the abdomen shows a left perinephric abscess *(asterisk)*, which is displacing the left kidney *(arrows)* superiorly and anteriorly.

9. **Describe the role of CT in the management of retroperitoneal abscesses.**
   CT-guided percutaneous drainage along with a proper course of antibiotics is the first line of treatment for retroperitoneal abscesses and has a high success rate. Operative drainage is the alternative treatment if the CT-guided drainage is unsuccessful or if percutaneous drainage is not possible.

10. **What are the causes of retroperitoneal hematoma?**
    Common causes include the following:
    - Trauma—blunt or penetrating (Fig. 29-6)
    - Abdominal aortic aneurysm (AAA) or visceral artery aneurysm rupture (Fig. 29-7)
    - Anticoagulant or fibrinolytic therapy
    Rare causes include rupture of a renal angiomyolipoma in to the perinephric space (Fig. 29-8), rupture of an adrenal cyst, and so forth.

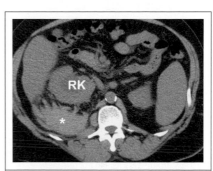

Figure 29-6. Perinephric hematoma secondary to trauma. Nonenhanced CT of the abdomen shows a retroperitoneal hematoma *(asterisk)*, which displaces the right kidney (RK) anteriorly.

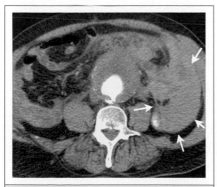

Figure 29-7. Aortic aneurysm rupture. Contrast-enhanced CT (CECT) of the abdomen shows a ruptured aortic aneurysm with a large retroperitoneal hematoma *(arrows)*.

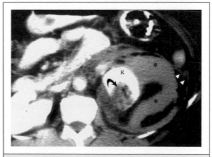

Figure 29-8. Perinephric hematoma secondary to angiomyolipoma. A left renal angiomyolipoma *(curved arrow)* with perirenal hemorrhage is seen *(asterisk)*. Note thickening of the lateroconal fascia *(arrowheads)*. K = kidney.

11. **What is the most common site for spontaneous retroperitoneal hemorrhage?**
The posterior pararenal space is the most common site for spontaneous retroperitoneal hemorrhage.

12. **Describe the CT appearance of retroperitoneal hematoma.**
CT of retroperitoneal hematoma demonstrates a nonenhancing high-density mass in the retroperitoneum with presence of stranding in the retroperitoneal tissue planes.

13. **Describe retroperitoneal fibrosis.**
Retroperitoneal fibrosis refers to the inflammatory condition resulting from proliferation of the fibrous tissue in the posterior aspect of retroperitoneum, causing encasement of blood vessels and ureters. It is usually bilateral.

14. **What is Ormond's disease?**
Retroperitoneal fibrosis secondary to an idiopathic etiology is termed Ormond's disease. It accounts for 70% of cases of retroperitoneal fibrosis.

15. **What are the causes of retroperitoneal fibrosis?**
   - Idiopathic (70%)
   - Drugs (ergot alkaloids, dopaminergic agonists)
   - Infections
   - Trauma
   - Retroperitoneal hemorrhage
   - Retroperitoneal surgery
   - Radiation therapy
   - Primary or metastatic tumors

16. **Describe the CT appearance of retroperitoneal fibrosis.**
Nonenhanced CT shows an isodense to hyperdense fibrosis in the retroperitoneum appearing like a mass over the aorta and the ureters with medial deviation of the ureters (Fig. 29-9). With intravenous contrast, early stages of retroperitoneal fibrosis show some enhancement owing to the higher vascularity at an early stage. At a later stage, fibrosis shows no enhancement. Malignant retroperitoneal fibrosis may involve the ureters, and this may lead to proximal dilatation of the ureters with hydronephrosis.

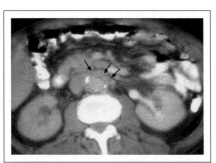

Figure 29-9. Retroperitoneal fibrosis. In this patient with mild left hydronephrosis, a rind of soft tissue is seen anterior to the aorta and inferior vena cava *(arrows)* from retroperitoneal fibrosis.

17. **Describe malignant retroperitoneal fibrosis.**
Malignant retroperitoneal fibrosis is a result of direct spread of malignant cells enclosing the ureter or a severe desmoplastic reaction in the retroperitoneum secondary to multiple metastases. Malignant fibrosis can be differentiated from benign fibrosis with biopsies performed under imaging guidance.

18. **What is the normal size of retroperitoneal lymph nodes?**
The upper limit of normal size of retroperitoneal nodes is as follows:
   - **6 mm:** Retrocrural and porta hepatis

- **9 mm:** Gastrohepatic
- **10 mm:** Lower para-aortic, celiac axis, mesenteric, and pelvic nodes

19. **Describe the CT findings in a malignant retroperitoneal lymphadenopathy.**
CT findings in a malignant lymphadenopathy are variable and can include the following:
- Single or multiple discrete enlarged lymph nodes
- Conglomeration of enlarged lymph nodes
- Large homogeneous mass that obscures the normal contours of surrounding structures

20. **Can benign and malignant lymphadenopathy be differentiated on CT?**
No. However, CT may be able to diagnose certain conditions:
- Whipple disease shows lymph nodes with a low attenuation from 10–30 HU secondary to deposition of fat and fatty acids.
- Lymph nodes with low attenuation <30 HU with peripheral enhancement due to central necrosis are suggestive of *Mycobacterium tuberculosis* infection.
- Calcified nodes are a feature of postinflammatory conditions, mucinous carcinoma, sarcomas, and treated lymphomas.

21. **What is the most common benign tumor involving the retroperitoneum?**
Lymphangioma. Other benign retroperitoneal tumors include lipomas, paragangliomas, neurogenic tumors, hemangiomas, and mature teratomas.

22. **Describe the types of retroperitoneal malignancies.**

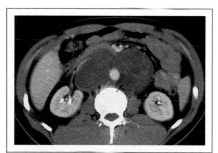

Figure 29-10. Retroperitoneal lymphadenopathy. In a patient with testicular cancer, enlarged para-aortic lymph nodes are seen *(arrows)*.

- Extracapsular growth of a primary neoplasm of a retroperitoneal organ, such as the kidney, adrenal, colon, or pancreas
- Primary germ cell neoplasm arising from embryonic rest cells
- Primary malignancy of the retroperitoneal lymphatic system, such as lymphoma
- Metastasis to retroperitoneal lymph node, as from testicular cancer (Fig. 29-10)
- Primary malignancy of the soft tissue of the retroperitoneum (e.g., sarcomas and desmoid tumors)

23. **Which is the most common retroperitoneal malignancy?**
Malignant fibrous histiocytoma is the most common primary retroperitoneal malignancy, followed by retroperitoneal liposarcoma.

24. **What are the histologic types of retroperitoneal sarcomas?**
Retroperitoneal liposarcoma, leiomyosarcoma, fibrosarcoma, and malignant peripheral nerve sheath tumor.

25. **Describe the CT findings of a retroperitoneal sarcoma.**
Retroperitoneal sarcomas are malignant tumors arising from mesenchymal cells and are usually located in muscle, fat, and connective tissues (Fig. 29-11). They appear as soft tissue density masses that displace, compress, or obscure the retroperitoneal structures.
CT of a retroperitoneal liposarcoma (Fig. 29-12) shows a mixed density mass with both fat and soft tissue components. This mass shows some enhancement on intravenous contrast administration.

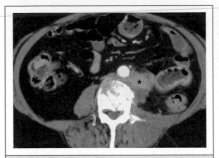

Figure 10-11. Retroperitoneal sarcoma. Contrast-enhanced computed tomography (CECT) of the retroperitoneum demonstrates a left para aortic retroperitoneal mass *(asterisk)* involving the left psoas muscle, confirmed on biopsy.

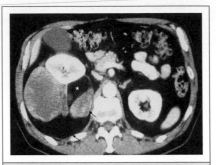

Figure 29-12. Retroperitoneal liposarcoma. The right kidney is displaced anteriorly by a large mass with solid and fatty *(asterisk)* components (retroperitoneal liposarcoma) confined to the perirenal space *(arrows)*.

26. **Which syndromes are associated with an increased incidence of sarcoma?**
    Von Recklinghausen's disease and Li Fraumeni syndrome have an increased incidence of sarcoma.

27. **What is the site of metastatic lymph node involvement in testicular cancers?**
    Nodal metastasis from the **right testis** tends to be midline, with primary areas of involvement being interaortocaval, precaval, and preaortic lymph nodes group.

    Left testicular cancer metastasizes to left para-aortic nodes, followed by preaortic and interaortocaval nodes. Left suprahilar lymph nodes are found to be involved even if the left renal hilar nodes are normal, whereas on the right side the right suprahilar nodes are not involved if the right renal hilar nodes are normal in size.

28. **What are the advantages of CT over lymphangiography (LAG) in detection of retroperitoneal nodal metastases?**
    - CT has a higher specificity than LAG but a lower sensitivity.
    - CT detects early metastasis to renal hilar nodes, which is not normally opacified by LAG.
    - CT can define the exact extent of the tumor mass, which is helpful to plan the radiation therapy.
    - CT can detect metastases to extralymphatic organs (e.g., liver, lung).

29. **Compare CT and magnetic resonance imaging (MRI) in the evaluation of retroperitoneal lymphadenopathy.**
    - MRI can distinguish vascular from soft tissue structures without use of contrast. This is of importance in pelvic lymphadenopathy.
    - MRI is helpful in the evaluation of postsurgical patients with surgical clips and prosthesis without causing streak artifacts as in CT.
    - CT can detect lymphadenopathy in patients with poor retroperitoneal fat.
    - MRI has poorer spatial resolution; as a result, a cluster of normal-sized nodes may mimic an enlarged node.
    - MRI does not detect minor calcifications in lymph nodes.
    - MRI is more expensive and less available.
    - MRI can distinguish residual fibrotic changes (postradiation therapy) from viable neoplasms, unlike CT.

30. **Define the term choleretroperitoneum.**

Retroperitoneal abscesses secondary to biliary tract disease are termed choleretroperitoneum and are hypothesized to result from rupture of the common bile duct or perforation of the gallbladder.

31. **What is pneumoretroperitoneum?**

Pneumoretroperitoneum is defined as presence of air within the retroperitoneum. It is a rare condition and results from air insufflation during laparoscopy. Air may also be seen in the perinephric space secondary to emphysematous pyelonephritis.

32. **What are the advantages of multidetector CT (MDCT) over single-detector CT in imaging of the aorta?**

MDCT allows increased longitudinal volume coverage and spatial resolution as compared with single-detector CT, which requires acquisition of multiple separate body parts, followed by the fusion of the slices, to get a longitudinal coverage of the vessel. With the help of MDCT, the entire thoracoabdominal aorta can be imaged using a single acquisition, capturing the entire contrast bolus. Shorter scan durations and high contrast sensitivity of MDCT also permit use of smaller volumes of contrast for imaging of the aorta and its branches.

33. **Describe the protocol for MDCT angiography/aortography.**

Aortography is performed using a bolus contrast administration in a single breath-hold of 15–20 seconds. Eighty to 150 mL of nonionic iodinated contrast are administered at rates of 3–5 mL/sec through an upper arm peripheral venous access. Images are acquired using a slice width of 1–1.25 mm.

34. **Describe the various postprocessing techniques used in aortic angiography.**

- **Multiplanar reconstruction (MPR) and curved multiplanar reconstruction (CMPR):** MPR reorders image building blocks to alternate two-dimensional planes but is limited by the vessel curvature. CMPR is a modification of the MPR that displays the entire vessel length in a single two-dimensional image.
- **Maximum intensity projection (MIP):** MIP is the closest to digital subtraction angiography. MIP shows vessel opacification and the caliber of the lumen without giving any depth information.
- **Surface shaded display (SSD):** SSD gives an anatomic overview but no information about the lumen of the vessel. It may overestimate stenoses.
- **Volume rendering (VR):** VR gives a three-dimensional representation of the two-dimensional images. These volume-rendered three-dimensional images can give important extravascular information, such as information about the structures supplied by the vessel.

35. **What are the indications of aorta MDCT angiography?**

- Aneurysm
- Dissection
- Trauma
- Inflammation (e.g., vasculitides)
- Congenital anomalies
- Postoperative evaluation (stents, grafts and by pass procedures)

36. **What is the normal size of the aorta?**

The aorta normally has a diameter of less than 2 cm. Normal size of the aorta is affected by the body surface area, age, and sex of the individual. CT measurement of normal aortic diameter at the level of the renal hila varies from a mean of 1.53 cm in women in their fourth decade to 2.10 cm in men their eighth decade. Normal infrarenal aortic dimension just proximal to the bifurcation is smaller and averages 1.43 cm and 1.96 cm, respectively, in the previous two groups. Abdominal aorta diameter of more than 3 cm in elderly people or more than 2 cm in people younger than 50 years or a diameter double the normal size of the aorta is considered an aortic aneurysm.

37. **Can you diagnose anemia on CT?**
Yes. Normally, blood in the aortic lumen has an attenuation of 50–70 HU and the noncalcified aortic wall is indistinguishable from its intraluminal blood. In patients with reduced hematocrit, the intraluminal attenuation reduces considerably, and the noncalcified aortic wall can be visualized; this finding is suggestive of anemia.

38. **What are the risk factors for an aortic aneurysm?**
    - Atherosclerosis (most common)
    - Hypertension
    - Trauma
    - Age > 60 years
    - Males
    - Smoking
    - Infection (e.g., mycotic, syphilitic)
    - Congenital anomalies (e.g., Ehlers-Danlos syndrome, Marfan syndrome)

39. **What are the types of aortic aneurysm?**
According to type of aneurysm
    - **True aneurysm:** Contains all layers of an aortic wall
    - **Pseudoaneurysm:** Absence of intima

According to shape of aneurysm
    - **Fusiform:** Circumferential involvement
    - **Saccular:** Involves a portion of the aortic wall

According to location
    - Infrarenal (90%)
    - Suprarenal (10%)

40. **Why are infrarenal aneurysms more common than suprarenal aneurysms?**
Approximately 90% of all AAAs are infrarenal in location. This is because of the highest applied pressure load at this location secondary to the reflected pressure waves from the aortic bifurcation.

41. **What is the role of CTA in the evaluation of an abdominal aortic aneurysm (AAA)?**
    - Evaluation of extent of aneurysm
    - Evaluation of involvement of branch vessels of the aorta
    - Monitor the growth increment of the aneurysm
    - Detection of complications, such as rupture and thrombus formation
    - Preoperative and postoperative evaluation

42. **Describe an aortic pseudoaneurysm.**
Pseudoaneurysms are saccular outpouchings from the aorta formed as a result of a "contained leak" from the aorta. They do not contain the intima and are commonly caused by trauma or infection.

43. **When should an aortic aneurysm be treated?**
An aortic diameter more than 5 cm should be treated because of a 20% increased risk of rupture. Other indications for surgical repair include the following:
    - Rapid growth rate of the aneurysm (increase of 5 mm or more in 6 months)

- Mycotic aneurysm
- Pain
- Concomitant occlusive disease
- Iliac or femoral artery aneurysm
- Distal peripheral emboli

44. **Describe the CT findings of a mycotic aneurysm.**

A mycotic aneurysm is saccular in shape with an irregular contour, with minimal or absent mural calcification, and shows similar enhancement as the normal aortic lumen. Presence of gas in the wall of the aorta is very specific of a mycotic aneurysm. Additional findings include splenic infarcts, absence of atherosclerotic changes, and rapid appearance of findings.

45. **What are the complications of AAA?**
- AAA rupture
- Dissection of aorta
- Peripheral embolization
- Aortocaval fistula (rare)

KEY POINTS: RETROPERITONEUM

1. CT is the gold standard for the imaging of the retroperitoneum.

2. The most common cause of retroperitoneal fibrosis is idiopathic.

3. Only retroperitoneal fibrosis causes medial deviation of the ureters. Other masses cause lateral deviation of ureters.

4. CT cannot differentiate benign from malignant retroperitoneal lymphadenopathy.

5. Aortic aneurysm more than 5 cm in diameter should be surgically repaired.

46. **Describe the CT findings of an aortocaval fistula.**
- Early equivalent enhancement of the aorta and the IVC
- Enlarged kidneys with poor function
- Perirenal cobwebs

47. **Describe the symptoms of an aneurysmal rupture.**
- Sudden onset severe back or abdominal pain
- Pallor
- Shock
- Dry mouth/skin, excessive thirst
- Nausea and vomiting

48. **What is the classic triad of an AAA rupture?**
- Abdominal pain
- Hypotension
- Pulsatile mass

Less than one third of patients with AAA present with this classic triad.

49. **Describe the CTA findings of aneurysm rupture.**

Aneurysm rupture on a CTA may be represented by an extravasation of contrast or in case of a sealed ruptured site; it may be seen as a retroperitoneal hematoma, more commonly in the perirenal spaces than pararenal spaces (*see* Fig. 29-7). Additional findings include anterior displaced kidney by the hematoma, enlarged or obscured psoas muscle, focally indistinguishable aortic margin or discontinuity in the calcified rim of aortic wall, and/or mural thrombus of the aneurysm.

50. How do you diagnose an impending rupture of AAA?
Presence of a high attenuation crescent shaped area within the aortic wall is suspicious for an impending AAA rupture.

51. What is the role of MDCT angiography in postoperative (aneurysm repair) changes/complications of the aorta?
- **Evaluation of integrity of endovascular stent and detection of graft occlusions:** Presence of thrombus
- **Detection of stent migration:** Higher or lower
- **Detection of endoleak:** Presence of contrast outside the lumen of the graft
- **Detection of infection of the graft:** Paragraft fluid collections with presence of multiple, posterior gas collections (compared with benign postoperative gas, which is solitary and anteriorly located)
- **Detection of aortoenteric fistula (AEF):** Presence of paragraft fluid and extraluminal air

52. How is aortic dissection classified?
Aortic dissections are classified anatomically using two different methods:
Stanford classification (more commonly used)
- **Type A:** The ascending aorta is involved (DeBakey types I and II).
- **Type B:** The descending aorta is involved (DeBakey type III).
De Bakey classification
- **Type I:** Involves both ascending and descending aorta.
- **Type II:** Only the ascending aorta is involved.
- **Type III:** Only the descending aorta is involved.
  - Type IIIA involves the descending aorta distal to the left subclavian artery up to the diaphragm.
  - Type IIIB involves the descending aorta below the diaphragm.

53. Describe the CTA findings in an aortic dissection.
- Classic feature—the presence of an intimal flap acting as a partition between the true and the false lumens (Fig. 29-13)
- Internal displacement of intimal calcifications
- Delayed enhancement of the false lumen
- Widened aorta
- Mediastinal, pleural, or pericardial hematoma

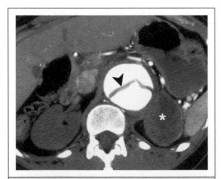

Figure 29-13. Aortic dissection. Contrast-enhanced computed tomography (CECT) of the abdomen shows a large intimal flap *(arrowhead)* within the aortic aneurysm. Also seen is a left adrenal mass *(asterisk)*.

54. What are the causes of pseudodissection?
CT artifacts, such as perivenous streaks and aorta motion artifact, may simulate an aortic dissection. Other causes that may simulate an aortic dissection include a mural thrombus in a fusiform aneurysm, periaortic fibrosis, retroperitoneal tumor, and anemia with hyperattenuating aortic wall.

55. What are the complications of an aortic dissection?

Obstruction of aortic branch vessels is an important complication of aortic dissection. There are two types of such an occlusion:

- Static obstruction: Intimal flap enters the branch vessel origin.
- Dynamic obstruction: Intimal flap covers the branch vessel origin like a curtain.

56. What are the types of arteritis involving the abdominal aorta?

Takayasu's arteritis (pulseless disease)

- Unknown cause
- Young women
- Asian descent
- CT: Thick enhancing aortic wall due to enlargement of vasa vasorum
- Later stages: Development of aneurysms, stenoses, occlusions of branches

Behçet's disease

- Affects small and large arteries and veins
- Young adults
- Medial hyperplasia and intimal fibroplasia in aorta

57. What is duplication of the IVC?

Duplication of the IVC (Fig. 29-14) is a congenital anomaly resulting from persistence of both supracardinal veins; it occurs in 0.2–3% of the individuals. There are two infrarenal IVCs and a single right-sided suprarenal IVC because the left IVC crosses over to join the right-sided IVC at the level of the renal veins. The left IVC is usually smaller than the right.

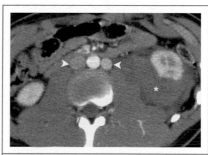

Figure 29-14. Double IVC. Contrast-enhanced computed tomography (CECT) of the abdomen shows presence of two IVCs *(arrowheads)* on either side of the aorta. Also seen is left perinephric hematoma *(asterisk)* after trauma.

58. What is transposition of the IVC?

Transposition of the IVC is a rare anomaly seen in 0.2–0.5 % of the population; it results from regression of the right cardinal system and persistence of the left cardinal veins. In this condition, a single IVC exists on the left side that crosses over to the right side at the level of the renal veins to follow a normal course cranially up to the right atrium.

59. What is a circumaortic left renal vein?

A circumaortic left renal vein occurs in 8.7% of individuals and results from persistence of the dorsal limb of the embryonic left renal vein and of the dorsal arch of the renal collar, resulting in the occurrence of two left renal veins forming a vascular ring around the aorta.

60. What is retroaortic left renal vein?

Retroaortic left renal vein has a prevalence of 2.1% and is caused by the persistence of the dorsal arch of the renal collar and complete regression of the anterior subcardinal veins. There is only a single left renal vein.

61. What is a circumcaval ureter?

Circumcaval ureter results from anomalous regression of the most caudal segment of the supracardinal vein and the persistence of the subcardinal vein. As a result, the ureter passes behind and around the medial aspect of the IVC as it courses to the bladder.

62. **Which malignancy involves the IVC?**

Leiomyosarcoma is a rare neoplasm originating from the wall of the IVC, commonly located between the diaphragm and the renal veins, and is seen in elderly women. CT shows a well-circumscribed, right-sided retroperitoneal mass inseparable from the IVC, with heterogeneous enhancement and displacement of the adjacent organs.

63. **What is the role of CT after IVC filter placement?**

CT helps to detect any complications associated with IVC filter placement, such as filter migration, caval perforation, and postfilter caval thrombosis. It also helps assess the structural integrity of the IVC filters.

BIBLIOGRAPHY

1. Gupta A, Cohan R: The retroperitoneum In Haaga JR (ed): CT and MR Imaging of Whole Body, Vol 2, 4th ed. St. Louis, Mosby, 2003, pp 1657–1709.

2. Lawler LP, Fishman EK: Multidetector row computed tomography of the aorta and peripheral arteries. Cardiol Clin 21:607–629, 2003.

3. Lee JKT, Hiken JN, Semelka RC: Retroperitoneum. In Lee JKT, Sagel SS, Stanley RJ, Heiken JP (eds): Computed Body Tomography with MRI Correlation, Vol 2, 3rd ed. Philadelphia, Lippincott-Raven, 1998, pp 1023–1085.

4. Nishino M, Haywkawa K, Minami M, et al: Primary retroperitoneal neoplasms: CT and MR imaging findings with anatomic and pathologic diagnostic clues. Radiographics 23:45–57, 2003.

CHAPTER 30

CT OF THE FEMALE PELVIS

Elizabeth J. Anoia, MD, and Jeffrey S. Palmer, MD

1. **What are the main indications for pelvic CT scan in a female?**
   Pelvic CT can be used to image the lower urinary tract and the gynecologic structures in trauma, infections, cancer detection/staging, or evaluation of lower abdominal pain.

2. **What is the rind sign?**
   The rind sign is enhancement of the rim of an abscess seen on a contrast-enhanced CT scan. Other features that are characteristic of an abscess on a CT scan are a well-defined, usually circular, lesion that has a low-density center with a thickened wall. An abscess may also contain gas, which is diagnostic.

3. **Describe the term "frozen pelvis."**
   It is a term that is used to describe the appearance of the pelvis when all fascial planes are lost resulting from extensive involvement of the pelvis by endometrial carcinoma or adhesion formation from longstanding pelvic inflammatory disease (PID). In these conditions, the pelvic organs are adherent to the side walls by the indurated supporting ligaments.

4. **Which is the most important measurement of the female pelvis that determines whether a pelvis is too small for vaginal delivery?**
   The most important one is the bispinous diameter measurement in the midpelvis extending from each ischial spine. If it is <10 cm, that pelvis will not accommodate a vaginal delivery.

5. **What are the CT size criteria that suggest lymph node involvement by tumor?**
   The lymph node size that suggests tumor involvement on CT is a maximal length of 1.3 cm and maximal width of 1.0 cm.

6. **Where does the anteflexed uterus lie in relation to the bladder?**
   The anteflexed uterus is posterosuperior to the bladder, whereas the retroflexed uterus projects into the cul-de-sac.

7. **Describe the clinical presentation of a uterine leiomyoma (fibroid) and its appearance on a CT scan.**
   Fibroids may present with pelvic pain, irregular or heavy vaginal bleeding, infertility, dyspareunia, or mass-related effects. A uterine leiomyoma gives the uterus an enlarged, homogeneous, globular appearance, which may or may not be heavily calcified (Fig. 30-1). It is well demarcated and may also exhibit intratumoral hemorrhage. The uterine leiomyoma demonstrates enhancement on contrast enhancement.

8. **Describe the appearance of endometrial carcinoma on CT.**
   Endometrial carcinoma is suspected when the uterus is enlarged and fluid-filled (Fig. 30-2). This fluid may be old blood or endometrial secretions. The endometrial cavity is usually occupied by multiple hyperdense nodules that can vary in size. However, it is difficult to differentiate these nodules from other benign uterine lesions, such as endometrial polyps or simply blood clots, and histologic diagnosis is needed.

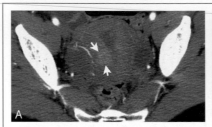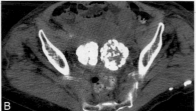

Figure 30-1. Uterine leiomyoma. **A,** Axial contrast-enhanced CT (CECT) of the pelvis demonstrates an enhancing intramural leiomyoma *(arrows)*. **B,** Axial nonenhanced computed tomography (NECT) of the pelvis reveals two calcified uterine leiomyomas in a different patient.

9. **When is CT scan appropriate in the evaluation of PID?**

   CT scan may be used in diagnosing PID in cases in which ultrasound provides inadequate information or if it is normal (up to one third of patients). The main findings on CT include *bilateral* adnexal masses that have low attenuation and thickened walls with an irregular border with distorted planes (Fig. 30-3). Other findings may include pelvic ascites, pelvic fat stranding, and ureteral dilation.

10. **How do you stage cervical carcinoma?**

    Cervical carcinoma is staged clinically, by physical exam and imaging (Fig. 30-4). It is not affected by operative findings. Hydronephrosis characteristically denotes a Stage III tumor and involvement of the bladder or rectum is Stage IV disease based on Federation of Gynecology and Obstetrics (FIGO) criteria.

11. **In cervical carcinoma, what are the advantages and disadvantages of CT scan versus magnetic resonance imaging (MRI)?**

    A pelvic CT scan is better able to identify any associated genitourinary (GU) tract abnormalities, such as hydronephrosis and hydroureter and the presence of lymphadenopathy. CT can also detect recurrence and aid in percutaneous biopsy of lesions. The disadvantage of CT is that normal uterus may be difficult to differentiate from tumor and treatment is partly based on tumor volume.

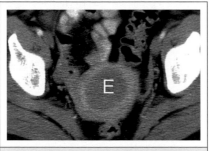

Figure 30-2. Endometrial carcinoma. Axial contrast-enhanced CT (CECT) of the pelvis in a 65-year-old woman demonstrates an enlarged uterus with a fluid-filled endometrial cavity (E). This was surgically confirmed to be an endometrial carcinoma.

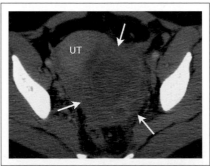

Figure 30-3. Pelvic inflammatory disease. Axial contrast-enhanced CT (CECT) of the pelvis demonstrates a low-attenuation mass *(arrows)* with thick enhancing walls located posterior to the uterus (UT) and pushing the uterus anteriorly and superiorly.

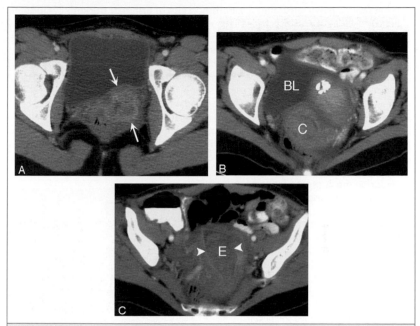

Figure 30-4. Cervical carcinoma. **A**, Axial contrast-enhanced CT (CECT) of the pelvis demonstrates an enhancing mass *(arrows)* at the level of the cervix confirmed to be a cervical carcinoma. **B** and **C**, Axial CECT images of the pelvis in another patient with a cervical mass (C) that extends superiorly into the endometrial cavity *(arrowheads)* and is seen as an endometrial mass (E) in part C. BL = bladder. Note left parametrial extension of cervical carcinoma in this patient.

12. **What is the differential diagnosis of hydrometrocolpos?**

The differential diagnosis of uterine or vaginal distention by blood or other fluid includes an imperforate hymen, longitudinal or transverse vaginal septa, vaginal atresia, and vaginal agenesis (Fig. 30-5). These disorders are a spectrum of canalization abnormalities of the vagina.

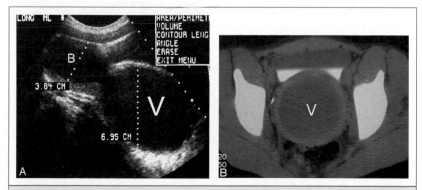

Figure 30-5. Hydrometrocolpos. **A**, Longitudinal gray scale sonogram shows a dilated fluid filled vagina (V). **B**, Corresponding contrast-enhanced CT (CECT) of pelvis in a case of interlabial mass demonstrates a dilated fluid-filled vagina (V).

13. **What female pelvic structure is a common site of origin of Burkitt's lymphoma?**

In women, the ovaries are a common site of origin of Burkitt's lymphoma.

14. **Name some common etiologies for ovarian cysts.**

Ovarian cysts can be physiologic, part of a syndrome called polycystic ovarian disease (PCOD), or a manifestation of a cystic malignancy. Physiologic cysts, such as the follicular, corpus luteum, and the theca lutein cyst, are usually small and asymptomatic unless hemorrhage or torsion occurs. Theca lutein cysts are usually bilateral and occur secondary to increased human chorionic gonadotrophin (hCG) levels. PCOD is a syndrome of chronic anovulation with the clinical presentation of amenorrhea, hirsutism, infertility, and obesity. The cysts of PCOD are much smaller than physiologic cysts and are usually found at the surface of the ovary. Cysts associated with malignancy may be larger or complex and associated with solid components.

15. **Describe the characteristics of physiologic ovarian cysts on CT imaging.**

These cysts are usually well demarcated with a homogeneous, low-attenuation appearance (Fig. 30-6). However, thin septa or solid debris from hemorrhage may be present. Theca lutein cysts may have a multilocular appearance in addition to their bilaterality. In some cases when there is a significant solid component present, these cysts may be difficult to distinguish from neoplasms.

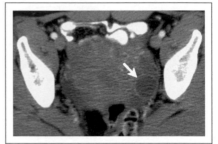

Figure 30-6. Ovarian cyst. Axial contrast-enhanced CT (CECT) of the pelvis demonstrates a left ovarian follicular cyst *(arrow)*.

16. **What is the Rokitansky protuberance in a mature cystic teratoma? What is its significance?**

The Rokitansky protuberance is the dermoid plug that is eccentrically located, projecting from the wall into the cyst (Fig. 30-7). The significance of this structure is that it is a site for the development of a malignancy in <1%, usually squamous cell carcinoma.

17. **Describe the appearance of ovarian carcinoma on CT scan.**

Ovarian carcinoma can be cystic or solid or have both components. The mass can be thick walled and contain septa or soft tissue. Psammomatous calcifications are present in up to 30% and can be seen on plain films, but they are best characterized on CT. Metastatic ovarian cancer is associated with ascites, peritoneal metastasis >2 cm, and liver lesions (Fig. 30-8).

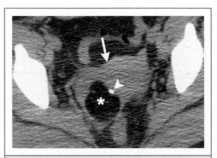

Figure 30-7. Mature cystic teratoma. Axial nonenhanced CT (NECT) of the pelvis demonstrates presence of a mass *(arrow)* with a fat density component *(asterisk)* and a focus of calcification *(arrowhead)*.

18. **Name the features of Meigs syndrome and Krukenberg tumor.**

Meigs syndrome is an ovarian fibroma that is associated with ascites and pleural effusion. Once the fibroma is removed, the ascites and associated pleural effusion resolve. The Krukenberg

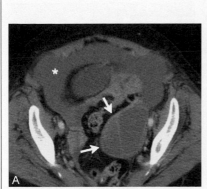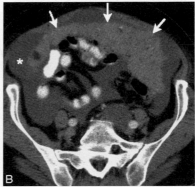

Figure 30-8. Ovarian carcinoma. *A,* Axial contrast-enhanced CT (CECT) of the pelvis demonstrates presence of a complex ovarian mass *(arrows)* with ascites *(asterisk). B,* Axial CECT in the same patient cephalad to the previous level demonstrates extensive omental metastasis *(arrows)* with marked ascites *(asterisk).* Patient also had metastases in the liver and spleen.

tumor is a metastatic tumor affecting the ovary with predominantly signet-ring cells and sarcomatous elements. It can be bilateral.

19. **Describe the appearance of a tubo-ovarian abscess.**
Approximately 1–2% of patients with PID may develop a tubo-ovarian abscess. On CT, there may be a round mass with multiple areas of low attenuation (Fig. 30-9). The wall may be thickened and contain septations or air bubbles. The fat planes between this mass and the adjacent normal pelvic organs may be lost. Hydroureter and adenopathy may also be present. These findings may also suggest an infected ovarian cyst or tumor, endometriosis, or a pelvic hematoma.

20. **What is adnexal torsion?**
In adnexal torsion, the ovary, ipsilateral fallopian tube, or both twist with the vascular pedicle, resulting in vascular compromise.

KEY POINTS: FEMALE GENITAL TRACT

1. Endometrial carcinoma cannot be distinguished from uterine fibroids by imaging alone.

2. Hydrocolpos and other similar conditions should initiate a search for a vaginal congenital abnormality.

3. Ovarian cysts are not uniformly benign; they may be part of a clinical syndrome or a component of a malignancy.

4. Dermoid ovarian cysts, although benign, may rarely degenerate into a squamous cell carcinoma.

5. Pelvic inflammatory disease must be in the differential diagnosis for bilateral adnexal masses.

6. An ovary that has the appearance of multiple cysts may actually be a torsion with dilated germinal follicles.

21. **What is the appearance of ovarian torsion on CT?**

   Ovarian torsion can cause significant pelvic pain and can be evaluated with multiple modalities. On CT scan, the ovary appears enlarged and the germinal follicles within it become dilated assuming a cystic appearance (Fig. 30-10). The ovary itself, due to its size, may cross midline and be found posterior to the bladder. It may have a beaked or a serpentine protrusion at the area of the torsion. After intravenous (IV) contrast, there may be prominent peripheral enhancement of the ovary and variable enhancement within it due to its inconsistent blood supply from the torsion.

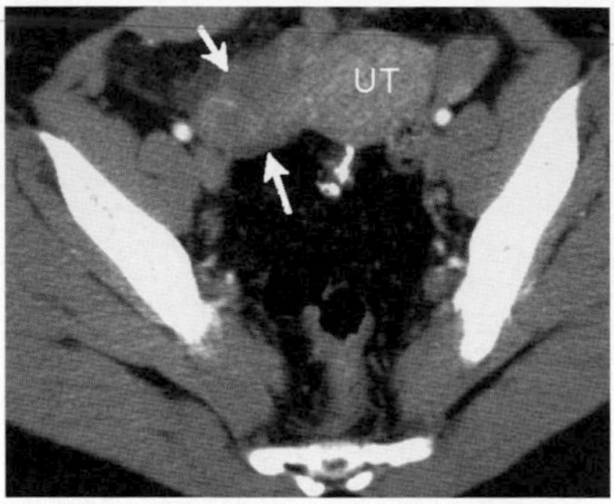

   Figure 30-9. Tubo-ovarian abscess. Axial contrast-enhanced CT (CECT) of the pelvis in a young woman presenting with spiking fevers and pelvic pain demonstrates a heterogeneous enhancing mass *(arrows)* in the right adnexa. Right ovary was not separately visualized from this lesion. UT = uterus.

22. **What is the CT appearance of ovarian vein thrombosis?**

   The characteristic CT findings consist of a tubular structure with an enhancing wall and low-attenuation thrombus in the expected location of the ovarian vein. This finding should not be confused with hydroureter, acute appendicitis, or a thrombosed inferior mesenteric vein. Thrombosis of an ovarian vein collateral vessel that is retrocecal in location, continues cephalad in the retroperitoneum, and terminates anterior to the kidney may be particularly difficult to distinguish from an inflamed appendix. However, careful assessment on multiple CT scans should facilitate diagnosis.

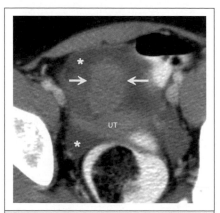

23. **What is the differential diagnosis of air in the urinary bladder on CT scan?**

   The differential diagnosis is a vesicoenteric/vesicovaginal fistula, emphysematous cystitis, or iatrogenic introduction of air by catheterization. A vesicoenteric fistula on CT scan has several key features in addition to the intravesical air—the

   Figure 30-10. Ovarian torsion. Axial contrast-enhanced CT (CECT) of the pelvis in a 13-year-old girl with acute pelvic pain reveals an enlarged ovary *(arrows)* located superior to the uterus (UT) and free pelvic fluid *(asterisks)*.

   presence of an adjacent structure containing air (i.e., bowel), thickened bladder wall >2 mm, and focally adjacent bowel wall thickness of >3 mm.

24. **What are the causes of bladder calcifications that are seen on CT?**

   A very common cause of bladder calcifications is stones (Fig. 30-11). These can either be stones that have moved down from the upper tracts or primary bladder stones as seen in patients with outflow obstruction or a bladder diverticulum. Bladder stones are usually free-floating and may change positions on different views. Stones within diverticula may appear close together and lateralizing. Other causes are a tumor that has calcified. This type of calcification may be linear or round and is usually associated with the bladder wall. Infections of the bladder, for example schistosomiasis or tuberculosis, can cause diffuse calcifications of the bladder wall. Foreign bodies (Foley catheter, ureteral stent, retained suture) can create oddly shaped areas of calcification within the bladder as can amyloidosis.

25. Characterize the findings of intraperitoneal and extraperitoneal bladder rupture on CT scan.
Generally bladder rupture results from significant trauma. Intraperitoneal bladder rupture results in a cloudlike appearance of the extravasated substance as it outlines the peritoneal organs. This fluid can collect in the lateral pelvic recesses or it may be midline and collect in the pouch of Douglas. With extraperitoneal bladder rupture, there is a symmetric compression of the lateral bladder walls and elevation of the bladder base. It gives the bladder a flame-shaped appearance. The extravasation is limited to the perivesical spaces (Fig. 30-12).

26. What is the differential diagnosis of a filling defect in the bladder seen on delayed images of a contrasted pelvic CT scan?
A filling defect of the urinary bladder may be due to multiple benign or malignant lesions. Some common lesions include carcinoma, stones, enlarged prostatic middle lobe, or blood clots. Less common etiologies are ureterocele, endometriosis, fungus ball, cystitis, or benign neoplasm. Benign neoplasms of the bladder include transitional cell papillomas, leiomyomas, polyps, hemangiomas, or, very uncommonly, pheochromocytomas.

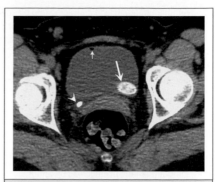

Figure 30-11. Bladder stone. Axial CT of the bladder demonstrates presence of a large bladder stone *(large arrow).* Also seen are a right ureterovesicular junction calculus *(arrowhead)* and some free air *(small arrow)* in the bladder secondary to prior Foley catheter insertion.

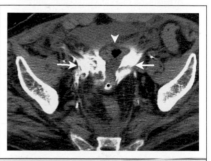

Figure 30-12. Extraperitoneal rupture of bladder. Axial contrast-enhanced CT (CECT) of the pelvis in a post-traumatic patient demonstrates presence of contrast *(arrows)* in the perivesical spaces. Bladder *(arrowhead)* is collapsed and shows absence of contrast.

27. How is CT scanning helpful in the evaluation of bladder cancer? What are its limitations?
A CT scan is not indicated for the diagnosis of superficial bladder tumors; however, it plays an important role in bladder cancer staging, which is the most important prognostic factor. CT allows for evaluation of bladder wall thickness to assess tumor involvement or gross tumor extension to adjacent pelvic structures. It can also demonstrate pelvic lymphadenopathy and distant metastases. The limitations of CT are that, in a postoperative or postradiation therapy patient, edema and inflammation resulting from treatment are indistinguishable from tumor.

Another limitation is that invasion into bladder muscle versus invasion into perivesical fat is difficult to differentiate on CT. Therefore, there is a degree of under- or overstaging. Overall, however, the mean accuracy of CT scan in staging bladder cancer is approximately 75%.

28. **What are the causes of a diffusely thickened bladder wall on CT scan?**
    Benign etiologies for a thick bladder wall are cystitis, trabeculations, or nondistention. Cystitis causing bladder wall abnormalities is usually chronic. Acute cystitis can have a normal appearance radiographically. Trabeculations are usually due to bladder outlet obstruction from prostatic enlargement or urethral stricture disease or neurogenic bladder. A less common and malignant etiology is infiltration of the bladder wall by tumor (Fig. 30-13).

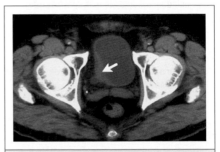

Figure 30-13. Transitional cell carcinoma (TCC) of bladder. Axial contrast-enhanced CT (CECT) of the bladder demonstrates an irregular thickening *(arrow)* of the right lateral bladder wall, pathologically confirmed to be a TCC.

29. **What is interstitial cystitis?**
    Interstitial cystitis is a voiding symptom complex that cannot be attributed to another cause; essentially it is a diagnosis of exclusion that can vary significantly from person to person. Radiographically, there can be nonspecific bladder changes that can be attributed to chronic inflammation. The hallmark of chronic cystitis on imaging is irregularity of the bladder wall usually associated with trabeculation and often with decreased bladder capacity.

30. **Describe the four anomalies of closure of the urachus.**
    The urachus usually closes by the middle of the second trimester and the median umbilical ligament is its remnant. The four closure defects are a patent urachus, an umbilical sinus, a diverticulum, and a urachal cyst.

31. **What is the clinical presentation of urachal carcinoma and its appearance on CT?**
    Urachal carcinoma can present as bloody or mucinous discharge from the umbilicus, or if there is still a patent urachus, mucus may be present in the urine. The most common histologic subtype is adenocarcinoma. On imaging, a midline mass just posterior to the abdominal wall and above the bladder may be seen. Calcification may be seen in some tumors, and if mucin is present there may be low-density components. Overall, there is a poor prognosis due to spread prior to diagnosis.

32. **List the pathologic types of urethral carcinoma and its clinical presentation.**
    Urethral carcinoma is more likely to occur in females. The most common histologic type is squamous cell carcinoma, followed by transitional cell, and least commonly is adenocarcinoma. These patients can present with any of the following symptoms—hematuria, dysuria with or without associated perineal pain, or irritative voiding symptoms, such as urgency/frequency.

33. **How is urethral carcinoma diagnosed and what important features may be seen on CT?**
    Urethrography is the best way to diagnose this condition; it will appear as a filling defect with an irregular border. However, a CT scan can be used to assess the degree of tumor extension and if lymph nodes are involved. The bladder neck may be superiorly displaced from the

mass, and it will usually have a lower density than the surrounding structures. Lymph node involvement is manifested as either enlarged inguinal nodes if the carcinoma arises from the distal third of the urethra or external/internal iliac nodes if it arises from the proximal two thirds of the urethra.

34. **Name other benign and malignant etiologies for female urethral filling defects.**
Urethral papillomas, also known as urethral caruncles, are benign lesions that are usually found in the distal third of the urethra. They are lined either by transitional cells or metaplastic squamous cells. Their associated filling defect is usually smooth in contour in contrast to urethral carcinoma. Another etiology of urethral filling defects is urethral stones. Urethral stones can be found within diverticula of the midurethra in female patients. These stones can be diagnosed with contrast studies of the urethra, with plain film imaging as most are radiopaque, or on CT as high-density lesions inferior to the pubic symphysis. Metastasis from adjacent organs can also involve the urethra by direct local spread resulting in a urethral filling defect.

KEY POINTS: FEMALE URINARY TRACT

1. Air in the urinary bladder may be infectious, iatrogenic, or due to a fistula.

2. In addition to stones, other etiologies of bladder calcifications are malignancy, foreign bodies, or infections.

3. A cloudlike appearance of extravasated contrast on a cystogram suggests an intraperitoneal bladder rupture, whereas a flame-shaped appearance suggests an extravesical rupture.

4. Blood clots from benign conditions may appear as bladder filling defects suggestive of tumor on CT scan.

5. The minimum size criteria for lymph nodes that may suggest tumor involvement are length of 1.3 cm and width of 1.0 cm.

35. **What is stress urinary incontinence (SUI)?**
SUI is the complaint of involuntary loss of urine during increases in intra-abdominal pressure, such as coughing, sneezing, sport activities, or sudden changes of position. The observation of involuntary urine loss from the urethra synchronous with the previously noted activities is the physical sign. Blaivas has devised a classification system of four types of incontinence based on the location of the bladder neck and proximal urethra relative to the inferior margin of the symphysis pubis during a stress maneuver.
- In **type 0** the bladder neck and proximal urethra are closed at rest and situated at or above the lower end of the symphysis pubis. During a Valsalva maneuver, the bladder neck and proximal urethra descend and open, but incontinence is not demonstrated.
- In **type I** the bladder neck is closed at rest and situated above the inferior margin of the symphysis. During stress, the bladder neck and proximal urethra open and descend less than 2 cm and urinary incontinence is evident.
- **Type IIA** again shows the bladder neck closed at rest and situated above the inferior margin of the symphysis pubis and incontinence occurs due to a rotational force.
- With **type IIB** the bladder neck is closed at rest and situated at or below the inferior margin of the symphysis pubis. During stress, there may or may not be further descent but the proximal urethra opens and incontinence occurs.
- In **type III** the bladder neck and proximal urethra are open at rest.

36. What are urethral bulking agents?

Urethral bulking agents are injectable materials that improve the ability of the urethra to resist increases in intra-abdominal pressure without changing voiding dynamics. The goal of these materials is to restore "mucosal coaptation" and its *seal effect* contribution to the maintenance of continence. The types of materials range from polytetrafluoroethylene to collagen to autologous substances.

BIBLIOGRAPHY

1. Bennett GL, Slywotzky CM, Giovanniello G: Gynecologic causes of acute pelvic pain: Spectrum of CT findings. Radiographics 22:785–801, 2002.

2. Blaivas JG: Classifying stress urinary incontinence. Neurourol Urodyn 18(2) 71–72, 1999.

3. Grainger RG, Allison D, Adam A, Dixon AK (eds): Grainger and Allison's Diagnostic Radiology: A Textbook of Medical Imaging., 4th ed. New York, Churchill Livingstone, 2001.

4. Squire LF, Novelline RA: Fundamentals of Radiology, 4th ed. Cambridge, Harvard University Press, 1988.

5. Walsh PC, Retik AB, Vaughan ED, Wein AJ (eds): Campbell's Urology, 8th ed. Philadelphia, Elsevier/Saunders, 2002.

6. Zagoria RJ, Tung GA: Genitourinary Radiology: The Requisites: The Lower Urinary Tract and The Female Genital Tract. St. Louis, Mosby, 1997, pp 192–302.

THE MALE PELVIC ORGANS

Kevin Garrett Miller, MD, and Vikram Dogra, MD

CHAPTER 31

1. **What are the indications of pelvic CT in a male patient?**
   The main indications are evaluation of the prostate gland, seminal vesicles, urinary bladder, and rectosigmoid region.

2. **What is the anatomy of the male pelvic organs?**
   The muscles of the urogenital diaphragm cradle the prostate, which is located inferior to the bladder base and anterior to the rectum. The seminal vesicles are paired structures superior to the prostate and posterior to the bladder base. The vas deferens courses from the internal inguinal ring to the seminal vesicle along the pelvic sidewall (Figs. 31-1, 31-2, and 31-3).

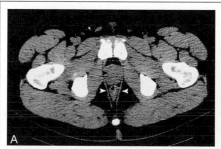

Figure 31-1. *A,* The muscles of the urogenital diaphragm *(white arrowheads)* cradle the prostate *(black arrowhead).* *B,* A more superior image in the same patient shows the relationship of the prostate *(white arrowhead)* to the bladder *(black arrowhead)* and rectum *(white arrow).*

3. **What is the normal appearance of the prostate and seminal vesicles?**
   The prostate is homogeneous and similar in attenuation to skeletal muscle. The normal prostate size is 2.8 × 2.8 × 4.8 cm. The simplest to measure on CT is the transverse dimension (4.8 cm). The seminal vesicles have a similar attenuation and measure approximately 14 mL in volume.

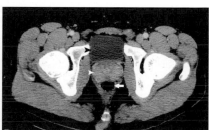

4. **What is the anatomy of the prostate?**
   The prostate has four zones. The peripheral zone is located under the capsule and formed of glandular

Figure 31-2. The vas deferens *(white arrowhead)* is demonstrated on this oblique axial CT image in its course from the internal inguinal ring to the seminal vesicle.

tissue. The central zone is deep to the peripheral zone and formed of stroma. The transitional zone surrounds the prostatic urethra. The periurethral zone is formed of short ducts. The central and transitional zones are found more superiorly within the gland. The gland tapers inferiorly.

5. **Can the zones of the prostate be distinguished on CT?**
   No. With other imaging, such as ultrasound (US) and magnetic resonance imaging (MRI), the peripheral zone can be seen with different characteristics than the other three.

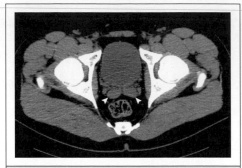

Figure 31-3. The seminal vesicles *(white arrowheads)* are paired structures superior to the prostate and posterior to the bladder base.

6. **What is the most common disorder of the prostate?**
   Benign prostatic hypertrophy (BPH) is the most common disorder. BPH is most commonly composed of fibromyoadenomatous nodules, which most commonly arise in the transitional and periurethral zones. This is distinct from prostate cancer, which arises in the peripheral zone in 70% of cases. The transitional zone increases in proportion as men age to form up to 95% of the prostate. Only 4–5% of cases of BPH require surgical treatment.

7. **What are the symptoms of BPH?**
   Patients with symptoms of BPH complain of a sensation of a full bladder, difficulty initiating urinary stream, decreased stream size and force, and dribbling.

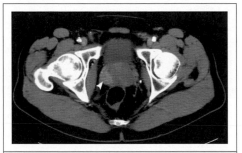

Figure 31-4. In this patient with prostate cancer, an arterial-phase enhanced CT image shows an enhancing nodule *(white arrowhead)* in the prostate. This corresponded to the patient's cancer. Unfortunately, this is not the norm in prostate cancer imaging.

8. **Can BPH and prostate cancer be distinguished accurately from each other on CT?**
   In most cases, diagnostic accuracy with CT is poor. Only stage T3b (invasion of the seminal vesicles) and stage T4 prostate cancer can be distinguished from BPH (Fig. 31-4).

9. **What is the American Joint Committee on Cancer (AJCC) staging system for prostate cancer?**
   See Table 31-1.

10. **What are the regional nodal groups involved in prostate cancer?**
    The first nodal group involved is the obturator group in the internal iliac chain. Both internal and external iliac chain nodes are considered regional spread of prostate cancer.

TABLE 31-1.	STAGING OF PROSTATE CANCER
AJCC	Description
T1	Clinically inapparent tumor not palpable or visible by imaging
T2	Tumor confined within the prostate
T2a	Tumor involves one half of one lobe or less
T2b	Tumor involves more than one half of one lobe
T2c	Tumor involves both lobes
T3	Tumor extends through the prostate capsule
T3a	Extracapsular extension
T3b	Invades seminal vesicles
T4	Tumor is fixed or invades adjacent structures other than the seminal vesicles
N1	Regional lymph node metastasis
M1	Distant metastasis
M1a	Nonregional lymph nodes
M1b	Bone
M1c	Visceral

AJCC = American Joint Committee on Cancer.

11. **Is imaging useful for the diagnosis of prostatitis?**
    The diagnosis of prostatitis is clinically based on pain, chills, malaise, and irritative voiding symptoms. Imaging is useful for the diagnosis of a prostate abscess, which is typically located in the peripheral zone. Transrectal US is the method of choice for abscess detection. The prostate can appear enlarged and ill defined on CT in cases of prostatitis. A prostate abscess on CT will appear as a hypoattenuating area when compared with the remainder of the gland (Fig. 31-5).

12. **What is cavitary prostatitis?**
    Cavitary or diverticular prostatitis is chronic prostatitis in which fibrosis causes stricture of the ducts. On imaging, the appearance is that of numerous small cysts within the prostate or a "Swiss cheese" appearance.

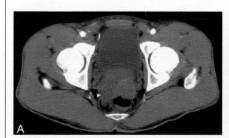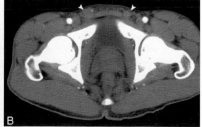

Figure 31-5. *A*, On this CT image, the prostate is enlarged. This young patient had symptoms and physical findings of prostatitis. Although not yet of fluid density, the hypoattenuating area *(white arrowhead)* is consistent with a developing abscess. *B*, In the same patient, enlargement of the spermatic cords *(white arrowheads)*, indicating edema, was also present. The same patient was also found to have epididymitis.

13. **What is a prostate utricle cyst?**
This is an enlarged müllerian duct remnant that arises as a diverticulum from the posterior aspect of the prostatic urethra. This is seen on CT as a fluid density structure in the midline of the prostate. The enlarged utricle can become infected, form stones, or cause obstructive voiding symptoms. This can cause infertility if it obstructs or compresses the ejaculatory ducts.

14. **What other disorders can have the appearance of a cyst in the prostate?**
Ejaculatory duct cysts and retention cysts also occur within the prostate. BPH can undergo cystic degeneration. Cavitary prostatitis and prostatic abscess also show cysts in the prostate. Prostate carcinoma can also be cystic.

15. **The vas deferens is embryologically what structure?**
The mesonephric duct forms the vas deferens, seminal vesicles, ejaculatory duct, and epididymis.

16. **What is the most common cause of vas deferens calcification?**
The most common cause is diabetes mellitus, in which the calcification occurs in the muscular layer. This is seen as tubular calcification on CT often at the seminal vesicles. Other causes include tuberculosis, syphilis, and nonspecific urinary tract infection (UTI). In these cases the calcification is intraluminal.

KEY POINTS: MALE PELVIC ORGANS

1. The main indications for CT of the male pelvis are evaluation of the prostate gland, seminal vesicles, urinary bladder, and rectosigmoid region.

2. In most cases of prostatic cancer, diagnostic accuracy with CT is poor. Only stage T3b (invasion of the seminal vesicles) and stage T4 prostate cancer can be distinguished from BPH.

3. The prostate can appear enlarged and ill defined on CT in cases of prostatitis. A prostate abscess on CT will appear as a hypoattenuating area when compared with the remainder of the gland.

4. A prostate utricle cyst is seen on CT as a fluid density structure in the midline of the prostate.

5. The most common type of prostate trauma is grade 3. Fluid (urine) is seen below the urogenital diaphragm on CT. This is inferior and lateral to the levator ani muscles cradling the prostate. In grade 2 injuries, fluid is seen above the urogenital diaphragm in the extraperitoneal space.

17. **What are the components of the male urethra?**
The male urethra is described as having a posterior portion, above the urogenital diaphragm, and anterior portion, below the urogenital diaphragm. The posterior urethra contains the prostatic segment and the membranous segment. The anterior urethra contains the bulbous and penile segments.

18. **How is male urethral trauma graded?**
Grade 1 trauma involves disruption of the puboprostatic ligament with elongation of the posterior urethra. Grade 2 is rupture of the urethra at the junction of the prostatic and membranous segments above the urogenital diaphragm. Grade 3 is rupture of the proximal bulbous urethra below the urogenital diaphragm. Urethral trauma is much more common in men.

TABLE 31-2.	STAGING OF TESTICULAR CANCER
AJCC	**Description**
T1	Tumor limited to testis and epididymis. Tumor may invade tunica albuginea
T2	Tumor limited to testis and epididymis with vascular/lymphatic invasion or invasion into the tunica vaginalis
T3	Tumor invades the spermatic cord
T4	Tumor invades the scrotum
N1	Regional lymph node metastasis with no single mass greater than 2 cm
N2	Regional lymph node metastasis with at least one mass greater than 2 cm, but no mass greater than 5 cm
N3	Regional lymph node metastasis with at least one mass greater than 5 cm
M1	Distant metastasis
M1a	Nonregional lymph node or pulmonary metastasis
M1b	Other distant metastasis

AJCC = American Joint Committee on Cancer.

19. **What is the most common type of urethral trauma?**
The most common type is grade 3. Fluid (urine) is seen below the urogenital diaphragm on CT. This is inferior and lateral to the levator ani muscles cradling the prostate. In grade 2 injuries, fluid is seen above the urogenital diaphragm in the extraperitoneal space.

20. **What is the AJCC staging system for testicular cancer?**
See Table 31-2.

21. **How is an undescended testicle evaluated?**
US is the first modality of choice, and if the testicle is not found within the inguinal canal, CT or MRI is then performed. This is an uncommon finding in adults because early surgical correction is the rule. Testicular cancer risk is increased in both the undescended and normal testicles.

22. **What disorders are related to a seminal vesicle cyst?**
A seminal vesicle cyst is related to congenital ipsilateral genitourinary disorders including renal agenesis/dysgenesis, ectopic ureter, collecting system duplication, and vas deferens agenesis. Acquired causes include BPH, autosomal dominant polycystic kidney disease, and infection.

23. **What types of malignancies are seen in the seminal vesicles?**
Primary tumors in the seminal vesicles are rare and include adenocarcinoma, sarcoma, and lymphoma. Other malignancies, such as melanoma and peritoneal cancers, can metastasize to the seminal vesicles.

BIBLIOGRAPHY

1. American Joint Committee on Cancer: TNM Schema Files. Available at www.cancerstaging.org/education/tnm-schema/tnmschema.html

2. Dahnert WF: Radiology Review Manual, 4th ed. Baltimore, Lippincott Williams & Wilkins, 1999, pp 723–821.

3. Davidson AJ, Hartman DS, Choyke PL, Wagner BJ: Radiology of the Kidney and Genitourinary Tract, 3rd ed. Philadelphia: W.B. Saunders, 1999, pp 637–648.

4. Spencer JA, Swift SE: Computed Tomography of the Pelvis. In Haaga JR (ed): CT and MR Imaging of the Whole Body, 4th ed. St. Louis, Mosby, 2003, pp 1715–1749.